639

**History of the American College of Physicians**

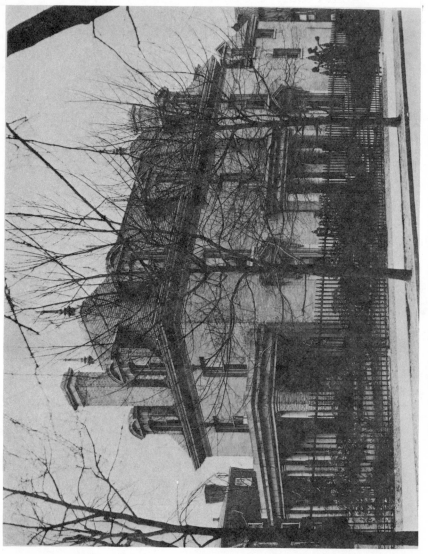

Plate 1. Eisenlohr Mansion (1905) - ACP Headquarters, 1936

History of the
American College of Physicians

# EXECUTIVE
# PERSPECTIVES
# 1959-1977

Edward C. Rosenow, Jr., MD, MACP,
*FRCP (London), FRCP, Hon. (Ireland), FRACP, Hon.*
*Executive Vice President Emeritus*

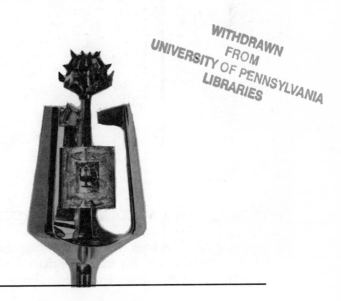

American College of Physicians, Inc.
Philadelphia, Pennsylvania
©1984

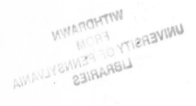
©1984, by the AMERICAN COLLEGE OF PHYSICIANS, INC.

Published in the United States of America

ISBN 0-943126-01-0

## DEDICATION

To Esther, my devoted wife

*"Chance cannot change my love, nor time impair."*
(Robert Barrett Browning)

# Foreword

This history of the American College of Physicians, written by Edward C. Rosenow, Jr., takes up where Dr. George Morris Piersol's *Gateway of Honor* ends, with the resignation in 1960 of Edward R. Loveland, the College's first Executive Officer.

From the time of its founding in 1915 by Heinrich Stern, the College, through teaching and research has had a profound effect on the shape of internal medicine and the manner in which internists practice. The present volume lucidly documents the continued influence of the College on medicine and its phenomenal growth during an 18-year span from 1960 to 1977, when Dr. Rosenow was its Executive Vice President.

Membership quadrupled from 10,000 to 40,000 with 15,000 young physicians in training, comprising a new category of Associates. Circulation of the *Annals of Internal Medicine* rose to 80,000, making it the third most sought-after journal in the medical world. The headquarters mansion at 4200 Pine Street had two additions, increasing working space over ten-fold for a staff that quadrupled in size. Attendance at Regional Meetings doubled and the number of postgraduate courses grew from 6 to 47.

The format of the Annual Sessions was altered to include "State of the Art" lectures, workshops, and "Meet the Professor" sessions. Most noteworthy was the development of the *Medical Knowledge Self-Assessment Program,* an educational tool that was subsequently adopted by many other specialty groups. In 1968, when the program was introduced, 12,000 physicians volunteered to take the test. In 1976, 38,000 subscribed to the fourth offering.

During this period, the College's main purpose continued to be promotion, improvement and advancement of teaching, research and practice in internal medicine. As the government and private insurers became increasingly involved in medical training, biomedical research and health care delivery, and as the public took more interest in medical care, it became difficult for the College to shun the socioeconomic aspects of medicine as it had steadfastly done in the past.

Recognition of the importance of political, social and economic factors to the assurance of high-quality medical care led to the unsuccessful attempt to merge the College with the American Society of Internal Medicine and ultimately to the reorganization of the ACP to fulfill a much broader mission. Marked changes occurred in its governance as Chapters were formed and relations between the Board of Regents and Board of Governors became closer than ever before. On major medical issues, its representatives began to speak out with increasing authority at all levels of government and at national medical meetings.

No one is better qualified to document the tremendous changes that occurred during these years than Dr. Edward C. Rosenow, Jr. The Board of Regents, in authorizing this volume, believed that the unique perspective of the first Executive Vice President would lead to a vibrant and exciting history of the College and its role in medicine during the explosive '60s and '70s. Edward Rosenow has fulfilled all of the Regents' hopes.

In the ensuing pages, the activities of the College and the parts played by its officers, members and staff in guiding internal medicine are clearly and accurately recorded in Dr. Rosenow's own personal way.

This history, coupled with Piersol's *Gateway of Honor,* gives us a clear picture of the College from its beginning to modern times. Together, they make it possible to understand something of our past and hopefully to be better prepared for the future. All of us are most thankful to Dr. Rosenow for his brilliant stewardship of the College and a job well done in writing this history.

Truman G. Schnabel, Jr., MACP

## About the Author

Son and namesake of a renowned Mayo Clinic microbiologist, and brother of two physicians, John and Frank Rosenow, Edward Carl Rosenow, Jr., received his undergraduate training at Carleton College (BA) in 1931 and his medical education at Harvard Medical School in 1935. While at Carleton, he spent two years teaching English in a Congregational Church mission in Shansi, China, where it was his good fortune to meet Esther Jane Church, his future wife.

Following an internship at Faulkner Hospital in Boston, he was a Fellow in Internal Medicine at the Mayo Clinic (1936-1940) and received a Master of Science in Medicine at the University of Minnesota.

In 1940, he entered private practice in Pasadena, California and was appointed Clinical Professor of Medicine at the University of Southern California. The next 17 years were noteworthy, the extent of his activities including service at various times as President of the Los Angeles County Medical Society, the Los Angeles County Society of Internal Medicine, the Los Angeles County Heart Association, the Huntington Memorial Hospital (Pasadena) and the Charles Cook Hastings Home (Pasadena). In 1958-59, he was appointed Clinical Professor of Medicine at the University of California in Los Angeles and the Loma Linda School of Medicine.

For nine years, from 1951 to 1959, he chaired the Postgraduate Activities Committee of the California Medical Association and served as Editor-in-Chief of *Audio-Digest* from 1954 to 1959.

In 1957, he was appointed Executive Director of the Los Angeles County Medical Association. Two years later, in 1959, he was designated Executive Director of the American College of Physicians, and assumed that position on January 1, 1960.

His professional society contributions were extensive. He was a member of the American Medical Association, American Clinical and Climatological Association, a Fellow of the American College of Chest Physicians, an Honorary Fellow of the American College of Gastroentrology, and a Fellow of the College of Physicians of Philadelphia.

He served as President of the American Medical Writers' Association, the American Osler Society, the International Society of Medicine, the Alumni Associations of both Carleton College and Mayo Clinic. In recent years, he has been a member of the Board of Trustees of Carleton College, Chairman of the Doctors Mayo Society (1978-1982) and was elected Emeritus Member of the Association of American Medical Colleges in 1978.

Elected a Fellow of the American College of Physicians in 1942, he was made a Master in 1976. During his tenure as chief executive officer (first as Executive Director, then as Executive Vice President), he was involved in every aspect of College affairs and personally knew hundreds of its members. He traveled widely, attending Regional Meetings and representing the College abroad.

In 1968, he was made a Fellow of the Royal College of Physicians of London; he is also a Fellow of the Royal Society of Medicine. In 1976 and 1977, respectively, he was made Honorary Fellow of the Royal College of Physicians of Ireland and the Royal Australasian College of Physicians.

Widely sought as speaker and lecturer, he was honored by both Carleton College (in 1967) and MacMurray College (in 1973) which awarded him Honorary Doctor of Science degrees. For his important contribution to ACP-sponsored postgraduate education in South America, he was made Honorary Professor of Medicine at the Universidad del Zulia, in Maracaibo, Venezuela, in 1976, and in 1977 received the Cruz del Sol of the Grand Cruz of Chile. He was also honored by election to Membership in the Chilean Academy of Sciences, the Medical Society of Santiago, and the Societies of Internal Medicine in Colombia, Argentina and Costa Rica.

His lectureships included the Amos R. Koontz Memorial Fund Lecture at the 173rd Annual Meeting of the Medical and Chirurgical Faculty of the State of Maryland in 1971 and the Arthur E. Mills Memorial Oration given at the Annual Meeting of the Royal Australasian College of Physicians in 1975.

Dr. Rosenow played a major role in the establishment of the Council of Medical Specialty Societies and throughout his tenure at the College, he was Clinical Professor at the University of Pennsylvania Medical School and taught at the Philadelphia General and Pennsylvania Hospitals. In the year of his retirement, 1977, he received both the ACP Alfred Stengel Award for distinguished service and the "Internist of the Year" Award of the American Society of Internal Medicine.

Since 1977, the Rosenow's have continued to travel and maintain their international friendships, attending Congresses of the International Society of Internal Medicine in Rome, Hamburg and Prague. In 1981, they joined a group from Oberlin College and returned to China, visited the schools in which they had taught and the house in which Mrs. Rosenow had lived. The house in which Dr. Rosenow had lived had been razed when the city wall of Fenchow was removed.

Continuing to teach first year medical students in history taking and physical examinations at Graduate Hospital, Dr. Rosenow also serves as Vice-Chairman of the Southeastern Pennsylvania High Blood Pressure Control Program.

# Preface and Acknowledgments

When Dr. Walter Frommeyer was President of the College, he suggested to the Board of Regents that a history of the College from 1959 until my retirement in 1977 should be written. The matter of authorship was discussed and the Board of Regents finally decided that most of the data and perceptions of what occurred during these years would need to be obtained from me and the records at the headquarters. For this reason, it concluded that I could bring to such a history a much more personal account, including my personal knowledge of each President and what he contributed to the College.

When I arrived in Philadelphia, Mr. Edward Loveland had been the administrative head for 33 years. This gave the College a very solid base in an outstanding period of growth of this educational organization. It was a base which I acknowledge with great respect. It was a great pleasure to have worked with Mr. Loveland for a year.

In this history, we have tried to show not only what happened each year, but how the events related to other things going on in medicine generally. For example, this was a great period of development of subspecialties. More and more doctors depend on their specialty society for education.

Similar changes have occurred in socioeconomic matters. Specialty societies have been active in these fields. The College has kept in the forefront of all these changes, taking action in health and public policy matters.

Continuing education in all fields of medicine has burgeoned and the College deserves great credit, especially in developing the new *Medical Knowledge Self-Assessment Program,* now in its 6th edition at the time of the publication of this history. The aim of all the College's educational activities, such as the *Annals of Internal Medicine,* postgraduate courses, Annual Sessions, and Regional Meetings, is to provide quality health care through education.

Miss Ott, who had worked with Mr. Loveland for 33 years, became my secretary. After a few years, she was my assistant editor for the *ACP Bulletin* and finally worked very hard in developing the base of information from which I traced the history of the College from its beginning in 1915, a most helpful contribution. Miss Ott retired at the same time I did in 1977. She had worked for the College for over 50 years.

All of the former Presidents of the College have been cooperative and were excellent sources of information and judgment.

For two years after my retirement, I worked at Graduate Hospital in Philadelphia and did not have time to begin the history. Dr. Robert Moser, currently the Executive Vice President, arranged for the College archivist, Miss Bernice Lemley, to provide research assistance and to edit the manuscript. She has been most helpful and much of the accuracy of detail is due to her painstaking work. She has also been most perceptive in reading what I have written and has made many suggestions which have all contributed to the value of the history. Thanks are also due to Mrs. Stella Neeson Moser for her valuable consultative help in reading and editing the manuscript.

This book is truly the product of many hands at the Headquarters. The College's excellent printing and production facilities made it possible to prepare this book almost entirely in-house, with only final printing and binding done by an outside firm. Lois Morgan's Communications Center staff, especially Sylvia Robinson, deserve thanks for patiently revising numerous "editions". John Campbell and his Graphic Arts staff are to be commended for their very careful work in production; Edie Stillman handled the tedious task of typesetting with great skill. Ellie Kuljian, proofreader and indexer for the *Annals,* was indispensible in the final deadline stages. Finally, both the Marketing and Circulation Divisions deserve thanks for planning and promotion and still have work to do after publication. Many others unmentioned here were nevertheless equally important to successful completion.

The list of acknowledgements would not be complete without naming my devoted wife, Esther. During our tenure with the College, she was a great influence and an indefatigible support. What Howard Lewis said in jest, when the Board of Regents urged me to take her with me on College business, "because much of the time, she does as much for the College as he does!" turned out to be true in every sense.

Edward C. Rosenow, Jr., MACP

# CONTENTS

# Illustrations

### Presidential Photographs Inset in Biographical Profiles

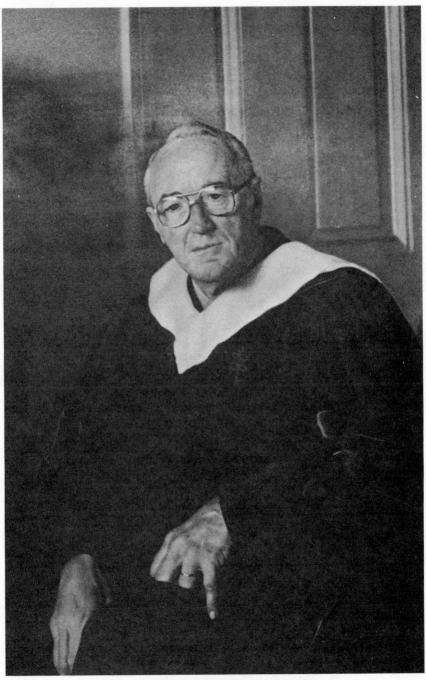

Plate 3.  Edward C. Rosenow, Jr., MACP
Executive Vice President, 1960-1977

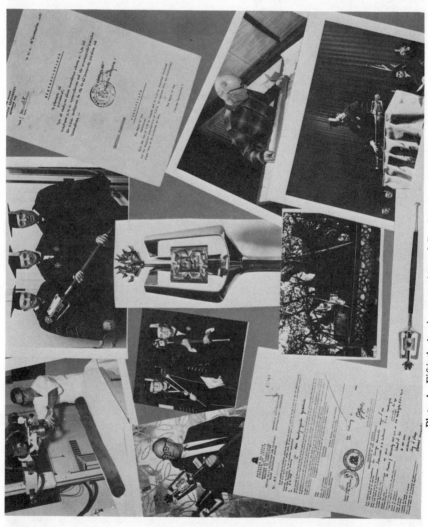

Plate 4.  Fiftieth Anniversary Annual Session, March 22-26, 1965
Montage showing history and first use of the College Mace

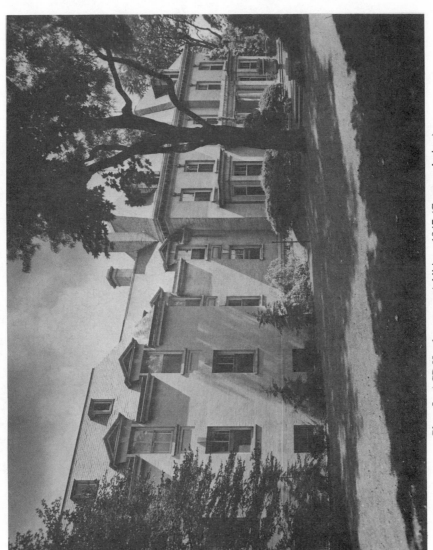

Plate 5. ACP Headquarters, Addition, 1947 (Courtyard view)

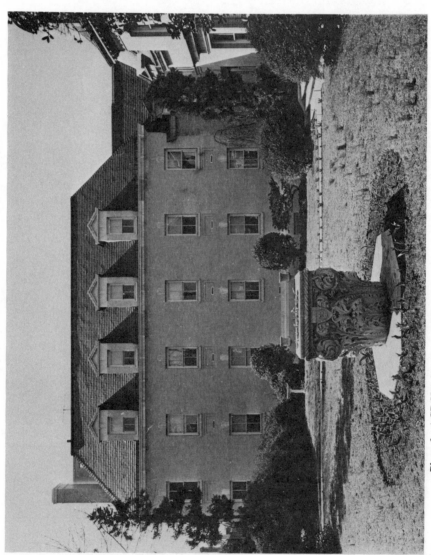

Plate 6. ACP Headquarters "West Wing" Addition, 1961 (Courtyard view)

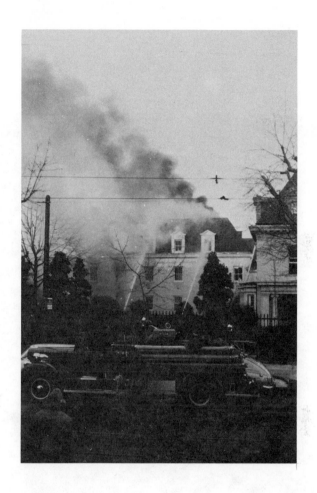

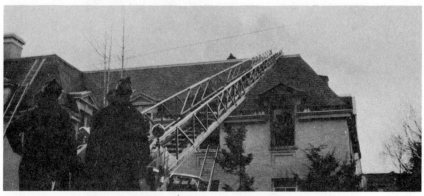

Plate 7. ACP Headquarters Fire, February 17, 1966

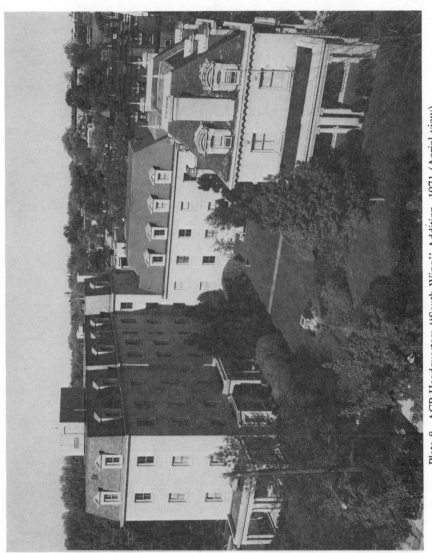

Plate 8. ACP Headquarters "South Wing" Addition, 1971 (Aerial view)

Prologue

# Enterprise in Internal Medicine

## 1915-1959

## Prologue

# Enterprise in Internal Medicine

### Beginnings - 1915-1926

In 1915, when the American College of Physicians [ACP] was founded, internal medicine was not a broadly recognized medical discipline. Membership in three societies founded prior to 1915 was limited to leaders in academic medicine. The American Clinical and Climatological Society was founded in 1884, the Association of American Physicians in 1886, and the American Society for Clinical Investigation in 1909.

Dr. Heinrich Stern, a New York internist, visited London in 1913 and attended a meeting of the Royal College of Physicians of London. He returned convinced that a similar college should be created in the United States. He presented the idea to a small group of physicians in New York City and in May, 1915, 14 physicians adopted the charter of the American College of Physicians.

Several months earlier, these same physicians organized the Congress of Internal Medicine for the purpose of sponsoring an annual clinical meeting. The Congress became the principal source through which members were recommended for Fellowship in the College. While the Congress involved a large number of practicing physicians, standards for election to College Fellowship were more selective; by 1922, only 597 physicians had been so elected.

Dr. Stern, the College's inspiration and its Secretary since its founding, died in May, 1918. Activity declined in the next few months and few Fellows were elected.

In December, 1918, a "Rescue Committee", composed of Frank Smithies of Chicago, Clement Jones of Pittsburgh, and William Gerry Morgan of Washington, regenerated interest. The former officers continued to serve, except Dr. Joseph H. Byrne of New York City, Secretary since Dr. Stern's death. He was succeeded by Dr. Smithies and the office was moved to Chicago.

In the succeeding years to 1926, the increase in membership was attributable to the energy of Dr. Smithies. Notably, however, academicians and the foremost leaders in internal medicine were not being attracted to the society. The subject of merging the Congress and the College was frequently debated.

The fledgling society, after sporadic publication of the *Transactions* of the Congress, published a journal, the *Annals of Clinical Medicine*, in 1922, which was very well received. Dr. Smithies served as its editor until 1924, when Dr. Alfred Scott Warthin of Ann Arbor, Michigan, assumed the editorship, continuing in this capacity until his death in 1931.

In 1922, significant changes in College government occurred. The Sixth Annual Clinical Session was held in Rochester, Minnesota, on April 3-6, and in Minneapolis on April 7-8. In what was recorded as the "Rochester Session" of the Council, proposed reorganization and a revised Constitution and Bylaws were approved and later submitted to the Fellows for adoption at the first Annual Business Meeting ever held by the College. The plan required the dissolution of the Board of Directors and Council and the creation of a governing body, the Board of Regents, and a Board of Governors to represent Fellows in each state and province. The Board of Governors was empowered to charge Fellowship dues. In fact, however, the Board of Regents continued to set the dues. This was formally adopted as a function of the Board of Regents in 1976.

In this historic first involvement of the full Fellowship in organizational decisions, the changes were approved unanimously. The Officers were empowered to appoint the Board of Regents and the Board was authorized to appoint the Board of Governors immediately, "in order to facilitate matters of reorganization". The Bylaws provided that certain special scientific societies could appoint representatives to the Board of Governors, but this provision was never implemented and the matter was later expunged from the Bylaws. The variety of societies was quite broad, including pathology, dermatology, radiology, and such organizations as the AMA, Southern Medical Association and the Association of American Physicians. Curiously, the American Gastroenterological Association was the only internal medicine subspecialty designated.

No set of circumstances of time and place could have been more propitious for the success of the plan. The Council held an informal meeting with Dr. William J. Mayo, a Fellow of the American College of Surgeons [ACS], in his office at the Mayo Clinic. He supported the plan strongly and assured the Council that if the membership adopted it, he would make every effort to promote the College among internists at the Mayo Clinic. The Mayo Clinic did, indeed, become a strong source of leadership over the years.

Several historical accounts detailed Dr. Smithies' efforts to persuade the Board of Regents to work closely with the ACS, which had been founded in 1913 and was also based in Chicago. Dr. Smithies' devotion to the growth of the College and the development of its prestige led him to promote cooperative intersocietal efforts in many directions without full approval of the Board, from which he received little encouragement to pursue closer cooperation with the surgical society.

In 1925, the Committee on Bylaws at last presented a plan to merge the Congress of Internal Medicine and the American College of Physicians. Members of the Congress were to be designated Associate members. This successful plan concluded several years of debate in which the regular agenda of the Board of Regents included proposals of methods to increase membership, improve standards for election and provide high quality educational programs. The Board of Governors nominated members for election to the Board of Regents, but it was relatively uninvolved in these other issues and in the promotion of the College's purposes until many years later.

## Reorganization - 1926-1930

The American College of Physicians underwent another series of changes beginning in 1926, spearheaded by Dr. Alfred Stengel, Professor and Chairman of the Department of Medicine at the University of Pennsylvania in Philadelphia. Elected to the Presidency of the College in 1926, he concluded, through input from friends and colleagues, that its development was being impeded. Membership nad increased since 1918 from 162 to 967, and there were 1,695 members in the Congress of Internal Medicine; the College's income had grown from $2,000 to $18,000; the journal was prospering, but there was much criticism of the College from the academic community because of its continued affiliation with the Congress. Fellows of the College did not include such leaders as department heads in medical schools, professors or distinguished research physicians. Dr. Smithies, Secretary-General for many years, was inclined to conduct a one-man show and largely dictated the decisions and directions adopted by the College.

Dr. Stengel appointed a committee to develop a plan to replace Dr. Smithies which would not peremptorily brush aside his long service and efforts. The committee suggested that Dr. Smithies serve another term, during the second year of which he was nominated President-Elect to serve the succeeding year as President. The tradition of long service in a given office was no longer deemed beneficial for the growing organization. Dr. Charles Martin of Montreal, Professor of Medicine at McGill University School of Medicine, succeeded Dr. Smithies as President. He accepted the nomination only after the Board of Regents agreed to meet five conditions for reorganizing the College:

1. A new Board of Regents with adequate representation from the academic leaders, and Dr. Martin to be given the privilege of designating at least four of these.
2. Such a new board must be given full power to raise the standards of admission. The present general policy of expansion was to be restricted so that the membership would be in keeping with the ideals of the College.
3. There was to be an entirely new and more appropriate application form.
4. The headquarters of the College were to be established in Philadelphia.
5. There was to be a readjustment of fees on a lower scale.''*

Dr. Martin emphasized the need for these changes by immediately presenting to the Board of Regents 20 Fellowship proposals received from medical school department heads, which would be submitted as formal applications if the Board adopted these suggestions.

Not the least of the reasons for the proposed move to Philadelphia was Dr. Stengel's advocacy of Mr. Edward R. Loveland as the College's first Executive Secretary. Mr. Loveland refused to accept the position unless the office was moved to Philadelphia.

The Board accepted Dr. Martin's proposals and immediately resigned as a body. The re-constituted Board included five additional members, whom Dr. Martin was given the privilege of designating. To minimize the "old guard" influences, Dr. Martin convinced Dr. Smithies that neither of them should accept nomination to the Board after serving as President, and neither did. However, thereafter, Past Presidents customarily returned to the Board for three years, until the duration was changed to one year in 1970.

*Piersol, George Morris, Gateway of Honor, Lancaster Press, c.1962.

The College enjoyed significant support and cooperation from the academic community following these changes, which introduced a new era with new priorities. The move to Philadelphia not only placed the leadership of the College firmly in the hands of academically oriented officers and Board members, but also introduced non-member lay executive administration. Edward R. Loveland was appointed Executive Secretary in 1926. Mr. Loveland had been Office and Personnel Manager of the University of Pennsylvania and was a personal friend of Dr. Stengel.

The publication of the journal also underwent important changes. In 1927, the contract with Williams and Wilkins was terminated and the College assumed responsibility for publication. Since Williams and Wilkins held the copyright to the title, the journal's name was changed to *Annals of Internal Medicine*. Thus was launched the journal that was to become one of the most prestigious publications in internal medicine. For several years, the printing contract was held by the University of Michigan Press in Ann Arbor. When Baltimorian Dr. Maurice C. Pincoffs was appointed editor in 1933, publication was moved to the Lancaster Press in Lancaster, Pennsylvania.

## Expansion - 1930-1940

By 1930, the College had consolidated its place among professional medical societies and stabilized its administrative and governance policies. In spite of the depression, it experienced a comparatively quiet and prosperous period. Membership increased rapidly and the College enjoyed financial stability due, in large part, to Mr. Loveland's sound fiscal and administrative management. An endowment fund was established, and in 1936 the permanent Headquarters building at 4200 Pine Street was purchased. Such stability characterized the 33 years of Mr. Loveland's service as Executive Secretary.

Annual clinical meetings had taken on increased importance by 1930. Responsibility for the Annual Session program was divided between the President and the General Chairman, who resided in that city where the Session would be held. Speakers for the general sessions were obtained by the President. All other aspects of the program were arranged by the General Chairman. This pattern continued until 1958, when the complexity of the scientific program and the size of the Annual Session necessitated the appointment of a Scientific Program Committee to assume responsibility for planning and supervision of the meetings.

The first Regional Meeting of the College was held in North Carolina in 1930. A modest beginning in grass roots activity, it nevertheless impressed the Governors of the College. Other state and regional meetings soon developed. During the same period, Bylaws changes enlarged the role of Governors in screening and endorsing candidates for membership in the College. These developments added to the role of the Board of Governors a new influence in the general affairs of the College. Since 1922, a Credentials Committee of the Board of Regents had nominated members for Fellowship, while a separate committee submitted applications for Associate Membership. In 1929, the Credentials Committee charge included recommendations for all classes of membership.

Governors, under these new provisions, assumed responsibility for screening proposals submitted to the Committee. Governors inevitably experienced the need for more personal acquaintance with physicians in their Regions, which fostered the increased organization of Regional Meetings.

In addition to these developments, joint meetings of the two boards added immeasurably to improved communications between Governors and Regents and with the membership. A joint boards' dinner was added to Annual Session events and proved to be highly useful. Very soon, this was changed to a luncheon which became a traditional part of the Annual Session.

The regularly recurring agenda of improvement in the standards of education in internal medicine was marked by two major developments: 1) In 1934, research fellowships were established. 2) In 1938, the first College-sponsored postgraduate courses were launched.

The first award of the College, the John Phillips Memorial Award, established in 1929, included a research fellowship and promoted further interest in this form of educational support, which has become a well established continuing program of the College.

Since 1927, the College had engaged in regular surveys of existing programs of postgraduate education in medical schools throughout the country. The Board of Regents determined that it need not create new education programs, but that the College should provide information about available programs by publishing a directory of courses for its members. By 1938, the Board determined that a more active role was required, and the first ACP-sponsored postgraduate course enrolled 116 members. The following year 120 were enrolled, and by 1940 registrations for the courses reached 144. These were offered just before the Annual Session. In the ensuing decade, having firmly established these courses as high quality education programs, the College expanded its activities by sponsoring courses in cooperation with medical schools.

Membership standards were a frequent subject of discussion between the Board of Regents and the Board of Governors. The recognition of specialists in internal medicine, as well as admission of allied specialists, presented particular problems. The Advisory Board of Medical Specialties [ABMS], a federation of medical specialty boards formed in 1933, suggested that examining boards should be established for all specialties.

In 1936, with the financial support of the ACP, the American Board of Internal Medicine [ABIM] was founded. It is interesting to note that the Board of Regents adopted a resolution several years earlier that passing a written examination was a prerequisite for Associate Membership. Anticipating the inevitable formation of a board which would administer examinations, however, the Board of Regents did not implement the resolution. Though the Board had considered for some years the possibility that the College could function as the board for internal medicine, as the Royal College of Physicians of London had functioned in England, it finally concluded that a separate board should be created to conduct examinations and voted funds for its creation.

With the establishment of the Certifying Board in 1936, it was generally agreed that board certification would be required for advancement to Fellowship in the College. However, the examination requirement was nullified for a two-year period, 1936-1938, when the ABIM decided to certify qualified physicians without examination. On application, the ABIM decided to certify, automatically, members of the Association of American Physicians over age 40, professors and associate professors in medical schools, Fellows of the College who had been in practice for 10 or more years, and practitioners in internal medicine for 15 years who were recommended by the Executive Committee of the American Medical Association's Section on the Practice of Medicine.

Steps taken to qualify candidates for certification inevitably stimulated hospital and other graduate training programs to conform to ABIM requirements. The Joint Commission on Accreditation of Hospitals [JCAH], founded in 1951 and the Residency Review Committee in Internal Medicine [RRC-IM] established in 1939, under the name of Conference Committee on Graduate Training in Medicine, were preceded by a series of ad hoc ACP and liaison committees. (In 1953, the Conference Committee's name was changed to the RRC-IM.) In 1938, the ACP Committee on Future Policy Development in Internal Medicine was appointed to study graduate training, and liaison representatives were appointed to the American Medical Association [AMA] Advisory Council on Education, Licensure and Hospitals.

The Board of Regents voted to continue admission of allied specialists such as pathologists, radiologists, neurologists, psychiatrists and dermatologists. In 1929, however, they had specifically excluded anesthesiologists from membership and this position remained unchanged until the 1970s when they were recognized as medical specialists and eligible for membership. Unrecognized also by the ACS as a surgical specialty, the anesthesiologists later refused an invitation to membership in that College and formed their own association.

In its third decade, the College continued to resist increasing pressures to respond to controversial medical practice positions taken by other organizations, particularly the AMA. An important precedent was set in 1938, however, when Dr. James H. Means stated his personal views on current controversies about state medicine and medical economics in his Presidential Address at the Convocation. Reaction was so strong that 150 Fellows who opposed his views submitted a critical resolution to the Board of Regents protesting public statements by the President on issues the College had chosen not to address. The Board upheld the right of presidents to speak on such subjects at their discretion without requiring Board approval.

In 1936, the administrative affairs of the ACP received a boost with the purchase of the permanent Headquarters. The Eisenlohr Mansion at 4200 Pine Street in Philadelphia was a distinguished architectural structure and served the College unchanged until 1947, when a new wing was added.*

*The Eisenlohr Mansion which currently represents approximately one-third of the total complex, was constructed in 1905 for the Eisenlohr family who were the owners of the Cenco Cigar Company. There were two brothers and a sister in the

Eisenlohr family and at one time, according to legend, the sister announced to her brothers that she was going to be married, because she wanted to have her own home. The brothers responded that it was not necessary to marry to obtain a home, because they would build one for her. The original mansion, now housing the offices of the Executive Vice President and other administrative offices, was that which resulted from the commitment by the brothers to their sister.

The architect was the very well-known Philadelphia firm of Horace Trumbauer. Another Eisenlohr house, designed by the Trumbauer firm is on Walnut Street, on the campus of the University of Pennsylvania. Other examples of Trumbauer's work can be found throughout Philadelphia and environs. Among the most noteworthy are the Free Library of Philadelphia, Union League, Racquet Club, Widener Office Building, Adelphia Hotel, Philadelphia Museum of Art (in association with others), Jefferson Hospital, Gray Towers-Beaver College Campus (former home of W.H. Harrison), and Lynwood Hall - Elkins Park. Horace Trumbauer (1868 or 69 to 1938) was the descendant of a colonial family. Self trained, he began his career as a draftsman with the Philadelphia architectural firm of H.W. & W.D. Hewitt.

In contrast to the changes of 1926, which markedly limited the periods of service in the Presidency, leadership stability in the third decade was reflected in the impressively long service of other College officers. In addition to Mr. Loveland's long tenure, the *Annals* enjoyed a long period of consistent editorial policy under the leadership of Dr. Maurice C. Pincoffs, Professor of Medicine at the University of Maryland. He was appointed Editor in 1933 and contined to serve with dedication and distinction until his retirement in 1960. When headquarters were moved to Philadelphia, the Board of Regents decided that the Treasurer should reside nearby and elected Dr. William Stroud, who served in that position from 1932 to 1958.

## National Crisis Spurs Internist Training - 1940-1950

The year 1940 marked the 25th Anniversary of the founding of the College and the Board of Regents authorized the publication of a history of the College. Dr. William Gerry Morgan was appointed as historian and *The American College of Physicians, Its First Quarter Century,* was published in time for the Anniversary celebrations.

The House Committee recommended the installation of a seal or painting over the fireplace in the Board Room. Many years later, an oil painting of Dr. Alfred Stengel and Dr. Charles Martin was placed there. The wrought iron gateway at the entrance to the mansion includes the Seal of the College.

The years of World War II wrought some far reaching changes in the College. Most prominent was the College's increased involvement in educational programs, brought about by the necessity for training military medical personnel. The role of the Board of Governors in College affairs increased fourfold as they assumed "front-line" responsibilities in sponsoring postgraduate courses all over the country. Regional activities were focused intensely on training, and the

Board of Regents formally transferred the work of the Postgraduate Courses Committee to the Board of Governors.

A Committee on War-time Graduate Medical Meetings arranged for consultants in various categories of specialization, and the Board of Regents created a Committee on Educational Policy to oversee all the work of committees engaged in education.

Contributing to this dissemination of educational activities was the Board of Regents' decision to discontinue Annual Sessions, and the traditional postgraduate courses associated with them for the duration of the war (from 1942-1945). By 1943, 20 percent of ACP members were in the military services. The College continued to hold Annual Business Meetings, termed the "wartime meetings". Dr. James E. Paullin, who was President Franklin D. Roosevelt's personal physician at Warm Springs, Georgia, presided over the first of these meetings on December 13, 1942, at College Headquarters. Dr. Paullin succeeded Dr. Roger I. Lee and served until 1944. Dr. Ernest E. Irons was elected ACP President in 1944 and served for the duration of the war. At the request of the US Government, the College cancelled plans to resume Annual Sessions in 1945. In 1946, Dr. Irons presided over the first Annual Session held since 1942, in Philadelphia.

The impact of wartime educational activity became apparent in the post-war era. It not only increased the scope of College sponsored courses, but intensified College responsibilities in evaluating the quality of physician training. The College had played a significant role in evaluating physicians for the Surgeons General of the Armed Forces. The work and status of the Credentials Committee of the College increased, and standards for membership were closely examined by both the Board of Regents and the Board of Governors, with frequent interaction between the two.

The war period generated considerable pressure to require ABIM certification for continued Associate Membership and admission of military physicians without certification was a subject of intensive debate. The Board of Regents affirmed that Associates could continue without term limitation and without certification, and that military physicians without certification could be admitted as Associates. ABIM certification would continue to be a requirement for Fellowship.

The 1946 Philadelphia Annual Session was a joyful occasion and heralded the establishment of two new awards, established by a gift of $10,000 from Dr. James Bruce in honor of his close friend, Dr. Alfred Stengel. The "Stengel Award" honored an individual who made outstanding contributions to the College in an official capacity. Dr. Bruce's gift also provided for a Lectureship in Preventive Medicine. Dr. Bruce died on September 5, 1946, and the Regents established the Lectureship as the "James D. Bruce Memorial Award", honoring distinguished contributions in the field of preventive medicine.

College educational activities became international in scope in 1948 when, with a grant from the Kellogg Foundation, the Committee on Fellowships and Awards announced the initiation of Latin American Fellowships and the formation of a committee to oversee this extensive project.

The burgeoning expansion of College activity required increased Staff support and expansion of Headquarters facilities. An addition to the mansion was occupied in 1948. The second floor auditorium of the new wing housed Board of Regents meetings and Regional Meetings. The former Board Room became a lounge which was used infrequently until after the fire of 1966. In 1967, it was remodeled and became the office of the Executive Director.

In 1947, Mr. Loveland completed 25 years of service to the College and was given a silver tray and cocktail cups. Miss Pearl Ott, his secretary, was given a gold pin and a $500 bond for her equally long service to the College.

## New Standards in a Technological Arena - 1950-1959

Postwar activities in education and development of standards in training resulted in the formation of three major organizations, which have continued activities to the present day in the areas of hospital accreditation, residency training program accreditation and medical audit and hospital utilization standards. The JCAH, incorporated in 1951, represented major cooperative intersocietal action and was sponsored and financially supported by the AMA, the American Hospital Association [AHA], the ACP, the ACS, and the Canadian Hospital Association.

The intersocietal Conference Committee on Graduate Training in Medicine formed in 1939 was discontinued in World War II and reactivated in 1946. In 1953, it was renamed the Residency Review Committee in Internal Medicine [RRC-IM] and empowered to accredit internal medicine residency training programs in hospitals. Its representation in equal numbers included the ACP, ABIM, and the AMA Council on Medical Education and Hospitals.

An outgrowth of the JCAH activities, the Commission on Professional and Hospital Activities [CPHA], incorporated in 1955, included representation from the ACP, ACS, AHA and the Southeastern Michigan Hospital Association. It was directed to develop and employ computerized techniques to acquire data for the evaluation of quality care, medical audits and utilization reviews in hospitals. Preceding this development was a three-year feasibility study in medical audit, initiated by the ACP and patterned after the ACS's techniques in tissue audit.

The American Society of Internal Medicine [ASIM] was organized in April, 1956. Its origins reached back to 1946 when a California Society of Internal Medicine was formed to address special problems which internists were experiencing regarding reimbursements from third party payers, such as Blue Cross/Blue Shield. The movement grew in other states and by 1956 medical socioeconomic issues were becoming strong concerns to many internists.

At the Annual Session in Los Angeles in 1956, an informal group of members of several state societies of internal medicine met to consider the possible formation of a national society of internal medicine. A deputation from this group, Drs. Lewis Bullock, George K. Wever, and Walter Beckh, pressed the College to support the recommendations of the "Cheney Committee Report" and establish a standing committee on voluntary health insurance. In 1954, the Board of

Regents had appointed a committee, with Dr. William C. Cheney as Chairman, to study Blue Shield and "related issues".

The Board of Regents, however, chose not to incorporate its recommendations into the framework of ACP purposes. The formation of a new society which would address medical socioeconomic problems moved ahead. In future years, the ACP was to find itself more and more deeply enmeshed in dealing with the problems of appropriate relationships with the ASIM, and by the 1970s could no longer ignore the necessity of addressing the impact of legislative activity on medical economic and social questions.

Wartime use of paramedical personnel gave impetus to study of its employment in peace time medicine and in 1957, Dr. Edward C. Rosenow, Jr., soon to be Executive Director for the ACP, was appointed ACP representative to an AMA sponsored joint committee to study uses of paramedical personnel. At that time, there were more than 60 paramedical organizations in the nation and the AMA initiatives were an effort to institute an advisory medical activity which would provide for better nationwide planning in the paramedical manpower area.

Attendance at Regional Meetings of the College was increasing and postgraduate courses were being offered through medical schools and other organizations. The trend reflected a rising tide of interest in continuing medical education as military physicians returned to civilian life and technological advances in medicine altered traditional training.

Mr. Loveland was approaching retirement and the Board of Regents appointed a Committee on Administrative Structure, chaired by Dr. Walter L. Palmer, to consider the leadership requirements of the College in view of drastically altered directions in medicine since World War II. Mr. Loveland announced that he would retire in January 1959, as required by the Pension Plan, unless he was specifically requested by the Board of Regents to continue. Early in 1958, he became quite ill. The Board requested that he remain until the end of 1959, but it directed the ad hoc committee, appointed June 1958, to press its deliberations to an early conclusion so the College could begin the search for a new administrative director. The Board approved the Committee's recommendation that a physician be hired as the chief administrative officer and that a financial assistant also be hired.

The Committee also recommended changes in the Pension Plan which were adopted by the Board: 1) Membership in the plan was not mandatory; 2) An employee should retire at age 65 and would receive 120 months pension. If the retired employee died before completion of the period, the remaining payments would be issued to the beneficiary, until the full pension was paid.

In November 1958, the Committee on Administrative Structure was discharged and a Committee on Personnel was appointed to initiate the search for a chief administrator and financial assistant. Dr. Walter L. Palmer, Dr. Howard Lewis and Dr. Richard Stetson were appointed to the new Committee.

Mr. Loveland's longtime physician friends expressed their gratitude in 1954, when they arranged to have his portrait painted as a gift to the College, to be hung in the Board Room. Two years later, on his 30th anniversary, the Board of

Regents, in an unprecedented motion, made him an Honorary Fellow.

An era of College history was about to close with Mr. Loveland's retirement. On his 30th anniversary of association with the College in 1956, Mr. Loveland reviewed the impressive changes he had witnessed.

In 1926, there were 1,000 members; in 1956, 9,200. *Annals* subscriptions increased from 14,000 in 1926 to 20,450 in 1956. The Annual Session attracted 800 registrants in 1926, showing a phenomenal increase to 6,380 by 1956. Technical exhibits were introduced in the 1950s and showed a net income in 1956 of $45,000. In 1926, when the endowment fund was established, there were three Life Members; in 1956, 1,388 Life Members.

During Mr. Loveland's tenure, the ABIM was established. ACP postgraduate courses in 1956 had attracted 1,400 registrants. The Headquarters building had been purchased and one new wing added. Regional Meetings were now being held on a regular basis in most of the Regions and were showing marked growth in attendance by 1956. A College directory was being published regularly and Group Insurance Programs had been established. A Residency Revolving Loan Fund was initiated and a strong research scholarship program was started. The College had its own journal which had achieved a prestigious place in the medical literature. The JCAH, RRC-IM, and CPHA were recent additions in the intersocietal cooperative scene. The financial assets of the College had grown since 1926 from $8,000 to over $1.3 million in 1956. The number of Staff had increased from the original two, Mr. Loveland and Miss Pearl Ott, to 25, including two aides to Dr. Pincoffs, the *Annals* Editor, who was located in Baltimore.

After my arrival as the new Executive Director, I had many conversations with Mr. Loveland and came to understand his unusual success in medical society management, in spite of the lack of a medical degree. From the time of his employment in 1926, with Dr. Stengel's mentorship, he was never without access to strong leaders in internal medicine and in the College. Located in Philadelphia were a succession of ACP Presidents with whom he worked closely: Dr. Stengel, Dr. Piersol, Dr. H. O. Perry Pepper, Dr. T. Grier Miller, Dr. Richard Kern and finally, Dr. Thomas Durant, who later served as President in 1964-65.

Dr. Piersol had served for many years as Secretary General and was author of the second College history, *Gateway of Honor*, published in 1962. Dr. William Stroud, who served for many years as Treasurer was also a Philadelphia physician. Dr. Durant became Treasurer upon Dr. Stroud's retirement. All of these physicians had been or were associated with the University of Pennsylvania. Dr. Durant and Dr. Kern were affiliated with Temple University's School of Medicine while they were active in the College. Dr. Wallace Yater was nearby in Washington, D.C., a frequent consultant and close friend of Mr. Loveland. Dr. Yater had served as Secretary General and succeeded Dr. Piersol as Chairman of the Credentials Committee. Mr. Loveland had ready access to all of these by phone and regular contact on very short notice. Over his years of service, he acquired impressive knowledge of the nature of the medical profession and its problems.

The eve of the new decade, 1960, presented major opportunities and problems for the College in intersocietal activity, and Dr. Howard Lewis's advice to me on my arrival at the College was that I commit my time to attend virtually all meetings of the RRC-IM and the JCAH, and to make myself available at all times to the ABIM and to the AMA and its Council on Medical Education. This advice emphasized the primary reason for the College's decision to hire a physician for the post.

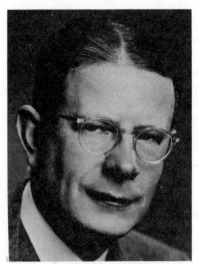

*Dwight Wilbur, MACP*

Dr. Dwight Wilbur, President of the College in 1958-1959, offered the following perspectives on the closing era in a recent interview.

When I became President of the College in 1958, my major concern was that the College was not attracting academically oriented physicians, and particularly, young internists. This was a time of a marked rise in the number of young academic people, because of the new funds being provided by the NIH and other health agencies for biomedical research. There was tremendous expansion in medical education after World War II, and officers getting out of the service and coming into the civilian life wanted to get residency training and become specialists. So the number of young internists in practice, in training and in the academic world was really growing very rapidly.

Dr. Wilbur asked these young men why they were not interested in the College and found that most of them felt they could get newer and better medical information by joining specialty societies such as the American Heart Association, more focused on their own specialty interest. While he thought the ACP programs were good, Dr. Wilbur also saw the need to provide something additional for these younger physicians. Through the help of Dr. Carl Moore, of Washington University in St. Louis, and Dr. Jack Myers, at the University of Pittsburgh, he developed sessions on clinical investigation. In addition, through the efforts of Dr. Robert Williams, of the University of Washington, Seattle, additional sessions in basic sciences were scheduled. They were very successful and eventually, when the Annual Session program was organized along subspecialty lines, the basic science and clinical investigation papers were integrated with clinical papers.

In the past, the Annual Session Program was pretty much the responsibility of the President and a Chairman of General Arrangements in the city where the session was held. At that time there were hospital clinics, TV clinics, and panel discussions. During Dr. Wilbur's term, the clinical pathological conferences were changed to clinical-basic science conferences to bring more physiology and biochemistry to the attention of the young clinicians. All of these new programs resulted in the formation of a standing Committee on Scientific Programs. This was the first time a standing committee was appointed for Annual Session matters.

One of the real problems confronting young internists that the College had to face was that when they finished their residencies, under the Bylaws of the College they were required to practice for two years in the community before they were eligible to become Associates of the College. During that two years these young internists directed their attention to specialty organizations, the county medical society, the state medical organization, the American Heart Association and similar groups. This was very unfortunate and it didn't tend to attract the younger internist to the College. This circumstance originated from the ABIM rule that you couldn't take the Boards until you'd had two years of practice.

The real key to involving these young people was having a good Annual Session program and getting the people you want means you must have a good program chairman who knows them and who'll talk them into participating, as Bob Williams did. Bob got on the phone because he had to do this in a hurry and as I think I mentioned to you before, he ran up a stupendous telephone bill over which Ed Loveland and I had quite a little battle, but he finally paid it. I think of things that I did in the College in my years of service and the Annual Session changes were the most important, but I think in the long run it brought into the College internists of a much broader base than had been interested in it before.

The time was approaching when Ed Loveland, who had been the one and only Executive Secretary of the College, was about to retire and Ed Loveland had done an absolutely remarkable job as Executive Secretary. He was very frugal in the days when the College was on a minimum budget and he had a very good concept, for a layman, of what the leaders in medicine and internists were interested in and what they wanted from the College. As the years went on, with his increasing experience, Mr. Loveland just became masterful at his job. I traveled around the country for a long time with Ed Loveland, going to Regional Meetings, which he knew how to run very well. He knew most of the Governors well and he could, therefore, go to Lexington, Kentucky or out to Montana, or wherever, and he felt right at home with a Governor and helped him tremendously in running a very successful Regional Meeting.

When the time came for a man of this importance in the College to retire, there were problems. It became quite clear to me and to several other members of the Board of Regents that despite what Ed Loveland had done as a layman, the College now really needed a physician, an internist and preferably a Fellow of the College in the chief administrative officer's role. It needed, as well, someone who was an expert in administration and financial affairs, which Ed Loveland had handled very successfully. One of the reasons for taking this stand was that the College was becoming increasingly interested in what today is called continuing medical education or as it was then called, postgraduate education. The College was also becoming increasingly active in things outside of Philadelphia, for example, the JCAH, relationships with the ABIM, the RRC-IM, the AMA, the National Research Council and the CPHA.

Ed Loveland was very opposed to the idea of a physician administrator. But our interest was not in obtaining an elder statesman symbol for the College, but in getting a really outstanding internist who had had experience with organizational affairs and in continuing medical education. In order that I, personally, would not be directly involved in the selection, I appointed a committee to study administrative structure and to consider this matter. When they submitted their recommendations, we changed the name of the Committee to the Committee on Administrative Personnel and Dr. Walter L. Palmer, who had been President of the College the two years before me, was appointed as chairman. Walter Palmer, I think, did an outstanding job on both committees.

I felt also at that time that the College was not doing what it really should do in terms of informing the public about the College or who an internist is, and what an internist does. There was a good deal of material that was developed that would be useful public information and I strongly urged the appointment of an assistant to the executive secretary for public information and the Committee on Administrative Structure agreed. Unfortunately, the individual selected for this job was unsatisfactory, and this function was tabled indefinitely. It is now an important part of the College's functions.

My other interest in organizational functions was to reactivate the Executive Committee and I think during my presidential year, the Executive Committee met on three occasions. Mr. Ed Loveland was opposed to this and thought the Board of Regents should meet twice a year, in November at Headquarters and at the Annual Sessions, and handle all of the College business. It was very obvious to me, however, that the Board of Regents was doing a lot of routine work that kept it from considering carefully more important problems that it faced.

The Executive Committee can't effectively meet at the same time as the Board meets, and during my time, we at least accomplished separate meetings of the Executive Committee.

At the Chicago meeting we decided to hold a luncheon for approximately 200 of Chicago's leaders in business, labor, education, commerce, government and so on. This luncheon was entitled, "The Care and Preservation of the American Executive". The subjects ranged from reducing the threat of cancer through the control of arthritis and rheumatism, the relationship of pressure and tension to high blood pressure, medical research, avoiding heart attack, emotional disturbances in business and finally, are ulcers necessary?

The members who participated were very distinguished people, such [physicians] as Harry Bockus of Philadelphia, William Menninger of Topeka, Kansas, Chester Jones of Boston, Philip Hench of Rochester, Minnesota, Howard Lewis of Portland, Sarah Jordan of Boston, Irving Page of Cleveland and Walter L. Palmer of Chicago. Each took about 10-12 minutes to discuss the subject and a question period followed. We had a very good attendance at that meeting and I thought it worked extremely well. It was carried on, I believe, for a few years after that and I guess it finally faded away.

In Philadelphia, we engaged the interest of the Greater Philadelphia Chamber of Commerce in a joint effort. It was as if the Chamber put on a program using the expertise of the American College of Physicians which happened to be meeting in

Philadelphia. The Chamber invited all the guests and the College provided the program. This was extremely successful, but in other cities we could not develop this kind of cooperation.

Now I should say a few words about socioeconomic affairs. The Society of Internal Medicine movement actually began at the Bohemian Club in San Francisco. My interest in this began when I returned from service in the Navy and began to practice again in 1946. I observed that an internist would get for an hour's work, involving a complete examination of a patient, in the neighborhood of $15. This was the amount paid by Blue Shield/Blue Cross or other third-party carriers. Well, it was simply impossible to do this, examining four new patients a day, winding up with $60 - if that much, paying the overhead and at the same time trying to carry the workload of old patients. I invited my friend, Ed Bruck, who was then one of the leading internists in San Francisco and Chairman of the Council of the California Medical Association, to lunch at the Bohemian Club about April 1946 and discussed this matter. He agreed with me completely.

We established a San Francisco Society of Internal Medicine and in a few months we met the leaders in California and established a California Society of Internal Medicine. We presented the idea that internists would be more effective in persuading the California Medical Association, particularly, to recognize the need for adequate compensation for what the internist did and that the solution was a relatively simple one. The physician need only to supply objective evidence that he had done a complete history and physical examination and provide a complete diagnostic review of the patient to the third-party carrier when requested. It was a good solution and it worked very well.

We succeeded in obtaining a re-evaluation of fee reimbursements. After this was accomplished, the Societies of Internal Medicine in a number of other states began to attempt the same thing. Some of the societies were purely scientific. The Minnesota Society, for instance, was probably the best Society of Internal Medicine of any state in the country at that time; others were established purely for economic and social reasons and finally the ASIM was established about 1956, ten years after these events.

The socioeconomic approach really began with the establishment of the California Society in 1946 and the individuals who played leading roles, at least in California, were Drs. Lew Bullock, Walter Beckh and George Wever. Well, I was really responsible for having started it here in California. I was very much interested in it and this is one of the reasons why I supported the Cheney Committee Report in the College. I felt the American College of Physicians should get into this activity and not confine its attention to the scientific and educational fields, but the Board of Regents did not go along with the Cheney Committee report, so I had two alternatives. One was to stay in the College and support its policies and the other was to resign from the College and get active in the ASIM movement and I chose the former.

The last point that I want to make is that in the time that I was President of the College, I went around to as many Regional Meetings as I could and my talk to them was almost always on the same subject. I called it "The Third Person in Medicine" and I discussed this to some extent in my Presidential Address at the Annual Convocation in 1959. I tried to point out that there was increasing interference in the physician-patient relationship by third parties. As the doctor sat by his patient's bedside or his office there was an increasing interference in that one-to-one relationship by third persons, some within the profession, but most outside the profession.

Within the profession there were such things as the growth of specialism. With some patients whom I saw as an internist, I had to consider what a specialist could do in this sort of a situation. Technology became increasingly important and there were more and more internists doing electrocardiograms, using fluoroscopic apparatus, taking X-ray films in their offices and performing other sorts of new things, such as pulmonary function tests. The tremendous growth of biomedical sciences and related technology that developed after World War II created the atmosphere in which the influence of third parties within the profession very significantly altered the one-to-one relationship of the physician and patient.

Another influence developing within the profession was the increasing hospital staff rules and regulations. But much more important influences from outside the medical profession came to sit at the bedside with the patient and the doctor. These included the media, because what the media wrote was a very important influence. Today internists are very much influenced by what patients read in the media or what they see on television and this, in turn, influences the practice of medicine and the physician-patient relationship. Furthermore, attorneys were becoming increasingly important in matters of professional liability and malpractice. Since that time these have just exploded all over.

I commented to Dr. Wilbur that when I first came to the College I stated to the Board,

> I think one of your objectives, among others, is that you'd like to make the College a truly national organization and not a Philadelphia based club, which it seemed to be in many ways. In order to make that so, you must agree to two things: 1) There should be no restriction on my travel when I think it is important for the College. 2) I don't want to hear anybody on this Board ever say that "so-and-so" can't be on a committee because he's west of Chicago and it would cost too much to bring him to a meeting. The Board agreed to that. Chester Keefer, especially, strongly supported it.

Mr. Loveland had helped to establish a solid and financially sound institution. Now, confronting the scene at the end of the 1950s, it was required to venture rather boldly into new and more uncertain waters than it had traditionally sailed. It was a good ship and ready for the high seas.

Chapter One

# Education and Research: Impetus for Growth

**1959-1964**

# I. Education and Research:
## Impetus for Growth

### Part One (1959-1960)

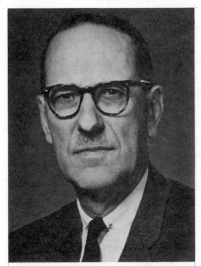

*Howard Phelps Lewis, MACP*

Howard Phelps Lewis, MD, was born in San Francisco, California, on February 18, 1902. He was married in 1927 to Wava Irene Brown. They are the parents of two children, Dr. Richard Phelps Lewis, and Thomas Howard Lewis.

Dr. Lewis received his Bachelor of Science in Chemical Engineering at Oregon State University in 1924. He earned his medical degree at the University of Oregon School of Medicine in 1930, where he also served his internship and residency from 1930 to 1932. During medical school he was an Assistant and Instructor in Anatomy and Instructor in Medicine. Following his training he joined the faculty, progressing to the rank of Professor and Chairman of the Department of Medicine in 1947. He served in that position until 1972, when he was appointed Emeritus Professor of Medicine.

He was a major and then a colonel in the US Army Medical Department from 1942 to 1946. He served at the William Beaumont General Hospital in Texas, the Holloran General Hospital in New York, and the Rhoads General Hospital in Utica, New York. He was a consultant in medicine, Second Service Command at Governors Island, New York. Following active service, he continued as a civilian consultant to the Surgeon General of the Army from 1947 to 1975.

Dr. Lewis holds membership in Alpha Omega Alpha and Sigma Xi. He was a charter director of the American Board of Family Practice and served from 1970 to 1978; a recertified diplomate of the American Board of Internal Medicine, he served as a member of the Board from 1952-1961, and its chairman from 1959-1961. He was a member of the American Clinical and Climatological Association, serving as its president from 1967-1968, and Governor for Oregon of the American College of Cardiology. He belonged to the American Federation for Clinical Research, the American Heart Association, the American Medical Association and the Association of American Physicians. He was a member of the Residency Review Committee in Internal Medicine from 1960-1965, and served as Chairman from 1963-1965. He was also a member of the Residency Review Committee for Family Practice from 1969-1976. He was a member of the Advisory Council of the National Heart Institute from 1956-1961.

Active in medical publishing, Dr. Lewis served as Editor of the American

Heart Association's *Modern Concepts of Cardiovascular Disease* from
1956-1961. He was also on the Editorial Boards of the *American Heart Journal,
Archives of Internal Medicine,* and *Circulation.* He published more than 150 articles and addresses, and one book, *The History and The Physical Examination,*
c.1979.

Dr. Lewis was a great admirer of Dr. Maurice C. Pincoffs, Editor of the *Annals
of Internal Medicine,* describing him as one of the wisest men he had ever encountered. Being conservative and not given to unconsidered change, Dr. Pincoffs often opposed Dr. Lewis's ideas. Nevertheless, Dr. Lewis remembered
him as unusually persuasive, reaching the heart of a matter in debate and expressing his opinions so incisively that he often carried the day, even in the presence
of strong opposition. Dr. Lewis received numerous awards, including an Award
of Merit from the American Heart Association in 1960; The Allen J. Hill Teaching Award, University of Oregon Medical School, 1966; Alfred Stengel Memorial Award, American College of Physicians, 1966; The Goldheaded Cane
Award, University of California School of Medicine, San Francisco, 1960.

He was the Goldheaded Cane Visiting Speaker, University of Texas Medical
School, Galveston, 1962, and the Donald Church Balfour Visiting Professor of
Medicine, Mayo Graduate School of Medicine in 1966. He was on the Board of
Overseers, Lewis & Clark College, Portland, Oregon, and received a Citation
for Distinguished Achievement in Medicine from Oregon Health Sciences Uni-
versity in 1980.

Dr. Lewis's leadership in the College began in 1948, when he was elected
Governor for Oregon. He then served as Third Vice-President from 1951-1952,
as Regent from 1952-1958, as President-Elect in 1958-59, and President in
1959-60. He was made a Master in 1964.

His recollections of those years highlighted some important innovations:

When he was Chairman of the Committee on Educational Policy, Dr. Eugene
B. Ferris, committee member, recommended that the Annual Session program
be changed to include basic sciences and clinical investigation in addition to the
usual clinical sessions. Dr. Lewis enthusiastically presented this idea to the
Board of Regents. The Board was resistant to the changes until Dr. Dwight
Wilbur, the President, simply introduced the new format in 1959 and demonstrated its success. Dr. Lewis's Presidential year was the second year of the new
program format. The basic science and clinical investigation programs drew
large numbers, which guaranteed their continued inclusion in the scientific program for several years. Later new approaches to programming were developed
based on specialty disciplines incorporating both research and clinical aspects.

The Annual Session program received special attention from Dr. Lewis. He
wrote to every Professor of Medicine at every medical school and stimulated the
submission of more than 500 abstracts.

Dr. Lewis also participated in the development of the American College of
Physicians Award, a proposal offered by Dr. Philip Hench which was adopted
by the Board, but with little initial enthusiasm. The Committee on Awards unanimously nominated Dr. Hench as the first recipient. He was unwilling, at first, to

accept the Award because of his role in proposing it, but yielded to the Committee's insistance that he ideally fitted the requisites defined in the award.

Dr. Lewis presided over the Convocation in Los Angeles in 1956, when academic regalia were first introduced. He recalled the lengthy debates which preceded its adoption. Dr. Richard Strong of Canada was the strongest proponent of replacing full dress and white ties with academic regalia and was largely responsible for its ultimate acceptance. Dr. Lewis recalled that this addition to the color and dignity of Convocation ceremonies was immediately appreciated by Board and College members.

The building program to add a wing to the Headquarters was also preceded by much opposition, particularly from the Committee on Finance. Dr. Lewis recalled,

> There was a lot of resistance to building this wing, which was greatly needed. As a way of putting this proposition over, I asked Richard Kern, who at the time was Chairman of the House Committee, to have some attractive architectural drawings made for the outside of the proposed wing and rough indications of the structure of the inside as well. I asked him to have these drawings on display in the Regents' room so all could see and then for him to explain in detail in his best style the need for such a plan. Dick really outdid himself and the idea was enthusiastically adopted even by Joe McCarthy, Chairman of the Finance Committee.

Dr. Lewis's greatest disappointment was the failure of the experiment with sectional meetings, but we shared some exciting times traveling to Regional Meetings, which were so often held in times of poor weather, in the days of propeller planes and poor navigational aids. One of the most memorable was an all night train ride to fogbound Columbus, Ohio, from Cleveland when a flight was cancelled.

On one occasion, we went to a Kentucky Regional Meeting which was a "stag" affair. During their business meeting, the matter of inviting wives to the dinner was discussed, and Dr. Lewis and I were asked to express our opinions. We spoke strongly in favor of inviting the wives and pointed out that Kentucky was the only Regional Meeting where this was not a tradition. Dr. John Scott, then over 80 years old, made a motion that Kentucky should get "in step with the rest of the College". The motion passed unanimously.

Our activities included meetings with convention managers from various cities in search of sites for future Annual Sessions and we were about to talk with the representative from Detroit when Mr. Loveland announced that he, Dr. Lewis and I were scheduled to drive to Newark, New Jersey, to a Regional Meeting and that Dr. Durant, our Treasurer, would continue the interviews. The gentleman from Detroit called me later to express his disappointment over this peremptory treatment. Thereafter, Mr. Dauterich and I conducted these interviews with convention managers in advance of Site Committee reviews for decision by the Board of Regents.

Dr. Lewis commented on the post convention tour to Honolulu,

> Our group was booked on a chartered jet, the other half traveled on a propeller plane. The thrill of my maiden jet voyage was dampened, however, when the plane developed engine trouble and was forced to return to Honolulu. However, we en-

joyed an extra free day in Honolulu while a replacement engine was flown in from the Mainland.

Throughout his career, Dr. Lewis especially loved teaching and working with medical students. While he was Head of the Department of Medicine at the University of Oregon, he considered history taking and physical examinations so important in training that he always participated in teaching the courses. I recall an AMA sponsored course on this subject which he taught. The course was oversubscribed by practicing physicians and was enthusiastically received.

On one occasion, he was scheduled to teach an ACP postgraduate course in Portland, Oregon. He called me to let me know of an error on the program, which described the five-day course as lasting for several weeks. His sense of humor soothed a most embarrassed ACP secretary, and the next time he was at the Headquarters, he sought her out and shared the humor of the situation with her. His generous and understanding attitude toward headquarters staff reflected a typical quality of those who served the College as President.

Dr. Lewis was the first College President with whom I worked as Executive Director. He was a stimulating person, patient and kind, and a good friend. We shared a love of golf and from time to time enjoyed the sport together. His inveterate teaching impulses led him to send me an article on proper golf stances, which actually improved my game.

## 1959-1960

Mr. Loveland and Dr. Pincoffs retire; Dr. Rosenow and Dr. Elkinton appointed. American College of Physicians Award. Teaching and Research Scholars. ACP Bulletin. ACP/ASIM Liaison Committee. Medical Audit. Essentials of Residency Training Programs in Internal Medicine.

The American College of Physicians had grown steadily in size and importance since its inception. Through the wise leadership of its Officers and Regents and the careful administration of its affairs by Mr. Edward Rutherford Loveland, the College also enjoyed a stable financial structure as it entered the 1960s.

After 33 years of continuous and devoted service to the College, Mr. Loveland retired as Executive Secretary on December 31, 1959. He had been appointed in April, 1926, at a time when the ACP was passing through one of the most turbulent periods in its existence. Prior to his appointment there had never been a chief administrative officer, and even though he knew little about the College, he undertook that responsibility, firmly establishing the Headquarters office in Philadelphia and developing an efficient administrative and financial program, both of which the College had previously lacked.

Mr. Loveland was responsible in large measure for the conspicuous growth of the College, the success of the *Annals of Internal Medicine,* the popularity of the Annual Sessions and other educational activities. His efforts on behalf of the ACP did not go unrecognized. At the 1956 Annual Session in Los Angeles, the Board of Regents had bestowed upon him an Honorary Fellowship. This was the first and only time in the history of the College that a recipient was not a physician.

The greatest honor paid to Mr. Loveland, and the one he valued most, was given at the 1960 Annual Session where he was presented the Alfred Stengel Memorial Award. This was particularly appropriate since Dr. Stengel had worked closely with him throughout the early, critical years of the College's development. In fact it was Dr. Stengel who had recommended Mr. Loveland for this position when he was Vice President for Medical Affairs and Mr. Loveland was in the business office of the University of Pennsylvania. About the time he was awarded Fellowship, Mr. Loveland was also elected a member of the Alpha Omega Alpha Honorary Medical Society in recognition of his contributions to American medical education.

After a long, trying illness, Edward R. Loveland died on October 14, 1960. A tribute in the *Bulletin of The American College of Physicians [ACP Bulletin]* written by his long time friend, Dr. George Morris Piersol, exhibited the depth to which Mr. Loveland had devoted his life to the College.

> So great was his concern in the affairs of the College that up until the last few weeks of his life, he worked, so far as he was able, upon the preparation of a Manual of Rules and Procedures for the College and was indexing all of the accumulated minutes of the Board of Regents from 1915 through 1959. It is no exaggeration to state that there has never been a more efficient or dedicated member of the College staff.

The permanent Headquarters of the College was established in Philadelphia with the purchase of the property at 4200 Pine Street in 1936. As membership increased and programs became more diverse, additional office space was required to handle the increasing work load. In 1947 a building addition was completed which adequately met the requirements for the operation of the office at that time.

### Physician Hired as Executive Director

It was obvious that if the influence of the College was to continue to expand, progressive new programs had to be initiated and successful activities augmented to strengthen its position in medical education, science and research. Primarily for this reason, the Committee on Administrative Structure recommended, and the Board of Regents agreed, that a physician with strong background in postgraduate medical education and administrative experience should replace the retiring Executive Secretary.

At this time I was the Executive Director of the Los Angeles County Medical Association and had a special interest in continuing medical education, having occupied such positions as Director of Medical Extension, University of Southern California; Chairman of the Postgraduate Activities Committee of the California Medical Association, and Editor-in-Chief of *Audio-Digest*. A graduate of Harvard Medical School, I also served an internal medicine fellowship at the Mayo Foundation. I was active in many medical societies and had been a

Fellow of the College since 1942. The Board of Regents appointed me Executive Director and I took office on January 1, 1960. In making the announcement, President Howard P. Lewis asserted that "Dr. Rosenow brings to the office many very important qualities which the professional man as the Chief Administrator of the College should have."

In California, in the Fall of 1958, Dr. Dwight Wilbur, then President of the College, had asked me whether I was interested in the chief administrative office of the American College of Physicians. Dr. Wilbur had known me for many years, including the time in Rochester, Minnesota, before I went to California. He knew that I had practiced internal medicine for almost 19 years in Pasadena and was also a Clinical Professor of Medicine at the University of Southern California School of Medicine during that time. He was aware of my work with the California Medical Association as Chairman of the Postgraduate Committee and of my activities as Editor of *Audio-Digest*. I had had experience in several organizations, having been President of the Los Angeles Society of Internal Medicine, the Heart Association and the County Medical Association. I served as Executive Director of the latter organization from 1957 to 1959.

During our conversation, Dr. Wilbur told me about the Regents' discussions regarding the type of physician they hoped to find. Some thought that an academician, such as a medical school dean or professor, would be best. Others preferred someone who was well versed in clinical practice, with a clinical teaching appointment in a medical school.

I expressed an interest in the position and in February, 1959, I saw Dr. Wilbur at a Regional Meeting of the College and he described the difference of opinion among Search Committee members on exactly what kind of physician they wished to employ.

In a recent discussion, Dr. Lewis recounted his memory of the final decision:

> We had an informal meeting with the Search Committee in Dwight Wilbur's suite at the Annual Session in 1960 to discuss possible candidates. I had met you at the Regional Meeting in Palm Springs in February and was much impressed with your suitability for the job. I was the one who moved that we seek you for the post. They all agreed.

I went to the Annual Session in Chicago in 1959, expecting that the Board of Regents or someone from the Committee might want to speak with me about this position. Only Dr. Howard Wakefield mentioned it, asking if I knew that they were considering hiring a physician to take Mr. Loveland's place. When I replied affirmatively, he asked whether I would be interested and opined that I would be a good candidate. It appeared that he did not know that I had already been suggested.

Having heard from no one, I was a little surprised when Dr. Wilbur called me after the meeting to ask if I was still interested. He explained that I had not been approached because of a fear that at the Annual Business Meeting some changes in the Bylaws might cause a year's delay in the appointment, engendering embarrassment. But neither the old Bylaws nor the changes appeared to prohibit employing a physician, and Dr. Wilbur suggested that I meet with the Search Committee at the time of the AMA meeting in Atlantic City in June of 1959. By that date, Dr. Wilbur had assumed the chairmanship of the Search Committee. Also attending my meeting with the Search Committee were Drs. Chester Keefer, Marshall Fulton, Marvin Pollard and Murray Kinsman. There was a man waiting to be interviewed by the Committee before my appointment with them who told me that he was a candidate for the business assistant position. I told the Search Committee that if I were hired, I would prefer to choose my own assistant. I also stated that, if appointed, I would be available by September in order to work with Mr. Loveland for several months before his retirement.

After meeting with the Search Committee I visited with the President, Dr. Lewis, in Portland, Oregon. We spent a long afternoon discussing the potentials of the position, and he offered me a three-year contract to be negotiated in November by the Board of Regents. I preferred a letter of agreement instead of a contract, however, feeling that neither the Board nor I should feel bound if things did not work out. In the letter I requested that I be permitted to attend all meetings of the Board of Regents and College committees, including executive sessions unless the meeting's agenda was to be a discussion about my own responsibilities, compensation, etc. In those instances, I expected to be informed of the decisions and to be allowed to respond to questions.

Dr. Wilbur suggested this inclusion, since he recalled that his father, who was President of Stanford University, found that at the very first meeting of his board he was excluded from an executive session. When he returned to the room, he submitted his resignation saying that no university president could do a good job unless he had the total support of the board. The board agreed and he withdrew his resignation. Dr. Lewis was especially helpful to me during my first year, and advised me about the Board of Regents' expectations on many subjects.

My employment required some revisions in the Pension Plan, which specified that employees must be under 48 years of age and had to work for two years before age 48 to qualify. I was 50 and the Board passed an exception to the rule. I reviewed the pension plan and concluded it should be uniform for all employees, varying only in the percentages to be applied to each cohort, with higher percentages based on age, especially for those over 40. The Regents agreed that because of my position and age additional annuities could be provided outside the pension plan. In 1960, the plan called for a 20 percent contribution by the employee. A number of years later it was revised to 100 percent contribution by the ACP. This forced full participation by all employees. The original plan, which allowed for voluntary participation, made preferential exceptions possible which could force the College to contribute additional funds for favored employees.

The Board of Regents, wishing to retain Mr. Loveland's useful services as long as possible, proposed that he be retained as a consultant. At my first Board meeting, I was surprised that the agenda item specified that he would be a consultant to the College and not to me. I told the Board that I would not accept this arrangement, but I would be happy to have him as my consultant. The Board agreed, and it proved to be a satisfactory arrangement.

In October of 1959, I noticed two men visiting in Mr. Loveland's office and asked the bookkeeper, Ms. Tyndall, who they were. Ms. Tyndall said they were architects for the new building addition. She was surprised that I knew nothing about a building program. It was obvious that the architects, Mr. W.E. Frank (who had designed the original mansion) and his son were making preliminary sketches to present at the Board of Regents meeting in November. They had not been apprised of my relationship to the ACP. I informed the son that on January 2nd I would assume the role of Executive Director and requested that he keep me fully informed of the building developments. The architects accommodated my request in a professionally sensitive manner which avoided intrusions on Mr. Loveland's authority during the remainder of his tenure.

During the time I was working with Mr. Loveland, we became good friends. We often ate lunch with Dr. Piersol and, later, with Mr. Fred Dauterich almost every day. He shared his enormous fund of knowledge with me, and I learned to appreciate this truly dedicated and able man. He knew what every employee did from day to day. He enjoyed repairing his own portable typewriter and other typewriters, and personally typed many of his own letters.

I recall an amusing incident when we were reviewing the first budget I would have to work with. Miss Pearl Ott was on his right side and Miss Hannah Tyndall on his left, and they were berating him about the old fashioned hand-cranked ditto machine. He replied, "The exercise is good for you." After a little more wrangling he asked me what I thought and I said, "I know what you are paying these women and I think the time they spend using a hand-cranked ditto machine is hardly efficient office operation." He responded, "Okay, put in an item for a new automated duplicating machine." It was incredible how much this loyal, hardworking staff managed to do with some pretty outdated equipment.

Miss Pearl Ott, who had been Mr. Loveland's secretary for 33 years, had assumed an enormous amount of responsibility, especially in the last year or two during Mr. Loveland's illness. It became apparent to me that she had difficulty accepting the new arrangements with a physician in charge. However, by January she had become accustomed to my presence, and while it was a difficult transition for her and to some extent for me, I decided that her past experience would be a valuable resource and retained her on the staff. After a couple of years, I appointed her to be my editorial assistant for the *ACP Bulletin*. This worked out well, since she was always an invaluable source of information. I extended her employment when she reached age 65 and she retired when I did in 1977. She had given a little more than 50 years of service to the College. She had had only one other job of short duration before joining Mr. Loveland in 1927 at the ACP.

During the months following my arrival. I consulted some friends about the best means of recruiting a business assistant. Dr. Blasingame, the executive of the AMA, recommended hiring a management consulting firm to seek out candidates. I obtained the services of a Philadelphia firm, Butterick & McGeary. Mr. McGeary spent a couple of days with me at the Headquarters before referring three candidates, two of whom were very promising and well trained in business management. Mr. Fred Dauterich was one of these. Following Mr. McGeary's suggestion, I invited each of them with their wives to our home for dinner a few days apart. Mrs. Rosenow's perceptiveness on these occasions foreshadowed her future role in our life with the College. We agreed that Mr. Dauterich would encounter no conflicts when College demands took precedence over his personal life. He wryly noted that his experiences with a large number of PhDs at the Academy of Natural Sciences made him certain that working for MDs couldn't be all that difficult.

One day I asked him to recommend a simple book I could study to understand the balance statement. He laughed and said he would be glad to, if I would recommend a simple book on medical terms that he could understand. I soon found him to be an ideal assistant. He liked detailed work, did not mind interviewing candidates for jobs and was always very supportive of what I was trying to do.

In 1959, our staff numbered 29, including two editorial assistants who had worked in Baltimore with Dr. Pincoffs. Several departments were big enough to require managers. Mr. Paul Cotton managed the Membership Department and the work of the Credentials Committee. The Advertising Manager, Mr. Andrew Philips, was very successful in increasing the advertising revenues for the College. Mr. Elmer Jones was manager of the Circulation Department, which maintained members' addresses and the *Annals* subscriptions. In 1964, I employed Miss Joan B. Murphy as my assistant. She was reliable and helpful to me, was well liked by the Staff as well as by the Governors and Regents, and remained my assistant until my retirement in 1977.

During Mr. Loveland's illness in 1958-59, Dr. Wilbur spent much time in Philadelphia. On his recommendation, the Board of Regents decided to employ a public relations officer. One was hired with Mr. Loveland's acquiescence, but not with his enthusiastic approval. When I arrived in September 1959, this appeared to me to be an unsatisfactory arrangement. Shortly thereafter Mr. Loveland terminated his employment, saving me a difficult problem.

Another somewhat embarrassing matter concerned a Mr. Higgins, whom Mr. Loveland had hired originally as a possible replacement for himself, before the Board of Regents had decided the chief administrative officer should be a physician. When I arrived, Mr. Higgins was compiling a new membership directory. Mr. Loveland suggested this might be a good experience for me and would improve my proofreading skills. After a week or so, I told Mr. Loveland he might be right, but that I intended to have people already expert in such skills do this kind of work. Mr. Higgins left shortly after I came and moved to an executive position in New England.

In the Fall of 1959, I attended my second Regional Meeting in Providence, my first having been in Indianapolis. In the course of a few "after dinner remarks", I recounted that Dr. Chester Keefer and I had shared a common experience, having both been in China from 1928 to 1930, but did not meet. He had also been my professor at Harvard Medical School. I also mentioned that I had had lobar pneumonia while in California, which had been treated with sulfamerazine instead of penicillin. At the time of my illness Dr. Keefer was in charge of releasing penicillin to investigators and to the Armed Forces in World War II. I told him and the audience I felt sure that if he had known I had pneumonia he would have released some for me. I expressed gratitude to Dr. Marshall Fulton for his impartiality during our interview concerning the Chief Administrative Officer's position despite having known me when I was a medical student at Harvard.

I thanked Dr. Jack Graham for helping me get a Pennsylvania license to practice. He was, at the time, Chief of Medicine at the Faulkner Hospital where I had served my internship. When he called me to ask what information was needed in his letter of reference, I asked him please to emphasize how well I had done in obstetrics during my internship. Although this had not been an official part of the intern program, I had helped deliver a few babies, and Pennsylvania very much emphasized obstetrics in granting a license.

At this dinner, I also met other medical school mentors: Dr. Richard Stetson, who had been one of my instructors at the Boston City Hospital, and Dr. Chester Jones, who had been one of my professors at the Massachusetts General Hospital. They all made me feel as though I had, in a way, returned to the fold.

I shall always remember the first year with the College as one of my best years. We were very busy, and I learned many important things. The support I received from the Officers and Regents was contrasted to my previous experience with the Los Angeles County Medical Association, where I always felt everyone wanted to tell me what to do and how to do it. The College Officers asked me what they could do to help. My wife Esther was also very enthusiastic about the College and made many friends everywhere. It is small wonder that after a few years the Regents directed me to take her with me whenever I felt it was in the best interest of the College.

### Annual Session 1960

President Lewis's report to the Combined Meeting of the Regents and Governors in April, 1960 indicated progress in a number of are as:

1. The transition of Headquarters administration had been remarkably smooth.
2. The Annual Session Program Committee had worked hard; more than 500 abstracts had been submitted from which excellent papers had been selected.
3. A committee to revise the structure of awards announced the American College of Physicians Award. First bestowed at the 1960 Convocation, it was given for contributions in basic science as related to internal medicine. Scientists from any country, and in any field, whether clinical or non-clinical, biochemical or sociological were eligible for this award.
4. President Lewis applauded the development of the revised version of Research Fellowships.

Dr. Lewis then recommended that the College augment its educational programs by developing a different type of meeting; sectional meetings similar to the Annual Sessions, but held in different parts of the country.

The idea was to present top-flight scientific meetings on an annual basis, preferably in the fall, to areas of the country remote from the Annual Session site. The program was to be similar to that of the Session, excluding exhibits, and would last approximately three days.

Dr. Lewis thought such a step was advisable because many members felt that the Annual Session had become so large that only a few cities could accommodate it, and many members of the College could not afford to attend on a regular basis. Furthermore, the quality of the Regional Meeting programming did not always meet their high expectations, and there was discouragingly low attendance by Associate members and Fellows in many areas.

After studying the suggestion, the Committee on Education recommended to the Board of Regents at its November, 1960 meeting that the College begin by establishing one annual Fall Meeting and if that proved successful, meetings would be organized in other areas. In addition, abstracts of papers read were to be submitted to the Editor of the *Annals* for possible publication, to stimulate an increase of interest among young men and women in the activities of the College. The Committee also recommended that postgraduate courses of a general nature be incorporated into the meetings to encourage medical schools in the vicinity to participate more actively in the College's educational activities.

It was not entirely clear which Committee should have the responsibility for this type of meeting, but the Committee on Educational Programs was charged with developing a preliminary plan for formal presentation to the Board of Regents in May, 1961.

The 41st Annual Session of the American College of Physicians returned, for the first time since 1948, to the popular convention city of San Francisco on April 4-8, 1960. The Mark Hopkins and Fairmont Hotels served as official College headquarters with the Civic Auditorium hosting the technical exhibits, clinical sessions, panel discussions and color televised clinics.

The Annual Convocation of the College was held on Wednesday evening, April 6th, in the Auditorium of the California Masonic Memorial Temple on Nob Hill. The ceremony featured the induction of the new Fellows, an address by President Lewis, and the Convocation oration, which was given by the world famous astronomer, Dr. Harlow Shapley, Professor Emeritus, Harvard University. His address was entitled "Galaxies and What They Do to Us".

The Alfred Stengel Memorial Award was presented to Mr. Loveland. This award was given each year to a Master or Fellow of the College who, by leadership or example, had furthered the aims and ideals of the College, as well as having maintained and advanced the best standards of medical education, medical practice and clinical research. Dr. Franklin M. Hanger, Chairman of the Committee on Awards, presented the citation which read in part,

It was while Dr. Alfred Stengel was President of the College that he selected Ed Loveland for his illustrious career as Executive Secretary of the College. How fitting it is that we honor the memory of Dr. Stengel this evening by saying, 'Well done,' to the man who had justified from every standpoint Dr. Stengel's great faith and confidence.

The first recipient of the new American College of Physicians Award, given in recognition for distinguished contributions in science as related to medicine, was Dr. Philip S. Hench of the Mayo Clinic.

In March of 1959, President-Elect Chester S. Keefer, wrote the Board of Regents and suggested that the ACP develop "a new kind of research fellowship program" as a contribution to the continuing refinement of its educational program.

As an experiment, he proposed that two men be selected each year, and be awarded three-year research fellowships. The recipients were to have been research fellows, or individuals recommended as especially promising by Chairmen of Departments of Medicine. The work of these fellows would be reviewed at the end of the first and second years, in order to decide whether a continuation of the award was justified. In addition, they were not to be considered by the Department Chairmen as substitutes for faculty personnel who would otherwise be employed.

The Committee on Fellowships and Scholarships supported this suggestion in a report to the Board of Regents in November, 1959, and recommended that the College establish three-year fellowships in lieu of at least some of the existing one-year research fellowships. The Board approved the recommendation in principle and charged the Committee to submit a detailed plan ready for implementation at the 1960 Annual Session.

In the months following the November, 1959 meeting, certain events strengthened the feeling of the Committee that it would be wise to discontinue the one-year research fellowships. Applications for the one-year program had dropped from a previous four-year average of 26 to 17. Furthermore, it was quite evident that the qualifications of many of the applicants left much to be desired. Of the six men finally selected, three declined the awards, including one designated for the Stengel Fellowship; and of the four alternates, two accepted, one declined, and one asked for deferment until 1962-63. (Appendix B)

Not only was there a decided disinterest of quality candidates in the College research fellowship program, but closer inspection by the Committee revealed that two of the current group of ACP Research Fellows were in the embarrassing position of working in research units with fellows whose stipends, derived from other sources, were appreciably greater than theirs.

As a result of these disconcerting disclosures, and also the very strong conviction among many College members that continuing fellowships, covering at least three years of uninterrupted research, would provide a far greater contribution by the College to educational programs, the Committee recommended to the Board at the 1960 Annual Session that no further one-year research fellowships be awarded. Instead, they called for the adoption and immediate establishment of the three-year program.

In the Committee's view, the purpose of the three-year fellowships, was to further in young physicians a major interest in research or medical education, in any science basic to medicine. To emphasize that purpose, they stipulated that the recipient would have to devote a minimum of 80 percent of his time to research, regardless of the type of appointment he held at the institution.

Applications were to be submitted for the candidate by the Chairman of the Department of Medicine in any institution in the United States or Canada with a recognized program of medical education and research. Only one name could be recommended by a chairman of any given institution in one calendar year and a complete and careful evaluation of any nominee was required from the proposer. The recommendations were to be accompanied by a letter from the ACP Governor of the State or Province.

The final plan called for the establishment of two fellowships starting in July of 1961, two additional ones to begin the following July, and two to start July of 1963. Thereafter, two new fellowships would be added each succeeding year upon the completion of each pair of three-year fellowships. The stipends were set at $6,500 for the first year, $7,500 for the second and $8,500 for the third.

No rigid geographical distribution of fellowships was to be imposed because the Committee believed that after a brief period of time, suitable applicants would be found to provide a satisfactory apportionment of awards throughout North America.

In his first address as President at the 1960 Annual Business Meeting in San Francisco, Dr. Chester Keefer applauded the plan, stating,

> The sole concern of this College is to foster the acquisition and exchange of knowledge which pertains to medicine and to the medical sciences . . . The state of the future progress of medicine will inevitably depend, as we are all aware, upon discoveries of a fundamental nature. One can scarcely overemphasize the value of the contributions of medical research to man's welfare, but what may be of far deeper significance is the probability that there have emerged or will emerge some research discoveries from daily reports, the importance of which cannot at present be ascertained.

In action related to the scholarships and fellowships, the Board of Regents adopted the suggestion that the Alfred Stengel Research Fellowship award be temporarily discontinued and in its place a stipend of $500 be set aside in Dr. Stengel's name as a traveling scholarship. This was to allow a third or fourth year resident of advanced standing to travel to a medical center for a short period of intensive observation or study.

A significant final report of the Committee on Hospital Standards in Internal Medicine was made by Dr. Arthur R. Colwell, Chairman, in April, 1960. Early in 1956, this Committee was asked to find a way to measure and evaluate the quality of practice of internal medicine in American hospitals. The sample and measures utilized in this four year study included:

| | |
|---|---|
| Committee members, directors and staff | 12 |
| College members as field workers | 33 |
| Total participating hospitals | 167 |
| Hospitals which tested an appraisal plan devised by this Committee | 56 |
| Local appraising Committee members | 580 |
| Individual patient records appraised | 17,048 |

Total expenses were estimated at $92,000.

The following conclusions were reached:

1. Direct assessment of patient care in Internal Medicine by an outside agency was not feasible.
2. Hospital staffs could judge the quality of their own performance by systematic study of records of typical patients. It was deemed their obligation to do so.
3. A specific appraisal plan could be used effectively by the hospital staff with reasonable expenditure of time and energy.
4. Such appraisal undoubtedly could lead to elevation of standards of practice, chiefly by an educational process.
5. It was considered feasible for an outside agency to determine whether hospitals conducted such appraisals and how well they were done.

The Committee recommended:

1. Two plans for appraising and reporting would be submitted to the Joint Commission on Accreditation of Hospitals by the ACP. The first was "The Medical Appraisal Plan," as published in the October 1959 *Annals.* The second was the "Medical Audit Program" model of the Commission on Professional and Hospital Activities, Ann Arbor, Michigan, as described in November, 1958, to the Board of Regents by ACP representatives to the Commission, Drs. Eisele and Foltz.
2. Several administrative moves should be made, effective December 31, 1959.

The Board of Regents commended Drs. Arthur R. Colwell, Chairman and G. Karl Fenn, Director of the Study, for a "really colossal and outstanding piece of work".

The Secretary General, Dr. Wallace M. Yater, reported the number of members in the College: Masters 31; Fellows 6,881; Associates 3,831; for a total of 10,743. Among these were 1,472 Life Members.

The recurrent problem of the two classes of membership, Associate Member and Fellow, continued to generate controversy. It came into sharper focus with the initiation of the ten-year rule which stipulated that any Associate who failed to advance to Fellow after ten years would be dropped from the rolls. Various solutions had been offered from time to time ranging from the establishment of two classes of permanent membership, as the Royal College of Physicians of London had done, to that of a single class, Fellowship.

The Executive Committee of the Board of Governors passed a resolution in November, 1959, recommending to the Regents through the Board of Governors, that the term of Associateship, (later known as Membership) be extended indefinitely and that the ten-year limit be abolished. Opinion was considerably divided. Some were concerned that, obviously, most of the dropped Associates no longer would take part in College activities and thus could not take advantage of the educational opportunities offered by the College. Others felt that standards would be lowered by keeping the Associates indefinitely. In any case, no action was taken.

The first issue of the new publication, the *Bulletin of the American College of Physicians,* appeared in February, 1960. Its primary function was to keep the membership of the College acquainted with new developments, not only within the structure of the ACP, but in other important allied medical areas. Material previously published in the "News Notes" section of the *Annals,* including announcements of College meetings, statements relating to fiscal matters, and obituary notices, were incorporated into the publication. Included in the contents were news stories of importance about College members and Governors and information about fiscal matters.

Beyond a few specific directives, the guidelines laid down by the Regents were purposefully broad and elastic. It was their hope that the publication's ultimate form would be determined by input from its readers and by the imagination, ingenuity and guidance of the *ACP Bulletin's* Editorial Board and the Committee on Publications.

Dr. Thomas M. McMillan, of Philadelphia, was appointed Editor of the *ACP Bulletin* in April, 1959. He was made an *ex officio,* non-voting member of the Board of Regents at the Annual Session in 1960. Dr. Orville Horwitz, was named Associate Editor.

The *ACP Bulletin* followed the general format and page size of the *Annals,* but it contained no advertising. It was published bimonthly without page limitations. The publication was distributed to each member of the College and financing was obtained by allocating one dollar from each member's dues as a subscription fee.

Additional features included the "Executive Director's Page" in which I answered questions frequently asked at Regional Meetings concerning College policy and programs. A special section titled "American Society Of Internal Medicine News" was allocated to American Society of Internal Medicine [ASIM] communications. Dr. McMillan was given authority to accept, reject, or edit this section in keeping with the editorial policy relating to other copy.

In November, 1959, the Board of Regents asked the Committee on Liaison with the ASIM to make recommendations regarding the policy of the College with respect to Regional Meetings and the space allocated for ASIM news in the *ACP Bulletin.* In order to ascertain the feelings of the Regents and Governors in these matters, a survey of the two Boards was conducted.

The Boards agreed that the College should continue to devote its activities to scientific and educational endeavors and the Society to the field of economic and political questions.

The Committee offered the following fields of special interest which the ASIM should continue to pursue:

1. Economic and professional medical insurance matters
2. Political activities
3. Medico-legal considerations
4. Public relations
5. Office and practice management
6. Enhancement of the place of the internist in hospital affairs
7. Maintenance of standards of practice
8. Public education of the profile of the internist.

The Committee also favored the allotment of space in the *ACP Bulletin* for the ASIM and recommended that the Publications Committee handle details and policy problems.

The Liaison Committee decided that Regional Meetings were distinctive College functions and should remain so. The direction and arrangement of scientific programs should be solely the responsibility of the Governors. Authority for all decisions regarding the program, arrangements, and schedules should be vested in the Governors and integration of ACP and ASIM meetings was not to occur, although they had no objection to separate meetings held concurrently.

In accord with a suggestion from the Executive Committee of the Board of Governors at a November, 1958 meeting, a *pro tem* committee was appointed to "determine how much time the Governors spent, what direct expenses were incurred, together with their estimates of any indirect expenses involved in carrying out the duties of College Governorship". A questionnaire, designed to elicit the necessary information, was prepared and the response was prompt and informative.

The Committee reported to the Board of Governors meeting in 1960 that there was no indication of discontent or unhappiness among the Governors. There was even ample evidence suggesting that several Governors contributed time, effort, and money far beyond average levels. The factors responsible for these extraordinary contributions were directly related to a high concentration of medical populations in certain areas, Committee assignments which varied greatly in total number and type of responsibilities involved, geographic inequities in distance and time required for travel, and Regional Meetings in areas where single Governors held annual sessions.

The Committee recognized that in a few of the more populated areas, the load of work assumed by the Governors was so great that they recommended Governors be allowed to enlist experienced part-time secretarial help and develop an organization, including younger Fellows, to aid in the evaluation of proposals for membership. Although there were differences of opinion about the controversial suggestion of a Governor's fund, the majority of the committee favored arrangements that would provide to Governors money for secretarial help, Regional Meeting deficits and unusual expenses.

The Committee also exhibited strong support for the consolidation of several Regional Meetings, on the premise that it would relieve many Governors of the responsibility of meeting annually and facilitate the development of superior scientific programs.

During the meeting of the Board of Governors, Dr. Wright R. Adams, Chairman of the American Board of Internal Medicine [ABIM], made a report which had been requested by the Board of Governors, who were concerned about high failure rate and decrease in number of applicants. The report concluded that:

1. The large increase in applicants taking the written examination in 1953-54 was composed mainly of "repeaters", hence an apparent decrease in the number is accounted for by the drop in repeaters from the period immediately after the war. In the years since, there seemed to be as many as

ever who were taking the written examination for the first time.

2. Failure rate was higher for repeaters.
3. Those who qualified under Plan A, with three years of residency and two years of practice, did better than those who substituted other types of training. An exception was among those who substituted one year of research or teaching experience.
4. Obviously, the failure rate could be reduced by lowering the admission requirements.
5. The relationship of Board failure to College Fellowships was considered hard to appraise. For example, of the 60 most recently dropped Associate Members, about one-third could be attributed, at least in part, to failure to pass the Board examination. Many Associates did not apply to take the examination, hence the relationship could not be strongly established.

In making a motion to approve this report, Dr. William S. Middleton, Governor for the Veterans' Administration and former ACP President, said:

"The record of the American Board of Internal Medicine is a most predictable one and particularly in recent years had made a very strong contribution to the improvement in quality of care in internal medicine. It would be regrettable if the Board of Governors ever goes on record in opposition to the American Board of Internal Medicine . . ."

Dr. Middleton successfully urged the Governors to officially record the high commendation to the Board and thank Dr. Adams for an excellent report.

Two amendments to the Bylaws were passed at the 1960 Annual Business Meeting. The first revised the section on the Executive Committee of the Board of Regents. Membership was to consist of the President, President-Elect, Secretary General, Treasurer, Chairman of the Board of Governors, Chairman of the Committee on Finance and Budgets, and three Regents nominated by the President. The Committee was to be elected annually and members were eligible for reelection.

The function of the Executive Committee was to exercise all the powers of the Board of Regents in the management, direction and conduct of the affairs of the corporation during the interval between meetings of the Board and to act as an advisory body to the President.

The second amendment to the Bylaws specified that Masters, Honorary Fellows, and recipients of awards were to be elected by the Board of Regents upon recommendation of the Committee on Masterships and Honorary Fellowships and the Committee on Awards. Another section of the article specified that Governors, Regents and elected Officers of the College were not eligible during their terms of service for Masterships or for designated awards except under special circumstances, and then only by unanimous vote of the Regents.

Financially, the College continued to remain in excellent condition. The major funds gained slightly in 1960 and the investment portfolio increased. Dues, initiation fees, and subscriptions to the *Annals* all reflected a marked increase in membership growth.

The Committee on Administrative Personnel recommended, and the Board of

Regents approved, the appointment of Mr. Dauterich as Assistant Executive Director. I outlined the duties and responsibilities for this position. Under my direction, he would be the Director of Finance and Administration. He would have control and supervision of his staff. However, it was understood that supervision of the *Annals* and *ACP Bulletin* staff would be the respective Editors' responsibility.

Mr. Dauterich graduated from the Wharton School's Evening Division at the University of Pennsylvania. He worked for Jenkins Fetteroff, a large Philadelphia accounting firm, and the Thiokal Chemical Corporation. Just prior to the time of coming to the College he had acted as comptroller for the Academy of Natural Sciences.

The *Guide for Residency Programs in Internal Medicine* was approved by the Board of Regents at the 1960 Annual Session. It had been prepared by the Residency Review Committee [RRC-IM], which was made up of representatives of the American Board of Internal Medicine, the American College of Physicians, and the Council on Medical Education and Hospitals of the American Medical Association.

The guidelines were designed to assist program directors of internal medicine residencies in understanding and implementing the requirements set down by the AMA in the *Essentials of Approved Residencies*. This was the first time they had been prepared and they attempted to interpret and make suggestions regarding residency training with respect to the types of programs to be made available: subspecialty training, basic science instruction, outpatient department assignment, research, medical library, pathology and roentgenology services, neurology and psychiatry, practice, and responsibilities of attending and resident staff.

The first Group Life Insurance Program was made available to the membership of the College on February 1, 1960. The response to the program was so tremendous that the underwriters extended the enrollment period for members wishing to join the program, without evidence of insurability, for one month following the effective date of the plan.

Dr. Maurice C. Pincoffs retired as Editor of the *Annals,* having served from 1932 to 1960. In his last report to the combined meeting of the Board of Governors and Board of Regents, he said:

> . . . I leave the *Annals* in what I consider a flourishing condition. Dr. Clough and I have nursed it through these years and it has grown steadily from 1500 subscribers in 1932, to over 24,000. In its infancy, it always ran a deficit. With an active advertising committee and manager, the *Annals* is now the principal source of income for the College.
>
> I would like to say a few more words in parting from the Officers, inasmuch as I am perhaps a person who has held office longer than any other, starting as a Governor in the 1920s, elected a Regent and then through my editorship a permanent Regent, exofficio until now. The College honored me in various grades of Vice President, and finally with the Presidency and a Mastership. For all of these honors and distinction, I am grateful.
>
> One final word I'd like to say, don't underestimate young men. Do not make it easy

to get into the College. Do not mind turning away those who fail to measure up to standard. This College has progressed by making it more difficult to enter, because the higher the hurdle, the more men who seem anxious to show the stuff they have . . .

The College will progress best by keeping standards higher and higher as the level of the general education of the profession and as the ethical standards of the College increase.

Dr. Pincoffs was given a special Testimonial Certificate reflecting the appreciation and respect of the entire membership of the College for his devotion and stabilizing influence over the years.

At the Annual Session in April, Dr. J. Russell Elkinton's appointment as the new Editor of the *Annals,* effective October 1, 1960, was announced. Simultaneously, Dr. Edward J. Huth would become the Assistant Editor of the *Annals.*

## Part Two (1960-1961)

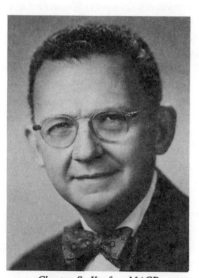

*Chester S. Keefer, MACP*

Chester Scott Keefer was born May 3, 1897 in Altoona, PA and died February 3, 1972 in Boston. His premedical education was obtained at Bucknell University and his MD degree was earned at Johns Hopkins University in 1922. He served residencies at Johns Hopkins from 1922-1926 and spent 1926-1928 as a resident physician in Chicago. From 1928-1930 he was Associate Professor of Medicine at the Peking Union Medical College in Peking. Upon his return from China he became Assistant and then Associate Professor of Medicine at the Harvard Medical School and Associate Physician at the Thorndike Laboratory, Boston City Hospital from 1930-1940. In 1940, he became the Wade Professor of Medicine at Boston University. He served in this position until 1964, when he became Emeritus Professor of Medicine. From 1940 to 1950, he also acted as Director of the Robert Dawson Evans Memorial Hospital at Boston University.

For many years he was a member of the Board of Directors of Merck & Company. In 1944-1946 he was a special assistant to the first Secretary of Health, Education and Welfare. In this position he controlled the distribution of penicillin in the early days of its use. He was Chairman of the Committee on Chemotherapeutics of the National Research Council. The China Medical Board sought his guidance repeatedly to the end of his life.

He was a diplomate of the American Board of Internal Medicine; a member of the Academy of Arts and Sciences; American Society of Clinical Investigation American Clinical and Climatological Association, its President in 1963; American Medical Association; American Philosophical Society; Phi Beta Kappa and Alpha Omega Alpha.

He was the recipient of many honors and awards, among them honorary Doctor of Science degrees from Bucknell University, Boston University and Bates College. The Chester Scott Keefer Auditorium at Boston University Medical Center was named in his honor.

His interest and enthusiastic support of the American College of Physicians was evident during his tenure as Governor for Massachusetts from 1944-1953, Regent from 1953-1961, and President-Elect and President from 1962-63 and 1963-64, respectively. In 1965, he was made a Master during the Convocation of the 50th Anniversary Session of the College.

Dr. Keefer was incisive and fair in his handling of difficult situations. This was best shown in a somewhat embarrassing situation which arose in Philadelphia while Dr. William Jeffers was the Governor for Southeastern Pennsylvania. Dr. Jeffers had written a letter to all of his constituents to express his feeling that the health of the candidates for President of the United States was of such importance that they should be screened prior to nomination to assure the state of their health. This was during the campaign in which John Kennedy was running for President. There had been some speculation that because of his having been treated with cortisone he probably had adrenal insufficiency. In his rather specific letter, Dr. Jeffers also mentioned the health of various other candidates, some of whom were later elected President. This letter was sent out on American College of Physicians' stationery, and one of the copies went to the ACP President, Dr. Keefer. It was our custom at that time that all correspondence initiated by Governors in which they used College stationery would have copies sent to the College President. This was not ordinarily done on local affairs, so this was a special case.

Dr. Keefer called and asked me to arrange a lunch meeting with Dr. Jeffers as soon as possible so that he could come down and discuss the matter with him. The three of us dined together the following day. Dr. Keefer did not ask his reasons for sending the letter, but merely told him that it was not possible for a Governor to use the College banner to promote some particular interest of his own. Dr. Keefer said that in his opinion, it would be impossible to get an unbiased medical opinion on the health of any Presidential candidate. I agreed with this viewpoint. Dr. Jeffers was embarrassed that he had caused any difficulty for the College President and immediately agreed that this had been an improper action and would not be repeated.

Another time, in connection with the Miami Annual Session, ACP Member Dr. Schmidt, of Miami, called me to report that one of the local professors who was to be a panel moderator at our Annual Session, had been arrested for drunkenness and, even more embarrassingly, for entering the home of and assaulting an elderly woman. Dr. Schmidt felt that the College should not have a person like this on the program. I told him I did not know whether we could make an immediate change. We inquired and ascertained that the accused physician was not in jail but out on bail. I called Dr. Keefer who, having heard the story, said he didn't think we should do anything because nothing we did could cause this professor any more trouble than he was in already.

With Dr. Keefer's strong interest in the best in medical education, his year of Presidency helped to consolidate our activities in that direction. It was also a turning point in the final resolution of problems relating to the College the two classes of Membership, Fellows and Associates.

During Dr. Keefer's year as President, Dr. Pincoffs decided to retire from his many years as Editor of the *Annals*. I remember several meetings I attended when Dr. Pincoffs was still on the Board that were very illuminating. He had a wise perception of what should be done, and the Regents almost always took his advice. Years before, when I became Editor of *Audio-Digest* in California, I went to the Annual Session in Philadelphia and sought permission to tape record some of the panel discussions. I found Dr. Pincoffs both approachable and enthusiastic about the idea. He was very helpful to us when we were just starting and I have never forgotten it.

Some time later, when I accompanied Dr. Elkinton to Baltimore to discuss the editorial transition with Dr. Pincoffs, his kind and thoughtful suggestions and his delightful and wry sense of humor were both helpful and memorable to both of us. Dr. Elkinton had no trouble taking up the mantle. Dr. Elkinton had always lived around Philadelphia and had been east to Europe many more times than he had been in the West. He never had been very far west of Philadelphia. On the way back to Philadelphia from Baltimore, he commented that I might have to help him find editorial board members from the West because he did not know anyone there. He added, however, that he did know one professor in Cincinnati. I believe the San Francisco meeting in 1967 was the first occasion on which Dr. Elkinton ever visited the West Coast.

## 1960-1961

Edward R. Loveland Memorial Award. Governors attend Credentials Committee meetings. Program for Cuban refugee physicians, Miami. Annals Editorial Office moved to Headquarters, Philadelphia.

In his Presidential report to the Board of Regents in November, 1960, Dr. Chester S. Keefer announced the death of Mr. Edward R. Loveland, Retired Executive Secretary, and appointed a committee to develop a suitable memorial. This committee suggested naming the board room in the new building the Edward R. Loveland Board Room. The Board also approved the establishment of the Edward R. Loveland Award to be given each year to a layman or lay organization that had made an important contribution to the health and welfare of the public.

Dr. Keefer outlined a wide range of activities and suggestions for policy development and implementation. He appointed an ad hoc committee to study membership. He also commented on the smooth transition of the editorial offices from Baltimore to Philadelphia.

I reported that a secretary had been provided to help Dr. Piersol finish the last two chapters of the history of the College and assist in preparing the manuscript for publication.

I also reviewed a statement about my relationship to the pharmaceutical industry which the Board approved: It was inappropriate for the Executive Director to actively solicit funds for entertainment at ACP meetings or for financial support of parts of the Annual Session program. However, if pharmaceutical firms offered to contribute funds to the College, I would be willing to guide these companies to suitable projects they might support. I also expressed my gratitude for the Board's approval of a staff assistant in administration and finance and reported that Mr. Dauterich had proved to be an excellent choice.

A recurrent problem that had created controversy within the College was the question of the two classes of membership, Associate Member and Fellow. It came into sharper focus with the initiation of the ten-year rule which stipulated that any Associate who failed to advance to Fellow after ten years, would be dropped from the rolls. Various suggestions had been offered from time to time ranging from the establishment of two classes of permanent membership, as in the Royal College of Physicians of London, to that of a single class, Fellowship.

### Associates Receive Indefinite Terms

The Executive Committee of the Board of Governors passed a resolution in November, 1959, recommending to the Regents, through the Board of Governors, that the term of Associateship, (later known as Membership) be extended indefinitely and that the ten-year limit be abolished. Opinion was considerably divided concerning this matter. Obviously, most of the dropped Associates no longer took part in College activities and thus were not taking advantage of the educational opportunities offered by the College. Others thought that standards would be lowered by keeping the Associates indefinitely. In any case, no action was taken.

During extensive discussion by the Committee and the Board of Regents about whether or not Associates should be elected without limit of term, Mr. Dauterich wondered why they should be dropped. He pointed out that as long as they were Associates and paid their dues they would receive the *Annals of Internal Medicine,* which in itself was an excellent form of education. In addition, they would more likely attend Annual Sessions, Regional Meetings and ACP postgraduate courses, which they would be unlikely to do if they did not belong to the College. It was counter productive, he believed, to dismiss these physicians from the College. It took several more years, incidentally, for this idea to be finally adopted.

In 1960, a survey was conducted of the 60 Associate members dropped the previous year. The results indicated that roughly two-thirds did not advance for various reasons, including indifference, failure to submit adequate material in the form of a thesis or case reports, and insufficient documentation of professional activities. The other one-third had failed to pass the American Board of Internal Medicine [ABIM] examination, making advancement to Fellowship impossible.

It was generally agreed among the members of the Executive Committee that not enough effort was being spent encouraging newly elected Associates to begin their qualifications for Fellowship at an early date. It was their expressed feeling that this group was the responsibility of the Governors, and that they should take more active steps to urge candidates to advance.

In November, 1960, several members of the Executive Committee attended, for the first time, a Credentials Committee meeting and were deeply impressed with the information received. They concluded that it was valuable to obtain first hand information about what the Committee expected by way of theses, case reports or published works. As a result of this learning experience, the Board of Regents passed a resolution requesting that each new Governor, early in his term of office, attend one meeting of the Credentials Committee at College expense. Furthermore, it decided that all future meetings of the Credentials Committee would be scheduled at ACP Headquarters in Philadelphia. Prior to that time the Committee had met during the Annual Session and during the Board of Regents Fall Meeting.

The immediate question of the classes of membership was not resolved, but investigation into the matter continued with the appointment of a subcommittee of the Executive Committee of the Board of Governors. They were to consider the problem of membership for those candidates who did not or could not qualify for advancement to Fellowship.

## Annals Moves to Philadelphia

October of 1960 marked the retirement of Dr. Maurice C. Pincoffs, another man who had become a legend in the history of the American College of Physicians. When he was appointed Editor of the *Annals* at the Annual Session in San Francisco on April 4, 1932, the journal was little known and comparatively insignificant in the field of internal medicine. Under Dr. Pincoffs' guidance the circulation increased from 3,000 to over 24,000, and it became one of the most prestigious medical journals in the English-speaking world.

The phenomenal growth of the journal was due in large part to consistent adherence to the policies that he set forth in his initial editorial in the January, 1933 issue of the *Annals* which read in part: "The scope of internal medicine should not be defined too narrowly; it blends without sharp boundaries into all the medical sciences and clinical specialties. Nothing in science or practice is truly foreign to its interest."

Dr. Maurice Pincoffs was elected a Fellow in 1923 and served the College in various capacities for the 37 years he was associated with the organization. In addition to being Professor of Medicine at the University of Maryland, he was ACP Governor for that state and later became a member of the Board of Regents. Dr. Pincoffs was elected President of the American College of Physicians in

1951 and, after his presidency, by virtue of his editorship of the *Annals*, he remained on the Board as an ex officio member. In recognition of his manifold contributions to the College, a Mastership was conferred upon him in 1947, and in 1955 he received the coveted Alfred Stengel Award.

Dr. Pincoffs tendered his resignation as Editor in November, 1958. It was his expressed desire that he be relieved of all duties no later than August, 1960. Dr. J. Russell Elkinton was appointed Editor at the Regents meeting in November, 1959.

The Publications Committee advised that the new Editor be located in Philadelphia so that the editorial operations of the journal could be in close proximity to the headquarters building. Space, however, was limited, and in the interim the editorial offices were housed at 404 South 42nd Street, in the Group Insurance Administrators building, pending completion of the planned expansion.

Dr. Elkinton assumed the Editorship of the *Annals* on October 1, 1960. His desire to continue to supervise the work of his laboratory at the University of Pennsylvania was honored by the Publications Committee, who recommended that the position of Editor could be a part-time job. Dr. Edward J. Huth was appointed Assistant Editor of the journal by the Board of Regents at the April, 1960 Annual Session in order to facilitate the smooth transition of the editorial operations from Baltimore to Philadelphia and to assist in reducing the significant backlog of manuscripts that had accumulated.

On December 8, 1960, Dr. Maurice C. Pincoffs died in the Johns Hopkins University Hospital in Baltimore at the age of 74. He was a man of many talents and interests and a prodigious worker. The value of his contributions to the American College of Physicians will never fully be assessed. Dr. Samuel P. Asper, then ACP Governor for the State of Maryland wrote in the March, 1961 *ACP Bulletin*, "Let those who read of this learned man learn his way of the complete physician; let those who knew this wise man be the wiser for their experience."

At the November Board of Regents meeting, the Postgraduate Courses Committee reported on the situation of ACP postgraduate courses as they related to the College and to other organizations, including the Association of American Medical Colleges [AAMC] and the AMA as well as medical schools. At their recent meeting, the Committee considered whether the College should be sponsoring postgraduate courses at all.

Discontinuing postgraduate courses was an appalling idea to me because I felt this was one of the very good programs of the College. I exclaimed quite forcefully that had I known that they were thinking of terminating sponsorship of postgraduate courses, I probably would have thought twice about whether I wanted to work for the College. The Committee discussed this at some length and concluded that because the College had an enormous audience for whom we had to provide a medical faculty, we could program some very specialized areas in considerable depth. This was never possible in the local areas for most medical schools because there might not be sufficient physicians with highly specialized interest to make it worthwhile to present a course. This was a turning point in the mission of the Postgraduate Courses Committee, and the program grew remarkably through the next several years.

As a result, the following College policy was established: 1) Postgraduate courses could be co-sponsored with medical schools and occasionally with other scientific organizations. 2) Fewer general review courses were to be scheduled because many medical schools contributed considerably in this area. 3) The emphasis of ACP courses would be directed toward more limited subject matter which was to be covered in greater depth.

The planned assimilation of the editorial operations of the *Annals* into the headquarters operations, coupled with the normal expansion of the Administrative Staff, made construction of an addition to the headquarters building one of the most important projects to engage the attention of the American College of Physicians for the following two years. The House Committee received initial authorization to select an architect to prepare specifications and plans, and secure bids for the proposed addition from the Board of Regents in November of 1959. Fortunately, the Board had already purchased the property directly adjacent to the headquarters building expressly for the purpose of future expansion.

The proposed addition was to extend south from the west end of the existing structure and originally was to consist of two stories and a basement. The Board finally decided that the cost of adding another floor at a later date would be more expensive than completing the structural and rough work at the time of initial construction. As a result, a three-story structure was planned.

Preliminary plans, along with the architect's tentative estimate of cost, were presented to the Board of Regents in San Francisco at the 41st Annual Session in April of 1960. The Board voted to proceed on the recommendations and approved a total cost of up to $350,000; appropriating $100,000 to be utilized as needed during 1960.

Bids were opened in August of 1960 and found to be far in excess of the initial estimate. The lowest bid, including the architect's fees, construction, grading and landscaping, exceeded $425,000. Consequently, the House Committee instructed the architect to revise the plans and specifications to come more within the means of the College without sacrificing the essentials in the function of the building.

In October the Committee received a new bid from the R. M. Shoemaker Company, low bidder in the first instance, which amounted to $330,727, a reduction of about $46,000 from their previous bid. Chief among the revisions was the installation of a less expensive heating and air conditioning unit, the substitution of wood floors for concrete, and a modification of the grading and landscaping of the parking lot and driveway. These changes were achieved without jeopardizing the College's insurance risk, but as time would reveal, a tinderbox had been substituted for a relatively fireproof building.

The Board of Regents gave final approval to the revised plans at their November, 1960 meeting. I was instructed to sign the agreement and work began early in 1961.

## Annual Session 1961

The 42d Annual Session of the College was convened in Bal Harbor, Miami Beach. This was the first time that the ACP had met in the popular South Florida area and the Americana Hotel served as official headquarters, and also accommodated the technical exhibits, clinical sessions, basic science programs, color televised clinics, and committee meetings. The Annual Convocation, President's Reception, and the Annual Banquet were also held in the hotel.

In my Executive Director's report, I had a few words to say about membership. In a recent analysis, I became quite aware of several trends. There had been a gradual increase of physicians but more and more were going into specialties. According to some reports, internal medicine was the fastest growing specialty, up 113 percent since 1949. There were, at that time, about 24,000 physicians who listed their specialty as "practicing internists." The exact number of the subspecialties was not known, but there was a real shift, particularly in academic circles. It seemed safe to predict that many of the professors of medicine at that time were subspecialists and perhaps in the future even more of them would be. It seemed desirable in some ways to take positive steps to make it easier to elect some of these men to membership, inasmuch as many of them did not take Board examinations, either by choice or by ineligibility.

Another striking fact was apparent. During the previous few years the proportion of Associate Members to Fellows had increased. The Associates (later designated as Members) were comprised of three basic groups: There were 1,800 Associates who paid reduced dues; 650 of these had received dues waivers. Of those 1,800 Associates who were in a reduced category, only 200 were listed as full-time faculty members. A second large group was in the military service, but the largest group, which was surprising, was 1,800 College members who were working for institutions. This was a characteristic I felt should be studied.

I also reported that I had attended many Regional Meetings and had found the American Society of Internal Medicine [ASIM] holding meetings at the same time. Two levels of activity were occurring. It was probably at the state level that most economic problems for internists were going to be solved and every encouragement should be given to these groups at that level. At least two functions lent themselves to solution at the national level. One of them was to furnish a forum for the exchange of information between state ASIM societies and the ACP; this forum should also serve to make internists aware of non-scientific matters of interest to all internists. Ordinarily, this had more to do with standards of practice than economics. The second function a national organization should be performing was to present nationally an authoritative voice or image promoting internal medicine in the public interest in every way possible. I felt the College should review its relations with ASIM in these different aspects.

An interesting sidelight was that inasmuch as the College only included 11,000 of the 24,000 practicing internists at that time, there might be a real possibility that the ASIM would eventually outnumber the College.

Dr. Kampmeier and I had attended a meeting at AMA headquarters where societies interested in continuing medical education were represented. Most of us favored formation of some joint commission to coordinate activities in education. Some, however, thought the joint sponsorship of the AMA and the AAMC would be preferred to setting up a completely autonomous national academy of continuing medical education as proposed by Dr. Ward Darley, former head of the AAMC. Dr. Darley, incidentally, was at the meeting and was quite agreeable to the idea of setting up such a joint commission. A later meeting of a smaller group was held, and the AMA established an Advisory Committee to its Council on Medical Education, but no further action on a joint commission was taken for a number of years.

Following my report, Dr. Howard P. Lewis, Chairman of the Committee on Educational Program, discussed two matters in some detail. One concerned the suggested interim or section meeting, and the other was the functions of the Program Committee in connection with the interim meetings. The Committee made the following recommendations:

a) One session should be held each year, although in the future, as needed, two such sessions might become necessary.

b) The interim session would be held in the fall of the year, and appropriate dates to be set by the Executive Director in consultation with the President and the Committee on Program.

c) The session should be held in an area which is most remote from the last Annual Session.

d) The cities used ordinarily for the Annual Session should not be used for these interim meetings.

e) The first session might be held in Portland, Oregon.

f) Program arrangements would be the responsibility of the Committee on Program and the Executive Director in consultation with the President.

g) The session should be of three days duration, preferably on Thursday, Friday and Saturday, and it should retain the same quality and general format as the Annual Session. It was not anticipated that television or hospital clinics would be used nor that there would be a technical exhibit.

h) No social events would be scheduled for those sessions, except perhaps for a subscription dinner to be arranged for those members in attendance.

i) Mr. Dauterich and I estimated that such a session might cost the College about $55,000 and about one half of that could be defrayed by having a technical exhibit, but at least for the first three years this was not considered advisable. This proposal was referred to the Committee on Finance and Budgets for study before final action.

In the Fall of 1960, important changes in the system of handling the College investment portfolio took place. In previous years the portfolio had been looked at only twice a year at the time of the Regents meetings. It was decided that the Investment Committee would meet with Drexel & Company on a monthly basis and report recommendations to the Finance Committee.

Another change empowered the Investment Committee to authorize Drexel to make transactions and then to report such actions to the Finance Committee. This seemed a much more logical way of proceeding than to wait for letters from the Finance Committee, and it has worked quite well ever since. The Investment Committee consisted of Mr. Dauterich, Dr. Sodeman, Treasurer, who was Dean of the Thomas Jefferson School of Medicine, and myself.

In Amendments to the Bylaws made operative at the Miami Beach Session, the Treasurer was made responsible for the receipt and disbursement of all College funds. Prior to that time the Bylaws stated that he collected and disbursed all funds. A synopsis of the duties and responsibilities of the Chief Administrative Officer was outlined; the composition of the Board of Regents was set forth; the membership and functions of the Executive Committees of both Boards were restated; and the terms of Associateship and eligibility for Fellowship were clarified.

The Ad Hoc Committee on Membership reported the following to the Board of Regents:

1. The membership structure had served the College well in accomplishing the objectives of the ACP and the Board of Regents firmly believed that the standards for election to Fellowship should not be lowered, nor would it be in the best interest of the organization to limit membership growth by altering the requirements for Fellowship. Rather, it was agreed that long range plans should be developed which would provide for an effective organization of more than 20,000 members by 1975.

2. The Committee was not persuaded of the advantages of a single category of membership, a proposal advanced by some members; nor did they see any justification for the establishment of a category of permanent Associateship which they envisioned as catering to a relatively small number of individuals who could not achieve full Fellowship in the established time limits. The Committee recommended the abandonment of the ten-year rule in favor of a return to the five-year maximum period of Associateship.

3. Further, it recommended that Associates would be eligible for advancement to Fellowship after two years rather than three.

4. The Committee was not impressed with the need to establish "Junior" Membership for individuals in internal medicine residencies or near the termination of their training. They did recommend, at least in principle and subject to further study, the establishment of a category of Affiliate Membership for colleagues from South America.

5. The Committee, in considering the place of the allied specialists, recommended that these individuals should continue to be eligible for membership, inasmuch as the College benefits from association with these allies.

6. The policy of reserving direct election to Fellowship as a mark of distinction for individuals with established national reputations in teaching, research, and clinical practice was also examined. The Regents concluded that there was no justification for a "waiting" period as an Associate, if the individual already had professional accomplishments sufficient for

election to Fellowship at the time of first review by the Credentials Committee. Bylaws changes were suggested at this time and approved in 1962 which provided for the direct election to Fellowship of those individuals who had satisfactorily fulfilled the requirements at the time of initial review.

The Mead Johnson Residency Scholarships had been limited to a single year. In response to an inquiry into the feasibility of renewing the grant for an additional year, the Fellowships and Scholarships Committee was of the opinion that the policy should remain the same but, under unusual circumstances, exceptional candidates could reapply and compete with new applicants for the positions. Further, it was decided that qualified noncitizens who had passed their Educational Commission for Foreign Medical Graduates (ECFMG) examinations could be included in the program subject to approval by Mead Johnson.

In regard to the new Research Fellowship program of the College, initiated the previous year, the Committee was requested to clarify whether a preceptor was allowed to augment the ACP stipend with outside funds. The prevailing feeling was that the university could supplement the fellowship grant, within the institution's salary structure, but the grant was still to be identified with the ACP and not to be shared with another in name. Furthermore, the supplement was not to imply other or additional duties, nor take the research fellow away from his research.

Many Cubans were forced to leave their country as a result of the revolution. The largest single group of exiles emigrated to the Miami, Florida, area and nearly 300 physicians had to be assimilated into the community. At least 10 full professors of recognized international stature in their respective areas of medicine, from the School of Medicine of the University of Havana, were among the group.

The University of Miami School of Medicine gave each of these men an appointment as a Visiting Professor in their specialty. An intensive postgraduate course, covering all of the clinical disciplines of medicine and the basic sciences particularly pertinent to clinical medicine, was formulated and a corps of bilingual tutors were employed to assist as necessary.

Believing that these Professors should be supported by Fellowships, the University of Miami turned to the national medical societies for help in producing the needed capital to support the program. The Board of Regents, in an attempt to alleviate the situation, approved a recommendation that $6,000 be appropriated for the support of an Instructor of Medicine, Dr. Jose Centurion, who was a displaced physician and a former Governor of the College for Cuba.

The College had engaged, to some extent, in programs of medical interest to business executives. These had been held at the time of the Annual Session. There were other areas, including Regional Meetings and the proposed "Interim Session", where guidance was needed in devising the best possible mode of informing the public as to the functions of the specialist in internal medicine and also the role of the College in the delivery of health care. The Board of Regents, therefore, established a standing Committee on Public Information and assigned it the task of developing a continuing program of information and education for the profession and the lay public regarding the activities and aims of the American College of Physicians.

This Committee was to be responsible for the preparation of guidelines and helpful suggestions for the use of regional and local committees at the time of the Annual Session and provide for the arrangement of an adequate press room at the Annual Session. It would also initiate advance contact with science writers and press representatives, arrange press conferences with key speakers and issue press releases pertinent to the announcements of the meeting, including the election of national officers and similar activities, and develop and coordinate all public educational activities as they related to regional and interim meetings, postgraduate courses, and the publications of the ACP.

The College, at that time, did have a Professional and Public Relations Committee which was concerned primarily with the review of membership relations within the College structure. It dealt mainly with controversies, complaints, resignations, recommendations of members, applications for waiver of dues, and review of relations with other scientific and non-scientific organizations in respect to membership in the College. This Committee was incorporated into the framework of the Membership Committee one year later.

In 1960, there had been considerable discussion about the Committee on Public and Professional Relations, which had previously only considered membership problems, and some members of the Board of Regents thought there should be a regular public relations department. As a result, an ad hoc committee to study the public relations problem was appointed and Dr. Irving Wright was its chairman.

This was an important year in another way. The Joint Commission On Accreditation of Hospitals [JCAH], for the first time, was considering a study on the appraisal of medical care in hospitals.

## Joint Boards Review Objectives

In the President's report at the joint meeting of the Board of Governors and Regents in Miami, Dr. Keefer made some remarks about the general objectives of the College. He believed that the College had always held firmly and exclusively to the main purpose and aim of its founders, namely, to promote and improve the practice of internal medicine. Its record was remarkable. The Board of Regents had always held, often against temptation and sometimes against coercion, that the function of the College was solely the improvement of medical practice through advancing medical education. However, the time might come, when it would be desirable and wise to depart from such an established course, even though such a departure might quickly change the character of the College. He was confident that the change would never be made lightly, but only if exigencies arose of such nature that the objectives which had thus far guided the College should be sacrificed to some worthier cause.

The College was constantly defining and redefining what it was trying to do.

The objectives were clear. This did not mean, he said, that there were no arguments about the objectives. Each change was adopted deliberately and pursued intentionally, instead of merely defending what the College had inherited from the past.

In this context, Dr. Keefer commented about membership. He thought that the continued success of the College depended chiefly upon a judicious and impartial choice of the members elected. The Committee on Credentials devoted all of its deliberations to these selections and the only criterion which had been used in its judgments was whether the candidate was doing good work as a physician and might be depended upon to do more. These assessments were made upon recognition by peers, colleagues, Governors and Fellows in addition to careful review of the candidates qualifications.

Dr. Keefer then offered some thoughts about the American Society of Internal Medicine and its multi-purpose aims. The College had elected to consider only scientific and educational matters and to use its meetings as a forum for reporting scientific advances. It had been the consensus of the governing bodies, heretofore, that discussions and studies of socioeconomic, political and undergraduate medical education problems should be left to other groups. He felt that socioeconomic and political ills could not be cured by doctors nor by medical science alone, because they were problems which do not fall within the domain of these sciences alone.

The general public had been led to believe that doctors were scientifically astute and humanely sympathetic. But they did not expect physicians to understand social questions too deeply. They held that opinion because, in general, they believed that professional classes were poor judges outside of their own professional expertise. And it was largely because they withdrew from one another that they lacked both professional and lay cooperation in developing better understanding. The ASIM had been making efforts to develop a better understanding of socioeconomic questions that concerned the organization. One of their main objectives was appropriate distribution and financing of medical care as practiced by the internist. The College was giving them support and advice. In Dr. Keefer's opinion, the College, as an organized body of physicians, could render the greatest public and professional service by adhering to its single-minded aim, and by cooperating with other groups which were more actively concerned with discovering methods which could happily and harmoniously direct and govern the communal life of the profession.

In his report, Dr. Yater, Secretary General, indicated that, at the time of the Annual Session in Miami, the Membership of the College was 33 Masters, 7,150 Fellows, and 4,088 Associates, with a total membership of 11,271.

During the Annual Business Meeting a number of amendments to the Bylaws were adopted. Briefly, the following changes were effected:

1. The Treasurer shall be responsible for the receipt and disbursement of all College funds. The Executive Director's proposed budget would be reviewed by the Committee on Finance and Budgets and then be submitted to the Board of Regents.

2. The Editors of the *Annals* and the *ACP Bulletin* shall be ex officio members (without vote) of the Board of Regents.

Advertising revenue for the *Annals* declined substantially in the first half of 1961, which was attributed to general economic conditions that existed early in the year and to effects of Congressional hearings relating to the drug industry. In the second half of the year, receipts ran ahead of the same period in 1960, but the volume of actual advertisements did not increase. The appreciation of advertising income was attributed to old contracts that were being renewed at new rates adopted in 1960 and put into effect on January 1, 1961.

The arbitrary allocation of one dollar of each member's dues to the *ACP Bulletin* for expenses covered approximately 50 percent of the overall cost of publishing and distribution and resulted in a $10,000 deficit in 1961. The burden of that deficit was to be assumed by the surplus from the *Annals*.

The Annual Session deficit had been steadily increasing from just over $900 in 1955 to almost $69,000 at the time of the 1960 San Francisco meeting. The net loss from the Miami Beach Session was $58,276, but during the past few years, the College had been able to pay only 50 percent of the cost of each meeting from income realized from exhibits and guest fees. The resulting deficit was covered with other College funds.

In considering financial actions for the future, the Treasurer pointed out that expenditures for existing services were rising at an appreciable rate. An Interim Session, estimated to cost from $50,000 to over $55,000, promised to be a very expensive addition to College activities. The estimated net income for 1962, after the appropriation of the usual $100,000 to the Endowment Fund and $75,000 to the recently increased Building Fund, was to be $50,000. Clearly, some priority decisions had to be made in regard to ACP programs, projects, and services.

In a report to the Board of Regents from the JCAH, Dr. Alex M. Burgess discussed several matters of importance to the College. The first was a report of the Committee on Research, dealing with the proposed study about how medical care could be appraised in a hospital. A second important question was the matter of how JCAH could deal with hospitals in which graduates of foreign medical schools who had not been certified by the ECFMG were on duty. A secondary matter, but an interesting problem, was what to do about the status of "chronic disease hospitals"; whether or not they should be surveyed as hospitals, and if so in what manner. The Commission had voted to make a study of the development of improved criteria of medical care in these institutions with the University of Pittsburgh. This was to be a joint effort; the cost of the study to be borne by the University.

Regarding the foreign medical graduate problem, the Commission's surveyor would inquire about the presence of foreign medical graduates on the hospital staff and whether they could prove with documentary evidence that they had been state licensed or certified by the ECFMG. If not, the surveyor investigated the activities of those individuals to determine their involvement in patient care.

Dr. Burgess further reported that Dr. Babcock, Director of JCAH, had noted that podiatrists or chiropodists were considered as "technicians" and would not be privileged to prescribe or treat patients in hospitals, regardless of what local regulations allowed them to do elsewhere. Dr. Babcock reported that third, fourth and fifth year residents, if licensed, should be authorized to authenticate histories, physical examinations and discharge summaries, which now must be done by staff members. The Director also reported that more and more hospitals were calling themselves "chronic" or "geriatric" hospitals. After a considerable discussion in which the rehabilitation function of many of these hospitals was stressed, it was decided that they should be considered as "hospitals" and surveyed as such. Dr. Burgess cautioned the College and said that the Commission, of which the College is a parent, certainly deserved full participation on the part of the College; the representatives cautioned that if the College did not fully participate, it would lose control of that part of medical patient care in which it is especially interested: the medical care of sick people.

The Committee on Finance and Budgets recommended that the appropriation to the JCAH, which at that time amounted to almost $50,000 per year for the next two years, be discontinued after 1962. The College Commissioners were instructed to advise the members of the Commission that the College found this contribution a financial burden of such magnitude as to require it to withdraw in the reasonably near future. Parenthetically, this was the beginning of a change in financing the JCAH which eventually led to dividing the cost into an administrative cost which would be borne by contributions from the members and a surveying cost which would be charged to the hospitals being surveyed. This was approved by the Board of Regents.

In a report for the Cancer Committee, Dr. Samuel G. Taylor, III, described several ongoing activities. He spoke as Chairman of this Committee and also as a representative on the Joint Commission on Endocrine Ablative Procedures in Breast Cancer and of the Joint Committee on Cancer Staging and End Results Reporting.

The ACP Committee met in May, 1961, and made the following recommendations to the Board of Regents:

1. That the College distribute to heads of departments of medicine in institutions with ACS approved cancer programs the enclosure in the 1961 Manual for Cancer Programs which defines a suggested role of internists.

2. That the College recommend to departments of medicine that adequate instruction and diagnosis and treatment of malignant disease was an essential part of residency training. This should include active participation in a tumor clinic, the use of newer techniques for the early diagnosis of cancer, and active participation in cancer chemotherapy programs at the institution.

3. The Committee also requested permission from the Board of Regents to initiate an active program designed to encourage those agencies which provide financial support for advanced training of young physicians, to encourage them to provide more support to young internists in fields related to cancer.

Expressing concern over the length of time involved in publishing the bi-monthly *ACP Bulletin*, the Board of Regents instructed Dr. McMillan and me to review the costs of monthly publication, its preparation in Philadelphia and the possibility of publishing it in some other form. These findings were to be presented to the Board at the next Annual Session.

In his first year as Editor of the *Annals*, Dr. Elkinton had managed a significant reduction in the backlog of manuscripts. The time between receipt of manuscripts and publication had been reduced to 6.7 months, and between acceptance and publication, 3.9 months. In the year ending September 30, 1960, 68 percent of the articles received were rejected, as were 80 percent of the case reports. The total number of articles received was 722. Quality, in lieu of quantity, continued to be a hallmark in the pages of the *Annals*.

Construction of the Los Angeles Ambassador Hotel Convention Center, which was to have hosted the 46th Annual Session, April 5-9, 1965, was reported at a standstill with no likelihood that the facility would be completed in the near future. The Southern California Committee therefore, requested that their invitation be withdrawn temporarily and reactivated only when their city would be able to offer adequate facilities to host the meeting. (A few years later a new auditorium was built in Los Angeles. It was unsuitable for use by ACP, however, because ceilings in meeting rooms were too low to permit projection of slides to large audiences.)

The Chicago Hilton, previously scheduled for the 47th Annual Session, April 18-22, 1966, was available for the week of March 22-26, 1965. The Board of Regents decided to move the Chicago meeting forward to 1965 and schedule the 1966 meeting in New York City, where two hotels under construction would be completed by January, 1963. These two hotels they concluded, could serve the 1966 Annual Session jointly.

In an attempt to prevent the oral examination given by the ABIM from becoming overcrowded, a one year minimum time interval, beginning in 1961, was required between the written and the oral examinations. This was an attempt to obtain and schedule better oral examinations without undue hardship and continual delay. The ABIM felt that when the number of candidates exceeded both the clinical facilities and the capacity of the examiners, the quality of the testing suffered.

The Group Insurance Programs of the College were progressing extremely well and the carrier of the Life Insurance Program presented a 10 percent dividend in the form of increased benefits to the physicians who were participants in the programs.

# Part Three (1961-1962)

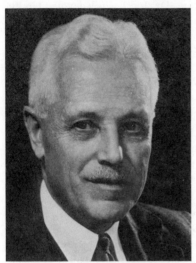

*Chester M. Jones, MACP*

Chester M. Jones, born March 29, 1891 in Portland, Maine, received a BS degree from Williams College in 1913 and an MD from Harvard Medical School in 1919. His graduate training was done at the Massachusetts General Hospital. He was a William Moseley, Jr., Traveling Fellow at Harvard Medical School in 1924-25, working for a year in France with Professor Leon Blum at the University of Strasburg. On his return to Boston, he served as Instructor in Medicine at Massachusetts General Hospital from 1925-1928, and remained as attending physician until 1954. He was appointed Physician-in-Charge of the Private Service Teaching Program from 1957 to 1964. During 1940-41, he was Acting Associate Professor of Medicine at Vanderbilt University. He was a member of the American Board of Internal Medicine from 1948 to 1957 and its Chairman from 1955 through 1957. He was a consultant to the US Public Health Service from 1943-1946. After the war he traveled with medical missions to Austria in 1947 and to Greece in 1948. He was President of the American Gastroenterological Association in 1936-37 and President of the American Clinical and Climatological Association in 1951-52.

Active in continuing medical education at Harvard, Dr. Jones served as Chairman of the Committee on Courses for Graduates from 1944 to 1956.

At various times, he served on the editorial boards of the *New England Journal of Medicine, Gastroenterology* and the *Annals of Internal Medicine.*

His honors and awards included an Honorary Doctor of Science Degree from Williams College; The Rogerson Cup & Medal for service, loyalty and wisdom, given to outstanding Williams College Alumni; the Julius Friedenwald Medal of the American Gastroenterological Association for distinguished service in gastroenterology.

He served the College as a member of the Board of Regents from 1957-1960 and 1962-1965. He was President-elect in 1960-61 and President in 1961-62. In 1967, he received the Alfred Stengel Memorial Award. For a number of years he was chairman of the Publications Committee and made a major contribution to the College as Chairman of the Search Committee which recommended Dr. J. Russell Elkinton to succeed Dr. Maurice Pincoffs as Editor of the *Annals.*

He married Kathleen Kohner of Seaforth, Ontario. They had three children. His son, Dr. Robert H. Jones, is Associate Professor of Preventive Medicine and Community Health at the University of Rochester Medical School. His daughter,

Elizabeth, married Dr. Samuel L. Clark, Jr., Professor of Anatomy at University of Massachusetts School of Medicine. Another daughter, Ann, is married to Dr. Ward Stoops of Petersborough, New Hampshire. Dr. Jones was a devoted family man and although he gave most of his time to his profession, he took time for reading and camping with the family in Maine, where they had a summer home on Lake Sebago. His favorite sport was tennis. He loved birds and flowers and was always inspired and renewed by nature's grandeur.

Dr. Jones died on July 26, 1972. His long and productive life was an inspiration to all who were privileged to know him.

During Dr. Jones's Presidency, an interesting episode occurred concerning the National Institutes of Mental Health [NIMH]. One of the NIMH staff members asked me if the College was willing to send out brochures about the mental health program being initiated by the Kennedy administration. After reading the brochure, I furnished the NIMH our mailing list, but an error was committed by the outside mailhouse. They sent out about a hundred envelopes bearing government franked postage marks which were filled with a commercial company's literature—not the NIMH brochure. We, and Dr. Luther Terry, who was Surgeon General of the US Public Health Service, and held jurisdiction over the NIMH and its literature, promptly heard about the *faux pas*. The NIMH person who had asked our permission to send out the mailing was irate and demanded that we send out another mailing. I was opposed, on the grounds that another mailing would assure that the recipients would notice the error, but reluctantly we agreed to repeat the mailing. As I predicted, many people called objecting to our support of a government program for mental health. It was interesting, however, that we received more letters and calls congratulating us for taking this step. Of those who reacted negatively, one doctor was so upset about it that I finally asked him if he had ever seen patients with Down's Syndrome; he said he had. I asked him if he knew of any effective treatment for this disorder; he was forced to reply, "No." I told him when he found out what to do for them, he should call again, but, at the moment I would like to get back to my other work.

I told Dr. Jones about this, because I was disturbed that I might have exceeded my authority in authorizing the mailing. He laughed and said that he well understood the embarrassment, but he knew that I would make occasional mistakes; the College hadn't hired me to make no mistakes, they wanted me to do things. Dr. Jones regularly displayed a very reassuring nature.

Another time, at a performance of the Philadelphia Orchestra, we had gone backstage during intermission to meet conductor Eugene Ormandy. Dr. Jones had the pleasurable duty to present the maestro with a gift and certificate from the College. Since I was not to appear on the stage, I was returning to my seat and was surprised to see Dr. Jones had followed me. He laughed and said that he had learned that he got along better at meetings if he followed me, rather than going in a different direction.

He was very fond of telling about his recurring embarrassment at Regional Meetings, when members introduced themselves by reminding him that he had administered their American Board of Internal Medicine [ABIM] oral examination. Always nonplussed, on a few occasions he remarked facetiously, "I guess I must have failed you." Once in awhile, the member responded, "Yes." Then he really didn't know quite what to say next.

In one of his characteristically humorous moods, during a Board meeting at the Headquarters, Dr. Jones remarked about the second floor men's room which had a chain-pull for flushing, "Ed, don't let anybody replace this. Someday you are going to have a Regent who never heard the expression, 'pull the chain'."

At a Virginia Regional Meeting, the Master of Ceremonies introduced him in an abrupt way. He had decided not to introduce anybody at the head table and said "We are all glad to see our President," and sat down. Dr. Jones promptly rose, dropped his pipe, bumped into the microphone and then gave a fairly long and not very exciting speech. The next day he asked me what he could do to improve his speech. Hesitating to instruct my former medical school professor in speech techniques, I responded that he should give the last ten minutes first and then he could eliminate as much of the rest as he wanted to. In the last few minutes of his speech he had given a superb statement, probably the best I had ever heard, about what it meant to be a Fellow of the American College of Physicians and what was expected of a Fellow of the ACP.

On a trip to Bermuda, Chester insisted that we go to a hotel for dinner where a hypnotist was billed as the entertainment. He was a wonderful person to be with and Esther and I enjoyed traveling with the Joneses.

## 1961-1962

New Headquarters Wing, Edward R. Loveland Board Room dedicated. Gateway of Honor published. Study of ACP/ASIM Relationships. New office of Governor-Elect. Membership and dues structure revised. Lifetime Learning for Physicians. Committee on Public Information.

In spite of a severe winter with nearly 50 inches of snowfall, construction proceeded on the new wing at the Headquarters, and it was occupied on October 1, 1961. Items of unexpected expense included the installation of a transformer to lower power rates; an ancient sewer line on the building site was discovered and had to be rechannelled.

The Finance and Budget Committee presented a supplemental budget appropriation to add furnishings to the new wing and renovate the original structure. The Eisenlohr Mansion was rewired, painted and plastered where necessary, and the heating system was modernized. A new kitchen and dining room, for employee use, was installed on the ground floor.

An amusing, but ultimately important, decision was made about the table and seating arrangements in the new Board Room. For a Board meeting on Saturday, a temporary 44-foot table was set up. This was the length necessary to permit the use of swivel chairs. The next day the table was set up to be 32 feet long, the length necessary if arm chairs were to be provided. The cost of the 44 foot permanent table and swivel chairs was $5,500 and the shorter table and straight chairs approximately $3,500. On the first vote, the Board approved the shorter table. Dr. Lewis, one of the tallest men on the Board, asked for reconsideration of the motion and asked the Board if they had really understood that if they voted for the shorter table, it would not be possible to use the much more comfortable swivel chairs. Obviously, the Board had liked the idea of a shorter table and overlooked the matter of seating. On a re-vote the Board changed its decision in favor of swivel chairs! In subsequent years, the long and tiring meetings of the Board proved this to be a wise decision. Many actions of the Board probably reflected the effects of the more relaxed and comfortable setting. The acoustics in the room turned out to be excellent and even with such a long table it was a rare occasion when someone could not hear.

In action related to the construction of the new wing, the Board of Regents established a separate account designed to finance future expansion.

The Regents Meeting was held for the first time in the Edward R. Loveland Board Room in November, 1961. The portrait of Mr. Loveland, painted in 1954 by Bjorn Egeli, was placed on the east wall facing the long walnut table, and a bronze plaque at the south entrance read,

> This room is dedicated with grateful appreciation to the memory of Edward Rutherford Loveland, BScEd, FACP (Honorary), 1893-1960. Executive Secretary of the American College of Physicians, 1926-1959, by the Officers, Regents, Governors and Fellows of the College, 1961.

In order to keep the College solvent while meeting existing obligations and providing for the future, a revised dues scale was adopted. Master, Fellow and Associate Member dues were increased to $40 per year for those out of medical school 10 or more years and $25 for those out 10 years or less. All other reduced-dues classifications were eliminated, including those of members in government service, public health, the Veterans' Administration, medical schools, and other nonprofit institutions.

At the November meeting in 1961, the Board of Regents made an important policy decision about a long standing membership question. In 1920 and 1960, the issue was the same: Shall we maintain high standards and limit membership or continue to receive members who cannot meet standards for Fellowship and emphasize the importance of continuing education as a College responsibility to this Associate group? In 1955, yet another proposal to eliminate Associate Membership had been rejected by the Board of Regents. The proposal of 1960 called for higher standards which would automatically limit membership. The Board concluded that with the rapid increase in fully qualified and certified internists, it could not maintain an exclusive posture. Long range plans were set in motion to provide for an effective organization of more than 20,000 members by 1975.

Bylaws adopted at the Annual Business Meeting on April 12, 1962, reflected these decisions:

1. Board certified Associates could be proposed for Fellowship after two years as Associate, provided the candidate had practiced internal medicine, a subspecialty, or an allied specialty, in one location for a minimum of two

years prior to proposal. The proposal should demonstrate strong interest in continuing scholarship and high standards of practice, evidenced in hospital or academic appointments, theses, contributions to scientific literature or a minimum of five well documented clinical case reports with literature reviews prepared during the Associate term. Proposals must be supported by the Governor, Masters, or Fellows from the candidate's jurisdiction, attesting to character, ethical standing and activities. Attendance at postgraduate courses was regarded favorably and attending at least one Annual Session was required during the Associate period.

2. Direct election to Fellowship without Associate term would be considered for candidates of age 35 and older, who were at least five years past the required graduate training with Board certification. Professional activity in the same locality for three years, in either private or institutional practice, as well as scientific contributions and accomplishments acceptable to the Credentials Committee, were also required.

3. Minimum qualifications for admission as an Associate required graduation from a Liaison Committee for Medical Education [LCME] accredited medical school five years prior to proposal and possession of a license to practice medicine. A fulltime Staff appointment in a medical or paramedical institution or practice limited to internal medicine or a related subspecialty, conducted in the same locality for at least two years, was required. Eligibility to take the American Board of Internal Medicine [ABIM] examination should be demonstrated.

The Credentials Committee was empowered to modify requirements in exceptional cases.

The Bylaws amendments rescinded the previous unlimited term for Associates and required that Associates, after their two-year term, should advance to Fellowship within five years or be terminated, emphasizing the College's strong commitment to professional progress.

Supporting these new approaches to membership, the Board also introduced a number of important decisions about the dues structure, designed to sustain current membership and encourage young physicians to maintain their association with the College.

Dr. William Middleton, former ACP President and then Director of the Veterans' Administration, gave strong support to the idea of basing the dues on time since graduation, rather than on titles and positions. He gave Mr. Dauterich information about the benefits that physicians in government services receive and how much a practicing physician would have to set aside to accrue the same benefits. This amount of money was substantial, and the facts confirmed that practicing physicians were not better able to pay higher dues.

The change in dues structure resolved a lot of problems. The previous method of basing dues on academic titles and positions were not interpretable or equitable in terms of seniority or income. These changes were adopted effective January 1, 1962.

The dues structure was amended to waive dues for members in all classes after age 65, who showed satisfactory evidence of retirement from active practice or other remunerative positions.

The Board of Regents also reserved its discretionary power to remit initiation fees or annual dues, without publicity, in whole or in part, for a member engaged in purely scientific research, full-time medical teaching, or active government service. These allowances were limited to individuals during the ten years following graduation from medical school. Waiver of dues was also a discretionary power of the Board in cases of financial reverses or serious disability. Dues were to be reinstated on resumption of practice or other regular professional activities after financial stability or reversal of disability had occurred.

The announcement of the general dues increases for all classes of membership was quickly followed by a number of resignations by young physicians in academic and research positions and in governmental services who found it difficult to afford such dues on limited incomes. The Board re-evaluated its position at its meeting in April, 1962.

Competing for these physicians' attention were a growing number of specialty societies and research organizations. The incomes of young full-time academic instructors, professors and basic scientists were limited. After a thorough review of the facts, the Board waived the dues increase for full-time basic scientists and clinical professors below the rank of full professor. The Board directed the Executive Director to write to those who had submitted resignations informing them of its decision and encouraging them to continue their association with the College at the lower dues rate of $15 per year, retroactive to January 1, 1962. This lower rate was also extended to members in Mexico and Latin America, excluding Puerto Rico.

About 650 members had received and would continue to receive dues waivers because they were 65 years of age or older, retired, or disabled. All reduced dues had amounted to over $32,000, with only approximately 7,000 of 11,000 members paying full dues.

Failure to increase revenue, of which dues were the most important source, would have resulted in a sharp curtailment of activities and growth of the College. Expenses continued to climb and one of these, Research Fellowships, was to increase from $8,000 in 1961 to $45,000 by 1963. The Board was also determined to maintain the regular office operations of the College out of dues income.

The Board also redefined the benefits of membership based on the new dues rates. Each member was entitled to a subscription to the *Annals,* postgraduate courses at $20 less than nonmembers, no admission fee for the Annual Session ($25 for nonmembers), participation in the Group Insurance Association plans of the ACP, and decreased assessments for future building expansion.

Initiation fees were also reviewed in November, 1962. No change had been made when the dues structure was altered in November, 1961. Consequently, the Board of Regents resolved that practicing clinicians depending upon private practice for income were to pay a fee of $80; full-time instructors or research workers in non-profit institutions, members of the Medical Corps of the Armed Forces, the Public Health Service, and the Veterans' Adminstration, were subject to a $50 assessment.

Registration fees for non-members attending the Annual Session were raised to $40. This registration fee was to include non-members, heretofore admitted without charge, from the Armed Forces, Public Health Service, Veterans' Administration, and non-ACP hospital staff members who were not participating in the Scientific Program.

A final item about membership was submitted by the Committee on Masterships and Honorary Fellowships. Dr. Irving Wright, Chairman, proposed the establishment of a new class of membership, to allow recognition of a number of distinguished physicians in foreign countries, who were really too senior to be considered as Affiliates and yet were not quite of the stature of those who in the past had been elected to Honorary Fellowship. No action was taken.

## Annual Session 1962

At the Annual Business Meeting, 1962, the Secretary General, Dr. Wallace Yater reported the current membership as follows: Masters, 29; Fellows, 7,262; Associates, 3,931; and a total membership of 11,222.

In the Treasurer's report, Dr. Thomas Durant reported that the total investments of the College as of October, 1961, were $2,969,456, about half of which was in the Endowment Fund and the other half in the General Fund. Total value of the portfolio had increased $456,265.

I expressed the gratitude of the entire Staff for the much needed new addition to the building. I recounted my own activities and said I had attended, over two years, all but seven of the Regional Meetings. I attended the White House Conference on Aging, representing the College. I was Vice President of a new organization, the National Association of Medical and Allied Journals, and had been appointed to the Advisory Committee of the Council on Medical Education and Hospitals of the AMA.

At the meeting of the Board of Regents, a resolution was adopted which transferred the authority to execute all contracts, agreements, and other documents under seal or otherwise necessary or appropriate for the regular and ordinary business of the College, from the Secretary General to the Chief Administrative Officer of the College.

At the conclusion of my report, I voiced my concern about the relationship of the College to the American Society of Internal Medicine [ASIM]. I indicated that there was a need to study future relationships and to develop a College position on these matters. From a strictly personal viewpoint, I said I would prefer that the College have nothing to do with socioeconomic and related issues. However, I had come to believe that the College was being placed inadvertently in a position of weakness. I reminded the Board that the College was a national organization with no local organizational structure. On the other hand, the ASIM was a confederation of dissimilarly organized state societies. Some more unified type of societies would certainly evolve in the future, but at present, they presented no unified picture, organizationally.

I felt that the ASIM demanded to be heard as spokesman for internal medicine because its membership was composed exclusively of internists. Many, if not all, socioeconomic problems faced by the physician would be solved at the local level, and the importance of the state Societies of Internal Medicine should not be ignored. Broad socioeconomic problems having more direct impact on the patient would need the attention of national organizations, making it imperative that the ACP and ASIM resolve their differences. I recognized the prerogative of many of the state societies to sponsor scientific meetings, and concluded that it would only be a matter of time before the ASIM might decide to sponsor national scientific meetings as well. Though I felt strongly that it was undesirable to have two societies acting in the areas of education and science in internal medicine, I presented no specific recommendations, but urged further study and development of policy positions.

The ASIM Liaison Committee reported to the Board of Regents in November that the ASIM had decided to initiate a general commercial exhibit area at its future annual meetings. There was also a distinct possibility that the ASIM might establish a scientific program at its annual meetings in order to foster membership interest.

The Committee conveyed three requests from the ASIM. First, the Society expressed interest in joining the ACP's health and accident insurance programs, excluding the liability coverage. Since the great majority of ASIM members were also College members (only 1,900 out of 8,000 were not) the Regents decided to make insurance coverage under the Group Insurance Administrators [GIA] programs available to all members of the Society, including non-ACP members.

Secondly, the Society requested that the ACP Directory designate those College Members who were also ASIM members. In response, the Board explained that the College did not, and had never, listed memberships in other organizations and was not prepared to establish the precedent.

In the third request, the ASIM expressed a wish to co-sponsor a Monday morning public information session with the College at the next annual ACP meeting. Although the Society did have a place in the general education of the lay public, the Board of Regents decided against such collaboration.

In view of these communications from the ASIM, the Board empowered the President to appoint an Ad Hoc Committee to Study the Relationship of the ACP to the ASIM. The Committee was directed to review the College's position, taken in April, 1960, which stated:

> The American Society of Internal Medicine is to continue in its field of endeavors the following: Economic and professional prepayment medical insurance; political activities; medicolegal considerations; public relations; office and practice management; enhancement of the place of the internist in hospital affairs; maintenance of standards of practice; and public education of the profile of the internist.

Following the report of the Ad Hoc Committee, the Board revised its position to state that

. . . Medicolegal considerations were to be performed as a joint effort of the ASIM in cooperation with the American College of Physicians along with public relations activities as they pertain to the internist. The enhancement of the place of the internist in hospital affairs was a primary activity of the ACP as exhibited in the College's support of the RRC-IM, the JCAH, the CPHA, and the ABIM. The maintenance of the standards of practice of internal medicine is of major interest to both organizations as each contributes in its own area (the College through postgraduate scientific education and the Society in socioeconomic matters as they relate to internal medicine).

I recall a conversation with Dr. James Hall of Traverse City, Mississippi, and Dr. Max Berry of Kansas City, at the Annual Session of the College in Philadelphia in 1962. Jim had been on the Cheney Committee (Committee on Prepaid Health Insurance) in 1956, which had recommended that the College establish a standing committee on health insurance and advised that if the College did not address socioeconomic issues, a national society of internal medicine would be formed to address them. In our conversation, all three of us agreed that it would be a good idea to merge the ASIM and ACP to create a unified organization speaking for internal medicine.

In 1963, Dr. Berry became President of the ASIM. Later he became an ACP Governor and then a Regent. He participated actively in negotiations in 1971 and 1972, when the attempted merging of the two societies was undertaken. He was devoted to the interests of internal medicine and worked hard to bring the two together. Dr. Berry also felt so strongly about internal medicine as a specialty that he had a medical student with him each summer working in the office, making calls with him, going to the hospital and, in general, showing the young physician the way he practiced internal medicine. He told me once that in the 12 to 15 years of these preceptorships, all but one of these students had chosen the specialty of internal medicine after graduating from medical school.

## Governors Review ASIM Relations

At the meeting of the Board of Governors in April, 1962, a wide ranging colloquium about the ASIM highlighted the following issues:

There was a general consensus that the greatest source of difficulty emerged from the fact that the ASIM, being a federation of state organizations, viewed policies from a different perspective than that of the College, which is national in character. The College, in the opinion of the Governors, had never set definite policies to deal with the ASIM, causing many misunderstandings and making it difficult for the Officers and the Executive Director to work closely with the new group.

Dr. Hugh Luckey, from New York, believed that the development of the ASIM was critically detrimental to internal medicine. He considered that placing the ASIM in a position to represent internal medicine in any area in this country was especially harmful to the ACP. Dr. Luckey suggested that the mistake might be corrected by some kind of alignment of the two organizations. Dr. Charles

Smyth anticipated that the ASIM would take over a major role in educational efforts eventually. As a Governor for the College, he expressed concern that he did not really have a good knowledge of his own constituency because of the absence of any formal organizations.

Dr. Walter Frommeyer, of Alabama, mentioned a certificate issued by the Alabama Society of Internal Medicine, which "certified" members as specialists in internal medicine. In effect, this action preempted the prerogatives of the ABIM. This matter was later settled with the ASIM as being inappropriate, and the practice was discontinued.

Dr. Roberto Escamilla and Dr. George Griffith, both Governors in California, favored a tolerant attitude toward the ASIM. The California Society of Internal Medicine, the first component society organized, always had a good relationship with the practicing internists in that state.

Dr. Chester Keefer felt that if the College took on some of the other issues being assumed by the ASIM, it would change the entire character of the organization which the College had become. The Conference endorsed the work of the Ad Hoc Committee, urging continued studies to develop a different plan of cooperation between the two societies.

The Board of Governors discussed how long a Governor's term should be. At that time Governors served three terms of three years each. Opinions varied and the debate addressed a proposal to change this to two three-year terms, a maximum of six years of service. By shortening the term, it was noted, the number of Fellows serving as Governors would increase by fifty percent. The shorter term was a disadvantage, some Governors asserted, precluding a period of getting used to the job and leaving office before a complete understanding of the duties was achieved. Other Governors countered that this problem could be easily solved by establishing a position of Governor-Elect, involving a one-year term before taking on the duties of Governor.

The Board of Governors finally voted to recommend to the Board of Regents that a change in the Bylaws be made providing that the term of Governors should not exceed two elective consecutive terms of three years each. By another motion, they recommended that a new office, Governor-Elect, be established. These changes introduced a necessary interim provision: A Governor who was already appointed to a standing committee of the College would be permitted to finish his term as the Governor representative, although his term as Governor had expired.

The Board finally granted approval for the implementation of interim sectional meetings after considerable debate covering a span of almost three years. The first Interim Session was scheduled for Detroit, Michigan, November 21-23, 1963, with the Annual Session for that year to be held April 1-5, 1963 in Denver. Responsibility for arrangements and program was to be assumed by the Program Committee and the Executive Office Staff. The general chairman was to act as local liaison for arrangements, other than those for the scientific program, and no exhibits were planned for the first three years. The same credit toward meeting the requirements for Fellowship given for attendance at an Annual Session would be allowed for the sectional meeting.

During preliminary planning, Dr. Irving Wright asked me to come to New York to dine with him and the public relations officer of the American Heart Association. The Association had drafted a job description for a public relations officer, which specified that he or she should be responsible to the Public Relations Committee and report to the chief officer on administrative matters. I had already stated my position; I was in favor of having staff support for an office of public information, but was not in favor of the usual kind of public relations program for the College. We were not likely to become involved in fund raising and there did not seem to be any impetus for deep involvement in public issues such as socioeconomics, politics, legislative matters or other activity that justified a broad public relations program. Later, I told Dr. Wright that I was so strongly opposed to having anyone on my Staff who was not completely responsible to me, that if the Board of Regents wanted to adopt this policy, I would have given up my position and returned to California.

As a result of the report of an Ad Hoc Committee to Study Professional and Public Relations of the College, the Board decided in November, 1961, that a standing Committee on Public Information should be appointed. This matter was continually discussed and tabled from the time Dr. Dwight Wilbur had pressed the Board to employ a public relations officer with unfortunate results. The new committee, specifically charged to relate to the membership, would have within its authority the following:

1. A continuing program of information and education about the activities and concerns of the American College of Physicians for the profession and for the lay public.
2. The development and coordination of all public educational programs and the preparation of guidelines and helpful suggestions for regional and local Annual Session committees.
3. The provision of instructions for local Annual Session committees; adequate press room arrangements; advance contact with science writers; arrangement of press conferences with key speakers and issuance of press releases.

The Committee would consist of seven members, at least two to be Regents.

I was authorized to employ staff as required to implement the program. In January, 1962, Mr. Stephen Donohue was employed as a part-time public relations consultant.

The Residency Review Committee for Internal Medicine [RRC-IM] recommended to the parent organizations that all two-year training programs be expanded to three-year programs by July 1, 1965, or be disapproved. They also recommended that all one-year programs, except for a small number of highly specialized ones, be discontinued as of July 1, 1965. These recommendations were part of the RRC-IM's efforts to upgrade the quality of residency training programs.

A careful survey of the one and two-year residency programs conducted by the RRC-IM showed that the majority were occupied almost entirely by graduates of foreign medical schools, decidedly below the professional quality desired. It was the Committee's opinion that any two-year program good enough to survive could combine with another stronger program, preferably university derived. The target date of July, 1965, would provide adequate time to make the transition.

The one-year programs were somewhat different in that there were very few specialty programs of the high caliber offered at the National Institutes of Health and Roswell Park Memorial Institute in Buffalo. Since those could provide an excellent one year program in research or in the specific clinical field involved, the quality and nature of the programs did not require three years. However, the Committee stipulated that this period of training was not to be considered as one of the physician's required two years of general clinical training.

At an important meeting of the Joint Commission on Accreditation of Hospitals [JCAH], Alex M. Burgess, Sr., described two reports that were given careful consideration.

1. The first was a report from the Committee on Research which had made a detailed study of the methods employed by the JCAH to investigate the quality of patient care in hospitals. The measures included everything pertaining to the care of the patient. This study, when completed, would merit a detailed report to the Board of Regents.
2. The second report stated that the JCAH was considering a new department for the survey and accreditation of in-patient care in institutions other than acute care hospitals, such as nursing homes and similar patient care facilities. The Commission passed the following resolution, with two ACP commissioners dissenting:
   a. that accreditation of in-patient institutions other than hospitals was desirable and necessary;
   b. that it could best be undertaken by a non-profit, non-governmental national organization of stature;
   c. that the JCAH was an appropriate body for this task; and
   d. that the Commissioners of the JCAH should be authorized to seek outside funding to establish this program.

Dr. Burgess stated the reasons for the ACP dissent: In its opinion, this added responsibility would constitute a definite handicap by placing an undue burden of responsibility on the JCAH Director, potentially jeopardizing the current work of the Commission. The ACP would be asked for financial and moral support. It was Dr. Burgess's belief that, in addition to the existing program, the survey and accreditation of nursing homes and similar institutions was a worthy objective, but the Commission should not be the responsible organization.

In the discussion, I pointed out the administrative problems of working with this complex body. The AMA and the ACP directly contributed their share for hiring the surveyors whom the JCAH Director appointed. The American Hospital Association [AHA] hired its own surveyors who did two jobs, one for the Hospital Association, doing inspections of a slightly different type; the other half of their time was made available to the Director of JCAH for survey duties. The American College of Surgeons also hired its own surveyors who also did two jobs. Part of their time was devoted to inspecting tumor clinics. It seemed desirable that some other way to finance the JCAH be developed. One plan, already suggested by members of the Executive Committee of JCAH, would divide the costs between running the central office and doing the actual surveys. At a later date, the JCAH adopted this approach to organization and financing.

In addition to the above JCAH issues, the College had been approached that year by the American Academy of Pediatrics, which asked whether the College would be willing to give up one of its three Commission seats to the Academy. The Academy would assume the cost of this position, approximately $20,000. The Board of Regents declined this offer.

Dr. R. H. Kampmeier reported on the Joint Study on Continuing Medical Education, formed after a meeting consisting of representatives from the AMA; the Association of American Medical Colleges; American College of Physicians, American College of Surgeons; American Academy of Pediatrics, American College of General Practice and other specialty groups. Dr. Bernard V. Dryer, of Western Reserve University, was employed to make a study of possible means to provide continuing education nationwide. The above organizations together pledged $40,000 for this study whose basic purpose was to set up communication in various fields and at various levels which could be conducted through a variety of media, e.g., television, printed material, etc.

Dr. Kampmeier indicated that the submission of its report, which was published as *Lifetime Learning for Physicians,* would complete the work of the Study Committee because the cost of implementation would be of such magnitude that it could not be financed by a few medical organizations.

The College Administrative Staff explored the possibility of having a more effective College Directory, published every two years instead of three. After studying their recommendations, the Board decided to accept a proposal to publish three issues of the Directory in a six-year period, which could be done at approximately the same cost as producing one every three years.

At the November, 1962 Board meeting, the Fellowships and Scholarships Committee related some difficulties in awarding traveling scholarships. While some had too many applicants, others might have none. The Committee, therefore, recommended that all applications be uniformly received, not for particular scholarships, but for an ACP Traveling Scholarship. The application form would list and describe each one available. The Committee might then be free to direct the applicant to an appropriate scholarship. Since the scholarships varied in the amount of stipend, the Board approved a uniform stipend for all traveling scholarships and raised from $400 to $500 the two Brower Scholarships and for the Bowes and Thompson Traveling Scholarships to conform with the new procedures. Since the awardees had already been selected for 1963, this new procedure was to take effect in 1964.

A questionnaire was sent out in 1961 by the GIA which attempted to ascertain the interest of the membership in a major hospital plan. Over 3,500 physicians responded; the vast majority favored the College sponsoring a contract of this character. Subsequently, the Insurance Committee reviewed the plans submitted and selected the one that provided the greatest benefits at the most advantageous premiums. Almost 400 applications were received in the first two weeks the program was offered and coverage became effective January 1, 1963. (Appendix F)

The Group Life Insurance Plan continued to enjoy favorable subscription and a poll of the members insured under the program indicated that many desired to obtain a higher level of insurance protection in lieu of the reducing term coverage that was then provided. The Supplemental Plan, as it was known, was adopted by the Trustees of the program in an attempt to make the Group Life Plan more attractive for members of all ages.

Philadelphia, home of the College Headquarters, was the site of the 43rd Annual Session, April 9-13, 1962. Total registration was over 7,000, making this session the largest up to that date.

One of the highlights of the meeting was the formal dedication of the newly erected wing of the Headquarters. More than 50 community and civic leaders were present and Dr. Gaylord P. Harnwell, President of the University of Pennsylvania, gave a short address of congratulations to the College for its continued involvement in the University City area of Philadelphia.

It was important that the members be apprised of the essential facts of College finances, to affirm that each dollar spent for dues was being utilized as efficiently as possible. An analysis of expenditures for 1961-1962 was prepared by the Treasurer. Continuing medical education, the primary purpose of the organization as stated in the founding constitution, accounted for 63.9 percent of the $1,192,000 of expended income. Of this, 37.6 percent was expended for publications; 9.4 for the Annual Session; 1.1 for Regional Meetings; 2.6 for fellowships; 7.3 for postgraduate courses and 5.9 for other medical programs. Of the remaining 36.1 percent, 17.2 represented administrative expenditures; 2.6 expended for building operations; 9.3 appropriated to the Endowment Fund, and an additional 7 percent was placed in the new Building Fund.

The Annual Session deficit was reduced markedly from $58,444 for the Miami meeting to $1,435 for the Philadelphia session. This remarkable improvement could be directly attributed to a reduction in travel expenses, but the Treasurer warned that larger deficits could be expected whenever the location of the meeting was distant from the areas in which the bulk of the membership resided. The Interim Sessions, the first scheduled for 1963, would also incur additional costs.

## ACP History Published

An honorarium of $1,500 was presented to Dr. George Morris Piersol as a token of appreciation from the College for his efforts in writing the history of the ACP, *Gateway of Honor.* The chronicle traced the foundations, accomplishments and personalities that had shaped the first 45 years of the organization, from its inception in 1915 to 1960. Over 3,000 copies were printed.

The total circulation of the *Annals* increased from just over 25,000 in January, 1962 to 26,600 in December. According to Dr. Elkinton, the Editor, this growth could be directly attributed to non-member subscriptions.

Dr. McMillan was reappointed Editor of the *ACP Bulletin* for a three-year term in 1962. He reported that, before the Board of Regents should consider changing the *ACP Bulletin* to a monthly publication, with a different type of cover designed to eliminate envelope mailing, further consideration should be given to such aspects as cover design, cover paper stock, separate publication of meeting lists, etc. He further stated that costs could not be reduced significantly by having the *ACP Bulletin* printed in Philadelphia.

## Part Four (1962-1963)

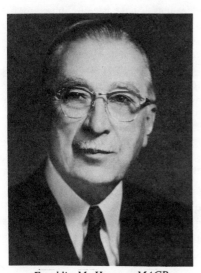

*Franklin M. Hanger, MACP*

Franklin M. Hanger, was born in Staunton, Virginia, September 6, 1894, and died there on October 10, 1971. He received a BS degree from the University of Virginia in 1916, and after graduating from Johns Hopkins School of Medicine in 1920, he obtained his graduate training at the Presbyterian Hospital and Columbia University College of Physicians and Surgeons in New York City. In 1926 he joined the faculty at Columbia, becoming Professor of Medicine in 1947. He spent his entire active career at that institution. Considered an excellent teacher and clinician, he was also a diligent researcher, with a special interest in the study of hepatic function. He was a member of the Society of Clinical Investigation; the American Association for Advancement of Science; the American Association of Immunologists; the Association of American Physicians and the New York Academy of Medicine.

Elected a Fellow of the American College of Physicians in 1937, he became an enthusiastic and supportive member. He was a Regent from 1957-1961; President-elect in 1961-62; President in 1962-63; Regent in 1963-1966. He was made a Master of the College in 1967.

A diplomate of the American Board of Internal Medicine, he was a member of the Board for a number of years.

Upon retirement he remained active, teaching at the University of Virginia in Charlottesville until his death in 1971.

In his Presidential Address in 1962, Dr. Hanger spoke about the many dislocations and transformations in modern society. He decried the growing tendency to attain objectives through mass alliances and through visionary regimentations as discordant to the homely tenets of our austere training.

> I think the concern of most internists over growing collectivism is due to their innate respect for individualism—the individualism of the patient, as well as their own. Our branch of medicine is not aggressively anti-social. We would all go along with John Stuart Mill who stated mildly, "The liberty of the individual must be thus far limited; he must not make himself a nuisance to other people."
>
> The internist selects his field of interest with youthful enthusiasm, and he continues in his later years to derive satisfaction through broadening his understanding of man as a "carrier" of physical and spiritual disorders. To uncritical outsiders, the success of his career might be measured by his worldly acquisitions, but within this College we know our sustaining contentment comes from being needed by others because of special knowledge and judgment.
>
> I think we represent a constructive force in the present day of oppressive tensions. Who is better qualified by training and human dealings than the internist himself to bring insight to his patients, and to others in his periphery, on the principles underlying medical efficacy? So many of those about us need guidance, not only in meeting the frustrations of health limitations, but in overcoming the feeling of futility that the swarming of humanity creates. The "potential individualists", who comprise the great majority of our countrymen, need to sense anew their own self-importance; their own nobleness. They should know the satisfaction of forming opinions, based on physiologic soundness and balance rather than giving repetitive voice to slogans and catch phrases. Let us in turn avoid sloppiness in our own thinking and callousness in our bearing. The physician by inspiring example, as well as by helpfulness, can create gallantry and toleration, and a sense of fair play in his fellow man. It is upon these [basic human attributes] that a sturdier social order can evolve.

Once during an active discussion about the possibility that the American Society of Internal Medicine [ASIM] might become involved in education, Dr. Hanger commented that the American College of Physicians should never be put in the position of opposing any organization wanting to do a job of educating physicians. For that reason he felt it improper for the College to tell another society what to do about educating the physician.

Apparently he was afraid I might become too interested in who might be elected President of the ASIM, for he voiced the opinion to me that a chief administrative officer should take no active part in determining who would be elected an officer of the ACP. I was in full agreement. I think that this incident illustrated how concerned he was that organizational business be conducted through proper channels.

During the Annual Session in Philadelphia in 1962, Dr. Hanger and I had breakfast with Dr. Charles Donegan and Dr. Bert Whitehall, President and Executive Director respectively of the ASIM. The atmosphere was pleasant, although there were strong differences of opinion on some subjects. After the meeting Dr. Hanger said to me, "The relations between ASIM and ACP will be a major concern to you and the Board of Regents as long as there are these two societies." He did not advise attempting a merger but did feel that it would be a continuing problem to make interrelations operate harmoniously.

Enroute by airplane to the Regional Meeting in Sun Valley, Idaho, Dr. Hanger told the flight attendants that we were on a skiing holiday. A few weeks later, I was on the same flight to Chicago and one of the flight attendants asked me where Dr. Hanger was. She wanted to know whether he really did any skiing in Idaho. She didn't believe he would, but her colleague had insisted he would. I explained that we did go to the top of the chairlift, but we did no skiing. One of the wives persuaded Frank to ride the chairlift at a place called Dollar Mountain, and equipped him with suitable attire. It was very cold and Dr. Hanger really looked amusing bundled into the extra clothes she had brought for him. He was always a good natured person and was very gracious in dealing with people.

On another of our trips together, we were discussing how we might shorten the Convocation. We asked his wife what she thought and she said shortening the citations would help; she commented that his citations had been even longer before she had read them and suggested cuts. Then she said, "It's just fine to shorten the ceremony, but keep it properly stuffy".

During his year as President, there was controversy among members of the profession about whether internists should be allowed to use radioisotopes. Dr. Hanger felt strongly that no one should use these materials without adequate special training. Eventually a conjoint Board examination was developed for Nuclear Medicine and a Board certified pathologist, radiologist or internist with special training could become certified in nuclear medicine.

In December, Dr. Hanger and I went to a clinical meeting of the AMA in Denver to survey meeting facilities, in anticipation of our own meeting in that city in April, 1963. We stayed several days and I took him to sessions of the House of Delegates, reference committees and hospitality suites. He had never belonged to the AMA and thanked me for showing him how it conducted its sessions. He commented: "I never really appreciated how hard these delegates work and how seriously they consider all matters. They are certainly a dedicated group."

During this time we went to Dr. Charles Smyth's house for dinner. He was the ACP Governor for Colorado at that time. There we encountered Dr. John Talbott, then Editor of the *Journal of the American Medical Association*. He had been a resident under Dr. Hanger and asked Frank what he was doing in Denver, as he was reputed to have little interest in the AMA. Frank, with a straight face, said he had become interested in the AMA and wanted to become more actively involved. Finally, he admitted that he really had come out to look over convention facilities for our April meeting. John replied, "I still don't understand why you are interested. Anyhow, what is the ACP up to now and who is the President?" Frank said he didn't know. Later John asked me and I told him Frank was. John's embarrassment amused Frank immensely; he said, "John, you haven't changed much since your residency."

At the end of the Annual Session, Dr. Hanger took me to lunch and was obviously very glad his term was over. When I asked him a few questions about the future he said, "My goodness, it never occurred to me that you were so far along in your planning that you're worrying about next year's meeting in Atlantic City and not about the meeting here in Denver."

## 1962-1963

Armed Forces Regional Meeting in Japan. Corresponding Fellows established. JCAH Division on Surveys. ABIM 12-year study of Board examinations. Federal legislation and ACP statements: FDA and "informed consent"; laboratory animal research bill; NIH and cancer research legislation.

At the November, 1962 meeting of the Board of Regents, Dr. Franklin Hanger, President, described a new ACP educational project, a Regional Meeting to be held in Japan. This was a cooperative effort involving the medical services of the Army, Navy and Air Force, working closely with local Japanese physicians. The services attached considerable importance to this event as manifested by their arrangement to have a greeting sent from the President of the United States to the meeting and their invitation to the Ambassador to Japan to be one of the speakers at the meeting.

The program, in Dr. Hanger's opinion, was outstanding. Participants were mostly young men; military medical officers from all service branches who felt themselves exiled far from their accustomed intellectual milieu. The meeting drew medical officers from Korea, the Phillippines and even Hawaii.

Dr. Hanger was impressed that there were over 120 Japanese physicians in attendance. Many of these were distinguished professors of medicine in Japan. Some participated in the program and the whole occasion was such a success that he recommended that it be repeated on an annual basis. The program was carried on for several years.

Dr. Wesley Spink, President-Elect, mentioned an educational opportunity which he thought would be appreciated by the Board of Regents: When a President or Officer goes to a Regional Meeting or postgraduate course held in the area of a medical school, quite often it is possible for him to spend some time at the medical school, and he urged that they be encourged to do so. For example, when he participated in a postgraduate course with Dr. Howard Lewis at Portland, Oregon; at the Regional Meeting in New England, in Hanover, New Hampshire, he spent a whole day at the medical school with students and faculty.

In my Executive Director's report, I described an important conference I had attended, sponsored by the AMA and the Association of American Medical Colleges [AAMC]. They had become interested in national health and international medical education. Clearly, the College would be asked to take a more active part in these areas. The United States government had discovered that aid in international health is one of the most important facets of our foreign policy. Unless high calibre people were found to operate some of these programs, these efforts could result in a great deal "of harm", according to the State Department.

Another interesting international subject came up at the AAMC meeting in the Fall of 1962. How could US medical schools help to staff the faculties of some of the foreign schools without jeopardizing the professional progression of young native faculty members who spend two years abroad in study? I asked the Board to consider whether the College should concentrate all of our international activities in one committee, pointing out that a special committee was working with

MEDICO and CARE and that special representatives were appointed for some other international activities. In addition, the College also had at that time a Latin American Committee.

## Kefauver Act - Drug Safety

Much time at several meetings of the Board was spent discussing the potential effects of the Kefauver Act and its regulations concerning the investigation and prescription of new drugs. These regulations, onerous to many physicians, eventually caused rather profound changes in drug evaluation procedures. For example, the Food and Drug Administration [FDA] drew up rules for journal advertising which placed the responsibility for truthful advertising about drugs on the manufacturers, who were required to document safety, and also effectiveness. Thus, the College's Journal Advertising Committee no longer needed to approve the information in each individual ad. Several years later, the FDA was given authority to regulate devices used in medical practice. On balance, these actions illustrated that government did consult and work with the professional societies in achieving objectives.

A critical event occurred during the summer of 1962. The FDA, as I mentioned, intended to impose new regulations which would cause problems to medical journals in the area of journal advertising.

1. The FDA intended to recommend taxing income from advertising in journals of tax exempt organizations, on the basis that it was unrelated to the purposes for which the organizations enjoyed tax exempt status.
2. Proposed new regulations would increase FDA monitoring and control of drug advertising. In particular, the FDA was proposing that advertising by trade name should be replaced by the use of generic names.

Subsequently, Dr. Keefer, Dr. Hanger and I appeared before the FDA's Commission on Drug Safety and pointed out the difficulty this might present to organizations such as the College which depended to some degree upon advertising in their journals. Our testimony notwithstanding, the FDA soon informed the College that proposed regulations had been approved; the scientific community had 60 days in which to comment. This period occurred when most of the medical community was on vacation, a particularly poor time; many physicians who would have commented could not. The FDA asserted, however, that they expected additional comments, and that the regulations which had been proposed in August had not been issued.

At the Board's request, Dr. Keefer again visited with the Commission on Drug Safety and also with HEW Secretary Celebrezze to discuss inherent problems which he recounted, in essence, to the Board in November.

1. The New Kefauver Act had been passed and signed by the President in October, 1961. The first problem arose in amending the regulations so that this Act could be administered realistically. Two provisions of this Act affected all doctors giving any drug not approved by the FDA. These provi-

sions concerned what is known as "informed consent". It was now required by law that any doctor who gave an experimental drug, or a new drug that had not been approved by the FDA, must obtain the consent of the patient before the drug was used. An exclusion clause in the law stated that the physician might not be required to obtain this consent if, in his judgment, he felt it would be unwise and, perhaps, when stated in explicit lay language, would ruin his experiment. The physician would, however, be required to document why he should not attempt to obtain informed consent.

2. A second provision in the law, important to all physicians, introduced the question of record keeping. All clinical investigators would be required to keep records and submit these records to the sponsor; the sponsor might be either in the drug industry, or an individual in a university who might develop a chemical and then ask the clinical investigator who might be outside the state to test the drug independently, or as part of a cooperative study. The investigator would then have to notify the FDA that he was engaged in such testing. The FDA did not have the authority at that time to visit a physician's office and inspect records, but it might do so upon request, if it were unable to get information from the sponsor or manufacturer, which was considered necessary under the provisions in the regulation.

Dr. Keefer mentioned that it would probably be a year or two before these regulations were adopted and before all clinical investigators would understand and feel the full impact of them. In his opinion, all physicians who were concerned with clinical investigation should study these regulations very carefully.

Regulations regarding control of advertising would not become effective until the Spring of 1963. The FDA would continue to monitor the advertising of drugs that go to doctors. Certain provisions about the use of generic vs. trade names would be more particularly defined.

One other provision in the proposed regulation essentially concerned censorship of scientific information and press releases from manufacturers or drug houses about new products before they had been released for sale in interstate commerce. These regulations provided that the manufacturer was forbidden to make public statements about the behavior of any drug, its safety or indications, until a New Drug Application [NDA] submitted to the FDA had been approved. A clause was added specifying that nothing in the regulation prevented a physician from disclosing his results on a new drug at a scientific meeting. This potential form of censorship had already evoked editorials and outcries in the public press. The clause was added subsequent to a hearing held by the Commission on Drug Safety, where apprehension about the regulation had been expressed.

The Residency Review Committee in Internal Medicine [RRC-IM] recommended to the ACP, the Council of Medical Education and Hospitals of the AMA, and the American Board of Internal Medicine [ABIM] that: 1) no new two-year internal medicine residencies be approved and that existing two-year programs be required to obtain three-year approval by July 1, 1965, or be discontinued; 2) approval of all one-year residency programs in internal medicine be discontinued after July 1, 1965, except for specialized programs of exceptional merit; and 3) that transportation and per diem expenses be allowed for regional consultants. The Board of Regents approved all three of these recommendations.

The problems of Governorship in the Eastern New York area, which had 1,275 Fellows and Associates, were made known to the Board of Regents at their November, 1962 meeting. The office was very time consuming, and it was becoming increasingly difficult for any one physician to do the job. An appropriate amendment to the Bylaws therefore, was ratified at the 1963 Annual Business Meeting which divided New York State into three Regions designated Upstate New York (including all the counties north and west of Albany in addition to Broome, Delaware, Schoharie, Albany, Rensselaer, Sullivan, Greene, Ulster, Dutchess, and Columbia), Downstate I (consisting of Manhattan, Bronx, Westchester, Rockland, Putnam and Orange) and Downstate II (which encompassed Kings, Queens, Richmond, Nassau, and Suffolk). In related action, the boundaries of California, Pennsylvania, and Illinois were realigned along county lines to conform with government postal zones and thereby facilitate College mailings.

At their Fall Conference, the Board of Governors had a long discussion concerning Governors' expenses. Some Governors were heavily burdened, especially if they did not have ready access to a duplicating machine and extra secretarial help. In larger areas with several hundred members, the administrative load was considerably heavier. To aid the Governors in the conduct of their office, the Regents elected to reimburse, upon request and submission of a detailed accounting, actual out-of-pocket expenses incurred in fulfilling the duties of the office. The maximum amount allowed was $2,400 to Downstate New York Region I. All other amounts were based on a ratio of the number of members in each Region to the number of members in the Downstate New York I district.

The Board of Governors also considered the question of charging registration fees at Regional Meetings. The Board of Regents did not think it was necessary, but advised the Governors that the College would pay administrative costs, excluding food and beverages, up to $250 for attendance of 200 or less and up to $500 for 200 or more. Such reimbursement required that detailed expense reports be sent to the Executive Director with each request for funds.

## ABIM Studies Exam Results

After a 12-year study of results of examinations from 1950-1962, the ABIM reported oral examinations had become so cumbersome and complex in administration that they recommended their discontinuance.

Results of the study showed that approximately 12,600 physicians had taken the written exam for the first time during that period; 11,250 passed, which was roughly 88 percent. First time takers of the oral numbered 9,100 with 8,010 or 88 percent passing.

The oral exam, consumed a great deal of the ABIM's energy, included 1,426 candidates in 1962. For each physician tested, one and three-quarter hours of examiner time was required. The ABIM was not suffering a loss of young physician interest, but it was finding it difficult to examine them all.

More than 2,100 physicians took the written examination of the ABIM in October, 1962; nearly 300 more than at any prior date. The ABIM's attempt to require a one-year waiting period between written and orals, which went into effect January 1, 1962, collapsed under a storm of protest. The number of candidates had far exceeded Board expectations and a tremendous strain was placed both upon examiners and host facilities.

At the Chicago site in early November, more than 900 patients were required for the oral examination of 436 candidates. This enormous examination load compelled the ABIM to drop the one-year waiting period and also necessitated adding another examination site, bringing to five the number planned for 1963.

The ABIM reported that the greatest number of oral exam failures occurred among candidates who did not demonstrate adequate ability in taking a history and conducting a physical exam. It was Board policy that the examiner not call to the attention of the candidate his errors, but notes were taken indicating the reasons for failure. If a candidate felt unfairly judged, upon writing the ABIM, he would receive from the senior examiner an explanation of the reasons for his failure.

The Publications Committee desired to stimulate student interest in the *Annals of Internal Medicine.* Upon their recommendation, the Regents elected to reduce subscription rates for students, interns, residents, and fellows-in-training to one-half the regular price. Effective January, 1964, the reduced domestic rate (in the United States, Canada, and Puerto Rico) would be $5, with foreign students paying $6 for all renewals and new subscriptions.

In November the Publications Committee regrettably accepted the resignation of Dr. Thomas M. McMillan, Editor of the *ACP Bulletin,* effective April, 1964. Illness in the family necessitated his leaving the Philadelphia area. Under his influence, the *ACP Bulletin* was becoming an increasingly important bridge between College administration and membership. In order to increase this interaction and insure that news about the College was given first priority, I was appointed Editor.

In action related to the *ACP Bulletin,* the Regents decided to gradually decrease, and eventually eliminate, the amount of space allocated to the ASIM. This decision was made in light of the Society's decision to inaugurate its own publication.

In recognition of his fine service to the *Annals,* Dr. Edward J. Huth was appointed Associate Editor by the Board of Regents.

This year also marked the beginning of increased local participation in College activities, directly resulting from changes made in the system of nominating Governors. The membership was polled locally and its choices were submitted to the central Nominating Committee which selected nominees and prepared the slate for elections.

I announced a new procedure to implement the plan to increase membership participation in the selection of College Governors. Henceforth, when a Governor was ineligible, or did not wish to stand for an additional term, his constituents would receive a card inviting suggestions for nominations. In those instances where the Governor was eligible to succeed himself, a similar card would be sent encouraging member comment. The cards were addressed directly to the Chairman of the Nominating Committee to be used in the selection process.

The Postgraduate Courses Committee felt that there should be a more realistic difference between tuition paid by Members ($60) and non-Members ($80) and that lower fees should be stressed as a benefit of membership in the ACP. As a result, members attending postgraduate courses would continue to be charged $60, while non-member fees were increased to $100.

In additional Regents' action, the composition of the Educational Program Committee was increased to four Regents, two Governors, and the Chairman of the Board of Governors. The Committee on Awards and the Committee on Masterships and Honorary Fellowships were merged into the Committee on Awards, Masterships, and Honorary Fellowships. Lastly, Governors were henceforth limited to two consecutive three-year terms, exclusive of any unexpired fraction of a term previously served, in order to broaden the base of member participation in organizational government.

The programs of the College were expanding steadily and with the addition of a Fall Interim Session, two large sessions a year had to be planned. For the efficient operation of both meetings it became increasingly imperative that full time Staff support be assigned the task. The Convention Department was organized at Headquarters to serve the local planning committees and assume responsibility for overall arrangements.

The new 1963 *ACP Directory* was made available, at $9 a copy, at the Annual Session in April, 1964. The biographical data was arranged geographically with an alphabetical index of members, and included spouses' names. In the future, the *Directory* would be issued bi-annually instead of every three years.

The program for Cuban physicians at the University of Miami School of Medicine continued with over 1,100 students having participated by 1963. The fifth short course had an enrollment of over 100. The ACP continued its support, but the Regents decided that the program should not be a protracted financial obligation for the College. Consequently, they voted that $4,000 be appropriated in 1963 and $2,000 in 1964, with the clear stipulation that ACP financing would then be terminated.

The ASIM's request to include its non-ACP members in the College's insurance program was accepted by the Board of Regents in 1962. Accordingly, resolutions were adopted establishing a new Trust and amending the existing Life Insurance Trust. As a result of these changes it was possible for the Chairman of the Committee on Insurance to render one report to the Board of Regents covering all of the Group Insurance Association Plans sponsored by the College.

On the 10th Anniversary of the ACP Health and Accident Plan, it was reported that over 14,000 individual Certificates of Insurance were in force, providing coverage under the several ACP plans. The total of benefits paid under these plans amounted to $4,267,119.98, covering the period from January 1, 1953 to February 28, 1963, a span of 10 years and two months.

The Joint Commission on Accreditation of Hospitals [JCAH] had been asked in 1961 to study the possibility of inspecting and accrediting inpatient care institutions other than acute care hospitals. This service was in great demand and the JCAH, by virtue of its experience, knowledge, and prestige, appeared to be the logical organization to supervise such an operation. Serious questions did arise, though, among the constituent members of the Commission with regard to the administration and financing of the proposed program.

The ACP's share of the total budget of the Commission at that time amounted to $54,000 a year. If a program of accreditation of inpatient care institutions were adopted, the College's share conceivably could increase by approximately $7,000 to $9,000 annually. The Board of Regents in November, 1961, had requested the JCAH to explore other means of financing its activities as supporting the Commission was becoming an increasingly burdensome financial drain on the College. Of the four member organizations the ACP, AMA, American College of Surgeons [ACS], and the American Hospital Association [AHA], the College was the smallest, and it was pointed out that the annual assessment to the JCAH was far in excess of what could be expected reasonably from a budget the size of the ACP's.

For several years, the College had instructed its representatives to JCAH to urge all possible ways in which the cost to the member organizations could be reduced. ACP's assessment of approximately $60,000 was unrealistic in terms of its resources as compared to the other members. Drs. Edwin Crosby, AMA; F.J.L. Blasingame, AMA; Paul North, ACS, and I, for the ACP, constituted the Advisory Committee to the JCAH and we agreed that administrative costs and the costs of conducting surveys could be easily identified, and that fees for surveys could be charged to hospitals. The JCAH previously had objected to charging hospitals a survey fee because this might make the survey less objective. During the time this was being considered, third parties, e.g., Blue Cross, private health insurers and the government were insisting that hospitals had to be accredited to be reimbursed. All of these agencies accepted the accreditation of JCAH. Thus, it was clear that it was financially important for hospitals to achieve and maintain accreditation.

In August, 1962, the Board of Commissioners of the JCAH accepted a proposed plan developed by the four chief administrative officers which was designed to reduce sharply the annual assessment made of each commission member organization. Subsequent to the above action, survey fees were accepted by all hospitals without any serious objection.

The fee scale for individual hospitals was introduced late in 1962 by the JCAH. Beginning January 1, 1964, a $60 charge plus $1 per bed (exclusive of bassinets) up to 250 beds would be assessed. This meant that the smallest eligible hospital of 25 beds would pay $60 plus $25, or a total cost of $85. A hospital of 250 beds or more would pay $60 plus $250, or a total of $310. The member organizations were to continue absorbing the administrative costs, but this new method of financing the activities of the Commission would save the College nearly $30,000, reducing its share to no more than $9,000 for each of its three seats on the Commission annually. The total budget requirements from the College for administration costs of both programs, therefore, was not to exceed $30,000.

The new division for the accreditation of inpatient care institutions other than acute care hospitals was to consist of a 15-member Board with representatives from inpatient care institutions, interested national health organizations, and one representative from each member organization of the JCAH. Two-thirds of the administrative costs were to be paid by the JCAH with one-third prorated among the other members of the division's board. The direct costs of the field survey were to be apportioned among the institutions surveyed.

At the November, 1962 meeting the Regents voted to approve the establishment of the new division of the JCAH subject to the concurrence of all four member organizations.

Meanwhile, the Board of Trustees of the AMA had voted at a meeting also held in November, that "negotiations be opened with the American Nursing Home Association [ANHA] with the idea of activating a National Council for the Accreditation of Nursing Homes." The AMA also instructed its JCAH representatives to oppose the accreditation of nursing homes by the Commission.

This action sparked the appointment of a JCAH ad hoc committee, which was instructed to obtain additional information concerning inpatient-care institutions other than acute care hospitals and to present further recommendations for policy and action to be taken by the JCAH. The Committee, consisting of one representative from each of the four member organizations, subsequently met in January of 1963 and urged the Board of Trustees of the AMA to reconsider its previous action. The Trustees respectfully declined, stating that they had no lack of confidence in the JCAH, but felt that nursing homes were different from hospitals and that accreditation was the responsibility of the American Nursing Home Association.

This activity on the part of the AMA and the ANHA in activating a National Council for the Accreditation of Nursing Homes, was accepted by the JCAH; the results to be reviewed with an open mind.

## College Mace

A committee of one, Dr. Irving S. Wright, was appointed in 1962 to study the question of procuring a suitable mace for use at the College Convocations. The Marshal was to carry it as he led the procession, establishing tradition and adding dignity to the ceremony.

The Garrard and Company, Ltd., of England was engaged as silversmith, and sketches were prepared and shown to the Board of Regents. After the selection of the design the next question became one of whether the shaft should be wood or silver. It was then that the idea of obtaining a piece of timber from the famous

Plane Tree on the Island of Cos was suggested by Dr. Wright, who attributed the idea to his wife, Lois.

"In cloakroom conversation after the Regents Meeting, I suggested to Irving Wright, somewhat in jest, that I might be able to obtain such a piece of wood," explained Dr. Theodore J. Abernethy, Regent from Washington, DC, in an article that appeared in the July-August 1963 issue of the *ACP Bulletin.*

Though he was a personal friend of the US Ambassador to Greece, Henry R. Labouisse, Dr. Abernethy did not fully anticipate the diplomatic protocol involved in accomplishing the quest. Preliminary negotiations revealed that the Plane Tree on the Isle of Cos was regarded as a Greek national treasure and that wood from it was almost impossible to obtain. The process involved not only some behind the scenes negotiations with the Ambassador and the Agricultural Attache, but also letters exchanged among the US Ambassador to Greece, a member of the Greek Parliament for the Dodecanese Islands, the Mayor of Cos, the Greek Phytosanitary Service, the US Department of Agriculture, the US Information Agency, and the Voice of America! As the Ambassador wrote Dr. Abernethy, "In connection with your request for a piece of wood from the Island of Cos to be fashioned into a ceremonial mace, the Parliamentary Deputy from the Dodecanese Islands has promised to try to get a branch from an old plane tree near the site where Hippocrates practiced. As soon as we have it, we will send it to you."

After some temporary delays, attributed to the lack of a phytosanitary certificate, the 5-foot 8-inch log arrived in Washington, DC, on March 20, 1963. A certificate accompanying the wood and signed by the Mayor of Cos, George Kaisserlis, attested to its authenticity.

". . . It didn't appear as weather-beaten as I had anticipated," Dr. Abernethy told the Board of Regents at the Denver Session. "A brownish-green bark had come off in irregular patches producing a colorful mosaic. It was straight, five inches at its greatest diameter and four inches at its smaller end, and weighed 45 pounds."

The matter of how best to handle such a piece of wood, in order to preserve it for years to come, became the next issue. Experts advised that the wood be soaked thoroughly for a time. "The wood is resting peacefully in a tub full of water in my basement", Dr. Abernethy proudly announced to the Regents.

Dr. Wright had considerable reservations about wood having the necessary durability required for the shaft of the mace, but the Board of Regents wanted very much to use this piece of wood and concluded that a shaft of silver could be made to replace it, if the wood deteriorated.

College regulations provided for reduced dues to all members from Mexico and the Latin American Countries. However, a reduced initiation fee of $50 had been extended to residents of Mexico only. In order to correct this inconsistency, the Board of Regents adopted a change in the regulations which authorized reduced initiation fees for all Latin American countries, excluding Puerto Rico.

The College's financial status was firm, but expenses and appropriations exceeded income by $10,000, decreasing the Operating Fund reserve. A new program had been initiated and several activities expanded. The Research

Fellowship Fund was enlarged from $28,000 to $45,000 per year, and the Residency Loan Fund was increased by $25,000. Money was also added to the Building Fund and the Endowment Fund, thus helping to secure future options.

The Finance Committee urged caution, lest the membership underestimate the Government's determination to obtain tax revenues from organizations like the College. Early in the year, the Regents were advised that the tax-exempt status of the ACP could continue, but the question of journal advertising was still being studied.

Although advertising revenues continued their downward trend, from gross billings of $480,000 in 1962 to $448,000 in 1963, *Annals* subscriptions increased, offsetting the deficit. Figures released by the Treasurer showed that approximately 24.3 percent of the total income of $1,178,379 in 1962 was contributed by dues income, whereas advertising and subscriptions accounted for almost 51.6 percent. Endowment investments amounted to 7 percent with another 8.5 percent derived from the exhibits and fees obtained at the Annual Session. The other 1.2 percent came from miscellaneous sources, including some gain from sale of stock.

An analysis of expenditures at that time revealed that of the total expenses of $1,101,861, publications represented 37.3 percent of the expenses, 9.2 for Annual Sessions, 0.8 for Regional Meetings, 2.5 for Fellowships, 5.7 for support of medical programs, 7.6 for postgraduate courses, 18.4 for administration, 2.6 for building operations; 9.1 percent represented appropriation to the endowment fund and 5.8 percent represented an appropriation to the building fund.

An analysis of the 1962 Annual Session expenses reported total expenses of $101,378.00, of which 62.2 percent of expenses were administrative, including salaries, printing, travel of Regents, Governors and Staff; 21.5 percent for the scientific program, including travel of program participants, rental of equipment, etc.; 3.8 percent was assigned to Convocation expenses and 7.9 percent was expended for social and entertainment features; 4.6 percent was spent for publicity and the invitation session for executives.

## Annual Session 1963

Coincidental with the 1963 Annual Session in Denver, I announced the formation of the new Headquarters Department for Convention Management, to be directed by Mr. Elmer Jones, who had previously managed the Circulation Department. At his first Annual Session as Convention Manager in Denver, Mr. Jones suffered the results of relying too trustingly on the hotel manager's assurances that all was in order. Before the Convocation, we had a formal dinner for the awardees and officers and their wives. This was always a very impressive and gracious occasion, but timing was critical, because all of these people had to be punctual for the Convocation immediately following the dinner.

About 15 minutes before dinner, I suggested to Mr. Jones and Mr. Dauterich that we check to see if all arrangements were in order. To our surprise, they were still setting the tables and the bar had not been set up yet. Mr. Jones took immediate action. By the time the first guest arrived we were almost ready. Fortunately, the first guest did not want a cocktail. Mr. Jones, henceforth, made detailed schedules very clear to the hotel people and convention management staff and expected everything ready as scheduled. He developed a written set of directions for all functions, sequentially organized from the first event of the week to the last. This supplanted the usually system of written directions based exclusively on room set ups. Most hotel people we dealt with said Mr. Jones's system was certainly a change for the better, and it relieved me of an enormous amount of detailed planning and checking at Annual Sessions.

Mr. Stephen Donohue, the new part-time public information staff consultant would handle the press room and all publicity for the Annual Session. In addition, he would report on various College activities, such as the Regional Meetings and postgraduate courses, publish articles of interest in the *ACP Bulletin* and *Annals,* and prepare press releases about appropriate activities to circulate to the press.

A new class of membership, Corresponding Fellows, was initiated with the idea of encouraging "friends of the College", physicians of outstanding medical achievement in countries other than the United States, Cuba, Canada, Mexico, or the Central American Republics, who would act in an international liaison capacity with the ACP. The intent was to foster the transmission of significant developments of scientific interest through correspondence and personal contact.

The Board of Regents made revisions in the committee structure of the College that were designed to retain experienced committee members, regardless of whether they were still on either the Board of Regents or Board of Governors, and also to broaden the representation on committees by members-at-large. Through Bylaws changes initiated in 1962, and approved at the 1963 Annual Session, the "hold-over" man on the Nominations Committee was to be a Regent. An additional amendment allowed members of the Executive Committee of the Board of Governors and the Postgraduate Courses Committee, who were on the Board at the time of their reappointment, to serve out their full committee terms.

After reviewing proposed legislation known as the Clark-Neuberger Bill, designed to establish a new federal regulatory agency intended to assure the humane treatment of laboratory animals, the College approved the following statement, at the 1963 Denver Annual Session:

> The American College of Physicians is deeply concerned about legislation introduced in the Congress of the United States for the avowed purpose of assuring humane treatment of laboratory animals. The proposed law would obstruct scientific research by placing undue restrictions upon physicians and other investigators who use animals in conducting their search for new ways to treat and cure diseases of both mankind and the animal kingdom. The great progress in the care of the physically sick and the mentally ill, developed so rapidly in the past several decades, has been the direct result of freedom of research and of freedom to make proper use of animals for research. Anything that would impair this freedom to advance medical science cannot be supported by this organization.

For this reason, the American College of Physicians, as representative of 12,000 physicians dedicated to the highest principles of medical care, strongly oppose any such legislation. It would greatly harm our country's outstanding medical research efforts and, thereby, handicap physicians in the care of the sick and suffering. It would also retard research in the care of animals of all types.

No action was taken; no hearings were scheduled by Congress in regard to this matter in 1963.

At an important meeting in Chicago, on August 5, the Ad Hoc Committee to Study the Relationship of the College to the ASIM, chaired by Dr. John C. Leonard, prepared a careful revision of the 1960 agreements of the respective roles of the ACP and ASIM. On November 15 in Philadelphia, the Committee presented the following recommendations to the Board of Regents:

1. That the American College of Physicians approve the present published goals of the ASIM, with the firm understanding that the ASIM will not enter into the educational and scientific fields on a national level.
2. That the members of the American College of Physicians be encouraged to take an active interest in their state society of internal medicine, and in the ASIM.
3. That the ASIM should not project long range objectives which could be in conflict with those of the American College of Physicians without prior consultation and with the approval of the American College of Physicians.
4. That the ASIM will continue to represent the viewpoint of its members in socioeconomic matters.
5. That the American College of Physicians support the efforts of the ASIM to improve medical care through an understanding of, and attempts toward solution of, the socioeconomic matters relating to internal medicine.
6. That the ASIM not lower its standards for membership.
7. That the American College of Physicians continue to publish pertinent material received from the ASIM in the *ACP Bulletin* at the discretion of the Editorial Board.
8. That the Liaison Committee of the American College of Physicians to the ASIM be increased to five members for geographical reasons. It is expected that whichever member(s) of the Liaison Committee of the American College of Physicians is (are) in attendance at the Board of Trustees meeting of the ASIM, will take an active part in the discussions to further effective cooperation between the two organizations. It is also understood that the member(s) of the Liaison Committee in attendance is (are) the only official representative(s) of the American College of Physicians at that meeting.
9. That it be the intent of these recommendations to modify the action of the April 1960 meeting of the Board of Regents, American College of Physicians.

The actions adopted by the Board of Regents at the April 1960 meeting had read:

The American Society of Internal Medicine is to continue in its field of endeavors the following:

1. Economic and professional prepayment medical insurance;
2. Political activities;
3. Medico-legal considerations;
4. Public relations;
5. Office and practice management;
6. Enhancement of the place of the internist in hospital affairs;
7. Maintenance of standards of practice;
8. Public education of the profile of the internist.

The Ad Hoc Committee recommended that the above be changed to read as follows:

a. That No. 3 read, "Medico-legal considerations are to be performed as a joint effort in cooperation with the American College of Physicians."
b. That No. 4 read, "Public Relations regarding the Internist are to be performed as a joint effort in cooperation with the American College of Physicians."
c. That No. 6, which read, "Enhancement of the place of the internist in hospital affairs," be omitted because, through the activities of the ACP in support of the RRC-IM, JCAH, the Commission on Professional and Hospital Activities, and the ABIM, it would seem that the enhancement of the place of the internist in hospital affairs is a primary function of the American College of Physicians.
d. That No. 7 read, "The maintenance of standards of practice in internal medicine is of major interest to the ASIM and to the American College of Physicians. Each contributes to this in its own area. Joint cooperation in this field may be engaged in, when necessary." The American College of Physicians believes that the ASIM can best work to improve medical care by working toward a solution of the socioeconomic matters relating to internal medicine.
e. No. 8, "Public education of the profile of the internist" is repetitious, but we can see no other objection to its inclusion.

The report was approved by Board of Regents and the Ad Hoc Committee was discharged with thanks.

These approved recommendations were subsequently reviewed by the ASIM Liaison Committee and on March 30, 1963, Dr. Charles Caravati reported to the Board of Regents that the Liaison Committee concurred with the recommendations, with one exception. He proposed that the following statement be reinstated, as amended, in the 1960 list of ASIM activities (originally No. 6):

Enhancement of the place of the internist in hospital affairs on a local level as this enhancement nationally is a primary function of the ACP through its activities in support of the RRC-IM, the JCAH, the Commission on Professional & Hospital Activities [CPHA] and ABIM.

The Board unanimously approved the reinstatement of this item as amended.

A statement of policy submitted by the Cancer Committee was also approved by the Board:

The American College of Physicians is primarily concerned with the maintenance of the highest standards in the practice of medicine and with the promotion of progress in the diagnosis, treatment and prevention of disease in man. The American College of Physicians is not an organization of scientific investigators but it affirms that the mainspring of the advances in medicine during the past fifteen years has been the growth and development of biomedical research. The creation and encouragement of the vast health research program in the United States has been a mandate of the citizens and it has been largely supported by the tax money of the American people. The National Institutes of Health [NIH] has been the instrument to implement the wish of the people for advances in the knowledge about disease and the National Institutes of Health and has done an outstanding service which has won for it confidence from both the lay and scientific communities.

Central to the philosophy of the NIH research program has been a policy of freedom to the investigator in his quest for knowledge. Creative thinking is best nurtured in an atmosphere of free inquiry. Restrictive policies narrow the pathways of investigation and limit the productivity of high quality research. In the opinion of the American College of Physicians, the revised Grants Manual of the NIH has changed the original policy of scientific freedom to one of greater federal control. The College recognizes the importance of careful administration of federal biomedical research grants and believes that this responsibility has been adequately met by the NIH. Efforts to introduce more restrictive regulations in the administration of grants may be detrimental to the purpose and aims of the research program. The American College of Physicians reaffirms its support of the NIH and its program and respectfully urges the Subcommittee on Intergovernmental Relations carefully to consider any recommendations which would interfere with, retard or discourage the rapid progress which is now being made in the preservation of health and the control of disease.

The Board of Regents accepted this report.

Following an executive session, the Board of Regents passed two resolutions. The first was to approve purchase of an annuity for me to supplement whatever College pension I would be entitled to receive. This was to be financed through an annual premium of $5,000. A second resolution expressed the Board's appreciation for my wife's efforts and strong support in behalf of the College in the following statement: "The Board of Regents shall direct the Executive Director to bring his wife, at College expense, to any meeting he deems wise and in the best interests of the College."

## Part Five (1963-1964)

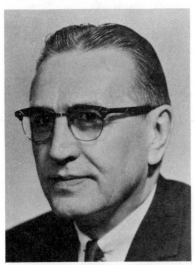

*Wesley W. Spink, MACP*

Wesley W. Spink was born in Duluth, Minnesota, December 17, 1904. He married Elizabeth H. Hurd in August, 1935. Two children, Helen and William were born in 1940 and 1946, respectively.

A graduate of Carleton College, Northfield, Minnesota, he received his MD in 1932 from Harvard Medical School. He was the Proctor Research Scholar, Department of Comparative Pathology, Harvard Medical School 1932-33, and served an internship in medicine at the Boston City Hospital (Harvard Services), and a three year residency at the Thorndike Memorial Laboratory of the Boston City Hospital, January 1933 to 1937. He was certified by the American Board of Internal Medicine in 1941 and by the American Board of Microbiology in 1961.

Following studies and research in Boston, he joined the faculty of the University of Minnesota Medical School in August, 1937. Thereafter, he advanced through Associate Professorship and was appointed Professor of Medicine at the University of Minnesota on July 1, 1947. He continued as full professor of medicine, and was named the Regents' Professor of Medicine, University of Minnesota in 1967, and Professor of Comparative Medicine in June, 1970. He was made Emeritus Regents' Professor of Medicine and Comparative Medicine in 1973.

Carleton College awarded him an honorary Doctor of Science degree in 1950. He received an award from *Modern Medicine;* other honors were: the Freeland Barbour Award and Lecture ("The Dilemma of Bacterial Shock") at the Royal College of Physicians of Edinburgh, 1964; the Chapin Medal for distinguished achievement in epidemiology by the City of Providence, Rhode Island, 1964; Award and Citation for Distinguished Achievements in Medicine at the Boston City Hospital Centennial, June 4, 1964; Alumni Achievement Award, Carleton College, 1968. In 1971, the "Wesley W. Spink Lectures on Comparative Medicine" were established, to be presented biennially at the University of Minnesota and at Carleton College, and published by the University of Minnesota Press. He received the National Library of Medicine Distinguished Scholar Award in 1973.

Membership in honorary societies included: Phi Beta Kappa, (Carleton College); Sigma Xi and Alpha Omega Alpha (Harvard). Honorary Memberships included the New York Academy of Sciences, 1955; Medical Society of Santiago, Chile; Royal Australasian College of Physicians; and American Veterinary Medical Association. Dr. Spink was a charter member of the American Board of Microbiology, founded in 1961. He was a member of the American Medical Association; American Association for the Advancement of Science; Association of American Physicians; American Association for the History of Medicine; American Society for Clinical Investigation, of which he was President in 1949; American Clinical and Climatological Association; American Association of Immunologists; the American Association of University Professors; and the Society for Experimental Biology in Medicine, of which he was President in 1950.

Always active in the American College of Physicians following his election to Fellowship in 1942, he was a Governor (1950-1959), a Regent (1960-1966), President (1963-64), and was made a Master in 1968.

He was consultant to the Secretary of War on Epidemic Diseases, 1942-1945; Member of the Commission on Streptococcal Diseases, 1942-1945; Member of the Agricultural Board, National Research Council; Chairman, Committee on Brucellosis, National Research Council; President, Inter-American Congress on Brucellosis in 1950; Member of the Panel of Expert Consultants on Brucellosis of the World Health Organization, and its Chairman in October 1957.

He was on the Board of Editors of the *Journal of Clinical Investigation, The Journal of Laboratory and Clinical Medicine,* and *Antibiotics and Chemotherapy.* He was also National Consultant in Internal Medicine to the Surgeon General, US Air Force (1959-64); a member of the Food and Drug Administration Advisory Committee to the Secretary of Health, Education and Welfare; National Academy of Sciences; Committee on Shock, National Research Council, 1963-1967; Harvard Medical Alumni Council (1963-1969), serving the latter as President in 1967-68; and United States Department of Agriculture National Advisory Commission on Brucellosis Control, 1976.

He was a visiting professor and lecturer at many medical schools which included: Jefferson Medical College; Mayo Memorial Lecturer at the University of Iowa School of Medicine; and Fourteenth Leo Loeb Lecturer, Washington University School of Medicine, St. Louis. He gave Alpha Omega Alpha Lectures at Emory University School of Medicine, Ohio State University College of Medicine; University of Chicago; University of Nebraska; University of Texas Southwestern Medical School. Other lectureships included General Lecture, St. George's Hospital and Medical School, London; University Lecture in Pathology, London University School of Medicine; The Gehrman Lectures (2), University of Illinois College of Medicine, Chicago, November 30 and December 1, 1949; James M. Anders Lecture, College of Physicians of Philadelphia, April 1, 1953; James Waring Lecture, University of Colorado School of Medicine, April 11, 1950; first Ellard M. Yow Memorial Lecture, Houston, Texas, March 24, 1966; Jenner Lecture on Intracellular Parasitism in Brucellosis, St. George's Hospital and Medical School, London, England, February 24, 1964.

In retirement Dr. Spink has continued his scholarly activities, and in 1979 authored a book: *Infectious Diseases: Prevention and Treatment in the Nineteenth and Twentieth Centuries.* It is described by one reviewer as a monumental storehouse of names, events and dates. It is divided into three sections: "Background of the Control and Treatment of Infectious Diseases", "The Development of Prophylaxis and Therapy in the Twentieth Century", and "Evaluation of Knowledge of Specific Infectious Diseases". It contains a very extensive bibliography and is a valuable source book for students and researchers.

I had known Dr. Spink at Carleton College and also at the Harvard Medical School. We were good friends and worked well together. He was a forceful, thoughtful person. He had much inner drive and strong feelings about many of his ideas.

He enjoyed Regional Meetings and could always find some special topic of interest. He also enjoyed having local Governors arrange a visit to the area medical school where he made rounds with students and residents. His enthusiasm for dealing with young physicians was contagious. He was especially pleased in later years when his appointment as visiting professor and lecturer at Jefferson Medical College honored the retirement one of his students, Dr. Robert I. Wise.

Dr. Spink and I went to the Royal Canadian College of Physicians and Surgeons meeting in Quebec. I suggested that the College mail his academic robe, to be packed with his baggage. He preferred that we ship it directly to Quebec. When I tried to pick it up I was told that it was being held in customs, and only Dr. Spink could claim it. It took him about two hours to do this and he was temporarily not very happy.

At the formal dinner during this meeting, the Premier of Quebec addressed the assembly in French. The talk was broadcasted on trans-Canada television. After he finished, Dr. Spink was called on to make remarks. He started, "Bon soir, monsieur et mesdames . . . , and now I will continue my remarks in English". This provoked laughter, and the rest of his talk was well received.

Dr. Spink was the College representative at the first Regional Meeting in New York City in January during a heavy snowstorm. Despite the snow and predictions by some that it was impractical to have yet another winter meeting in New York, there were over 400 in attendance. Drs. Victor Grover and Jeremiah Barondess, Governors for Downstate I & II, were congratulated by all. (Dr. Barondess later became President of ACP.) The Spinks had left Minneapolis the day before the meeting, circled stormy New York for awhile and landed in Chicago. The next morning they tried again and succeeded in landing in New York.

I remember also that Dr. Spink was greatly amused and pleased during one Regional Meeting in Philadelphia, held at the University Museum. Cocktails were served in the rotunda, among beautiful ancient Chinese art objects. The dinner was in the Egyptian Room where the tables were set among the sarcophagi and mummy cases. Dr. Spink commented after dinner, "We must be in the first half of Eden."

Dr. Spink is a true bibliophile. He once came to Philadelphia to speak at the College of Physicians of Philadelphia. After the talk he promptly went to Leary's Bookstore and spent his $100 honorarium on a rare Triton Edition of the works of George Santayana, the Harvard philosopher. He named Cushing's biography of Osler as the book which influenced him more than any other.

He told me of an interesting encounter he had with Paul de Kriuf, author of *Microbe Hunters*. Mr. de Kruif interviewed him on the use of Aureomycin, since

Dr. Spink and his coworkers had been among the first to use this antibiotic. The article appeared in *Readers' Digest.*

Several amusing things happened at the 1964 Annual Session. At the first meeting of the Board of Regents, Dr. Spink asked my new secretary, (of five or six weeks) "Who is the current President of the College?" She looked at the agenda and replied, "Dr. Hanger?" Wesley said, "That was last year and *I* am the President this year." She had copied the name from the previous year's agenda. However, she and Dr. Spink subsequently were on the friendliest of terms.

At the pre-convocation dinner, Lady Dodd, wife of Sir Charles, the president of the Royal College of Physicians on London, sat next to me and asked me how long my term would be. When I replied that I hoped I would endure until retirement, she exclaimed, "How perfectly ghastly!" She thought her husband, Sir Charles, who was serving a three-year term, was serving far too long.

I had arranged for a bus to take us from the hotel, after dinner, to Convention Hall for the convocation. To my chagrin, there was no bus, so we had to take taxis. Later I found that the hotel had indeed provided a bus, but no one told the driver it was for a special group. The new Fellows who were to be inducted at the Convocation had taken the bus. When it was loaded, the bus driver simply left for Convention Hall. Thereafter, the Staff always named the Atlantic City meeting as the one at which "Rosenow missed the bus".

It was at this session that the first meeting of the Regency Club was held. It was limited to officers and former Regents. It was rather a sad affair, because the few retired Regents who attended obviously felt that they did not have enough current information to take part in discussions. Those present urged that it be enlarged to include all former and present Regents. Since that time, the Regency Club Luncheon has included them all and has been a very pleasant and enthusiastically supported affair at the Annual Session.

Early in Dr. Spink's tenure as president, he told the Board of Regents he had some reservations about the way in which the ACP and the American Society of Internal Medicine [ASIM] were attempting to work together. He felt quite strongly that the ACP should be an independent organization with its own policies, doing what it felt like doing. He felt strongly that decisions by ASIM leaders should not affect the activities and policies of the College. This attitude was not well received by the ASIM leaders and was not universally accepted by the College Regents and Governors. His analysis of the problem of divergences seemed to be accurate, but despite this his suggested remedy of dissociation failed to convince those who favored a more cooperative liaison relationship.

Dr. Spink held a common perspective with many academicians in 1956, when the College decided that it did not want to be active in socioeconomic affairs. That decision opened the way for ASIM to fill the void. By 1963-64, the Society had become a strong and independent body. This created considerable confusion among the ACP members about the activities of both societies, because about half of the members of the Society were also members of the College. The time was not right for Dr. Spink's advocacy of mutually independent roles.

The year 1963-64, in some ways, can be considered a turning point in the policies of the College. From 1956 until Dr. Spink's term, there had been considerable discussion and widely varying reactions about what the relationship of ACP should be to ASIM. The Regents, although opposed to taking on socioeconomic matters as policy, nonetheless were not wholeheartedly in agreement that another society should assume that role. A good deal of committee and Board of Regents meeting time was spent trying to define what the role of the ASIM should be, instead of what the role of the College should be. Dr. Spink was the catalyst who brought this into focus. He felt strongly that the College should pursue an independent course and cooperate with ASIM on a case-by-case basis. He saw danger in two such differently organized societies trying to work out mutual policies. Subsequently, the Board of Regents decided to establish a Committee on Medical Services. This was certainly a departure from the original policy which prevailed at the time the American Society of Internal Medicine was formed in 1956. This move was designed to stimulate more active liaison efforts. The year, 1963-64, certainly could be called a decisive one.

# 1963-1964

Regency Club. Affiliate Members. International Medical Activities Committee. Educational Activities Committee. 25th Jubilee, Royal Australasian College of Physicians.

In the President's report to the Board in November, 1963, Dr. Wesley W. Spink recounted events of the 25th Jubilee Meeting of the Royal Australasian College of Physicians [RACP] held in Sydney, Australia in June, 1963. The Royal College of Physicians of London [RCP(L)] was represented by Sir Charles Dodds. In a morning convocation the president of the RACP received scrolls or gifts from representatives of other societies in various parts of the world in honor of the occasion. Unaccustomed to Jubilees, it had not occurred to us at ACP to prepare a gift. Dr. Spink was embarrassed, but thinking rapidly, he said that he would announce the College's gift that evening. At the dinner meeting he stated that the American College of Physicians was presenting to the RACP a very unusual gift: a gavel made from the branch of a tree under which Hippocrates had talked to medical students on the Island of Cos in Greece. The gavel had been carved from wood left from the branch used in fashioning a new Mace for the ACP. This was well received by everyone.

Continuing his report, Dr. Spink emphasized that the number one problem facing the College in that year concerned the relationship with the American Society of Internal Medicine [ASIM]. He announced this would constitute an important portion of the agenda.

Dr. Thomas M. Durant, President-Elect, indicated that the 1965 meeting in Chicago would be an important ceremonial event; the College would be celebrating its 50th anniversary.

The new Treasurer, Dr. William Sodeman, presented an optimistic view of the financial condition of the College: an estimated surplus of approximately

$292,000 by the end of 1963. In addition, the market value of operating fund investments over book value amounted to approximately $280,000. He reminded the Board that the Finance Committee intended to maintain the operating fund investment reserve at a level of income necessary to operate the College for one year. The Endowment Fund increased from $1,770,000 to $1,939,000 for the year ending September 30, 1963. On the negative side, he reported the possibility that the Internal Revenue Service might begin charging the College taxes on "unrelated business income" if they were able to interpret advertising in the *Annals Of Internal Medicine* as applicable.

In my Executive Director's report, I reminded the Board of Regents that they must act to establish two new Regents for the newly designated Northern and Southern Regions of Texas.

I informed the Regents of College activities in the Philadelphia community. The Philadelphia County Medical Society was undergoing a building program and the College had acted as host to their Building Committee to inspect the new wing of the College Headquarters.

In the Spring of 1963, the College had participated in a series of open house historic tours in the West Philadelphia area. The Headquarters building was one of a dozen or so of the houses on the tour. I also announced that I had offered the American Board of Internal Medicine [ABIM] temporary quarters if they moved to Philadelphia.

The College continued to support its membership in the West Philadephia Corporation, which was made up of universities and other institutions in this area, including the University of Pennsylvania, Drexel University, the Philadelphia Divinity School and the College of Pharmacy and Science. At Christmas time in 1962 a group of medical students used the reception and dining rooms of the College. This also seemed to be a good public relations effort.

The installation of floodlights to illuminate the facade of the building had been much appreciated by the neighbors, who thought it added to their safety when returning to their homes from the bus stop at the College corner.

My outside activities included participation in a discussion at a conference in Chicago sponsored by the Commission on Drug Safety.

At the AMA's meeting which I attended, progress was made toward improving the scientific programs and sections of the AMA, and I believed more improvement could be expected as the specialty societies became more involved.

My speaking engagements included addressing the North Dakota State Medical Association where I also conducted a panel on coronary artery disease; I also gave the convocation address at the 1964 Annual Session of the American College of Gastroenterology.

I continued some teaching service with medical students and residents at the Philadelphia General Hospital on the University of Pennsylvania service directed by Dr. Truman Schnabel, Jr.

After a report by the Executive Committee, the matter of the program for Cuban physicians at Miami was discussed extensively. While acknowledging that helping these displaced physicians had been very useful during a critical time, the Board of Regents decided it should gradually diminish the amount of stipend, and after 1964 provide no further support to the program.

At the Executive Committee's suggestion, the Board approved the sale of College hoods, which was previously not permitted. For a number of years, many Fellows of the College had been asking if they could purchase the hoods.

Dr. Irving Wright suggested that an informal club to be called "The Regency Club" be established; to provide perhaps a luncheon meeting during the Annual Session of the College. The Executive Committee proposed that it would be preferable to invite ex-Regents to "Sunday Night Family Dinner." It had no objection to the luncheon, but noted that including current Regents would represent an additional obligation for them. The Board, however, enthusiastically endorsed the formation of a "Regency Club". The first meeting was to include only ex-Regents and Officers. After the meeting in 1964, it was decided that all Regents should be invited because the older retired Regents particularly enjoyed meeting friends who were on the current Board.

## Interim Sessions

The first Annual Interim Meeting of the College was held in Detroit, November 21-23, 1963. Over 1,000 physicians, of whom approximately 667 were Fellows and Associates, attended the Clinical and Basic Medical Science/Clinical Investigation Sessions that ran concurrently for the two and one half days of the meeting. Panel discussions and symposia on general topics were scheduled daily with no formal ACP social functions planned. The Michigan Society of Internal Medicine, however, sponsored a banquet to which all registrants were invited. The next Fall meeting was scheduled for Los Angeles, October 8-10, 1964.

The tragic news reached the participants during the afternoon session on Friday, November 22 that President John F. Kennedy had been assassinated in Dallas. Dr. Spink sent a telegram to the White House expressing the shock and sadness of all members of the College.

In his report for the Executive Committee, which met in October, 1963, Dr. Spink reviewed in some detail ACP/ASIM relationships. He gave several examples of some problems in relationships at the local level.

1. The Liaison Committee, he thought, had not been given adequate opportunity to study at first hand how the two societies operated at the regional or local level.
2. In the area of economics, he asserted the College was engaged in some selected activities: the College endorsed the group insurance program for members; worked with other national organizations; co-sponsored the Joint Commission on Accreditation of Hospitals [JCAH], etc.
3. He thought the ACP should be the voice for internal medicine. The ASIM disagreed, and openly stated that ASIM was the spokesman for internal medicine and repeatedly emphasized that "the ASIM is the only organization which contains only internists".

He remarked that at times he had received no response to messages sent to ASIM. Discussion continued in the Executive Committee about the possibility of merging the two organizations. However, this would have to involve some method of offering the 40 percent non-ACP members of ASIM some form of membership in the College. The Executive Committee agreed that there should be no lowering of standards for ACP Membership to effect such an accomodation.

Other problems of interaction were emerging. I pointed out that at Staff level, communications tended to be one-way. The amount of news space provided ASIM in the *ACP Bulletin* caused some difficulty, and this matter was further discussed by the Public Relations Committee.

The Executive Committee suggested that communications might be improved in two ways: 1) the ASIM Liaison Committee should be enlarged if necessary and should be empowered to take a much more active part in regional and state meetings; 2) there should be improved communications between the Board of Regents, the Executive Staff and the ASIM Liaison Committee to the Governors about all matters pertaining to ASIM, at the national level. Governors should be urged to take complete charge of their own Regional Meetings and the ASIM should not meet during the entire length of the ACP portion of the Regional Meeting.

Since the meeting of the Executive Committee, Dr. Spink reported that he had seen a brochure recently printed by ASIM entitled "Aims and Purposes of ASIM". This had been sent to all College members. The implication in this brochure was that the ACP was not interested in the practicing internist and his problems, but only in scientific techniques and advances.

The relationship between ACP and ASIM had been reviewed by Dr. Franklin Hanger at the 1963 Denver Annual Session. The statement defining their respective roles which was approved by the Board of Regents in April, 1960, and amended in November, 1962, was further revised. In 1963, one part of the 1962 revision of the 1960 statement was deleted. In November, 1963, the Board approved the reinstatement of the following paragraph regarding the role of the ACP in the maintenance of standards in hospitals:

> . . . enhancement of the place of the internist in hospital affairs on a local level, as this enhancement, nationally, is a primary function of the ACP through its activities in support of the Residency Review Committee in Internal Medicine, the Joint Commission on Accreditation of Hospitals, the Commission on Professional and Hospital Activities and the American Board of Internal Medicine.

The relationship with ASIM was reviewed again and as a result, the Board unanimously adopted at this November meeting a recommendation to establish a standing Committee on Medical Services which was to replace the ASIM Liaison Committee. This action became clearer in light of the implications presented in the ASIM brochure, which stated:

> The ACP is rooted in academic internal medicine; ASIM is rooted in the practice of internal medicine. The American College of Physicians is the internist's instrument

to develop and improve the scientific and technologic substance of his specialty including the educational aspects of the discipline. The ASIM is his instrument to ensure that the internist himself is, and remains, qualified as an internist in his actual practice and that the circumstances of this practice are such that he is able to render the high quality of professional services for which he has been trained and which patients have the right to expect from him. Each organization has the appropriate structure for its purpose.

Through the College the internist speaks with a prestige which is rooted in the high echelons of academic and scientific medicine. Through ASIM his voice speaks with equal prestige and authority but reflects the experience of internists and the problems of the specialty in actual practice within the matrix of medical care in modern society. ACP is, therefore, authoritative for educational and scientific standards in internal medicine. ASIM is authoritative for socioeconomic matters and for the practical problems of the practice of internal medicine.

The Board of Regents in November, 1962, had outlined a working agreement of mutual interest to both organizations. This was accepted by the ASIM and constituted a basis for cooperative activities. In view of the ASIM brochure, the Regents expressed the opinion that the College should be the voice for internal medicine and that ACP should embark upon an independent program to provide the highest quality medical service possible.

Dr. Charles M. Caravati, Chairman, in his final report for the ASIM Liaison Committee read the preface, as follows, and then submitted some suggestions:

> In view of the happenings of the past few months, it is evident to the Liaison Committee that the current arrangements with the ASIM are unsatisfactory. The recommendation of the Committee is that the Regents reconsider their present policy and become active participants in a medical services program which will include among its principal activities public relations, maintenance of standards of practice, and possible liaison with third parties. The Board is faced primarily with the decision to take definitive and effective steps toward implementing policy with regard to medical services which are agreed to in principle in the November, 1962 meeting.

> If the Board of Regents decides to implement its decision of November, 1962, then it is proposed that a standing committee on medical services of the American College of Physicians be established. Its functions would consist of activities in the four fields of endeavor listed earlier and in any other area of activity that the Board of Regents so decides. These functions of the committee, once established, are not to be subject to any further negotiation with other organizations.

After prolonged discussion at the Board of Regents meeting, Dr. Caravati made the following motion:

> We move the establishment of a standing Committee on Medical Services.

> The major functions of this Committee will include in its scope expansion of our activities in the following areas:

> 1. Consideration of medico-legal problems.
> 2. Matters of public relations as they pertain to internal medicine.
> 3. The enhancement of the place of internists in hospital affairs.
> 4. Maintenance of standards in internal medicine.

In addition, this Committee will maintain liaison with other medical and lay organizations'.

When this was adopted, there was general agreement that no further official discussion should take place about this until Dr. Spink could present the entire matter to the Board of Governors and Board of Regents in April, 1964.

During the meeting of the Board of Governors in April, 1964, the Board received from its Executive Committee an expression of Governors' reactions about the manner of elections to Fellowship. There had been considerable misunderstanding, apparently, between the Credentials Committee and some of the Governors about how the College elected people to direct Fellowship. Eminent physicians, who would have been qualified under the old rules, sometimes failed in direct election to Fellowship because the Governor did not properly document the accomplishments of such a candidate. If any Governor thought the Credentials Committee should exercise its discretionary power, a letter from him should state this fact clearly and indicate his reasons. Frequently letters from Governors were too fragmentary.

ASIM also appeared on the agenda at this meeting of the Board of Governors. I made a few remarks about my own experiences and reactions to the ASIM:

1. Relations between the local ACP members and the members of state societies of internal medicine were usually satisfactory. This, however, did not extend to the national level, partly because each state (component) society of internal medicine was organized differently.
2. Most of the problems mentioned by Dr. Spink were symptoms of organizational differences between the two bodies with their separately organized Boards and Executive Offices.
3. Communication had been, more often than not, from the College to ASIM. We were seldom consulted about literature which referred to the College until after it was printed and distributed.
4. One example of the communications problem was that the Officers and executive office of ASIM had been given all the information sent to Governors and Regents in the Fall of 1963. In spite of being told, however, that the College would do nothing further until the April 4th meeting, much of this material was disclosed to ASIM members before it would appear through regular publication in the *ACP Bulletin.*
5. The stated result of a questionnaire which ASIM had sent out following the Board of Regents November 1963 meeting was to prove that from then on the ASIM would have to be considered an equal organization and not as a subsidiary of the ACP.
6. One great difficulty encountered by the ACP Liaison Committee had been the emphasis on solving ASIM's problems rather than articulating the ACP's position.

In conclusion, I stated 1) that ASIM state societies were effective and were in a position to do many good things; and 2) that it was paramount that the College should solve its own problems and establish a College position, rather than trying to solve all of ASIM's problems. If this could be done, other things might fall into place.

## Annual Session 1964

Rainy and unseasonably cold weather greeted those physicians attending the 45th Annual Session of the College held in Atlantic City in 1964. As a result, the turnout for the meeting was smaller than in Chicago for the 1958 Annual Session.

In Dr. Spink's report to the Board of Regents in April, 1964, he elaborated further on relations with ASIM. He announced that because of the amount of space allotted to ASIM in the *ACP Bulletin,* whose cost was borne by members of the College, the Board of Regents had decided in November 1963 to restrict the space allotted to ASIM and eventually to discontinue it.

The Liaison Committee had not been able to solve ASIM related problems, and for that reason, among others, the Board of Regents had set up a Committee on Medical Services. This action involved a series of important implications which Dr. Spink outlined as follows:

1. That ASIM had done a good job at the local level and this activity should be endorsed and continued.
2. The ACP is a strong central organization.
3. The College should represent internal medicine to other groups and to the public.
4. The ACP had made the right decision in 1956 not to go into socioeconomic matters, and this probably could have continued if better communication with ASIM had been possible.

In Dr. Spink's opinion, there is a characteristic difficulty whenever a strongly organized, long established national society tries to work with an emerging young national society which is reaching out for recognition. He did think that with action taken by the Board of Governors and with hard work by the new Committee on Medical Services things might work out satisfactorily. Dr. Thomas Durant, who would be President in April, 1964, described his plans for the Golden Anniversary Session in Chicago in April, 1965.

In the report of the Treasurer, Dr. William A. Sodeman gave some interesting comparative figures in membership statistics and financial statements. In 1926 there were 1,000 members; in 1951 there were 7,000; in 1963 there were 11,500. Total income in 1951 was $338,000; in 1963 it was $1,254,000. Total expenses were $222,000 in 1951; $1,550,000 in 1963. The circulation of the *Annals* in 1926 was 1,200; in 1951, 14,750; in 1963, 26,089. The Endowment Fund increased from 356,000 in 1951 to 1,888,000 in 1963.

In the Executive Director's Report, I gave some figures for Regional Meetings in the 1963-64 year. There had been 26 meetings, attended by 2,148 members, 1,595 non-members, and 151 visitors, for a total of 3,894. I emphasized that Downstate New York I and II had conducted their Regional Meeting for the first time. Having presumed that there were so many medical meetings in New York that few would attend a Regional Meeting in bad weather, they were pleasantly surprised by an attendance of 401 physicians.

The Northern and Southern California Regions met with the Nevada members in Las Vegas with 453 in attendance. There was a sharp difference in opinion about the propriety of the locale for a scientific meeting, but there was no question about the excellent attendance and the quality of scientific sessions.

I also announced that I had been named to the AMA's Committee on Continuing Medical Education. I had also been appointed President-Elect of the American Medical Writers Association and was the current President of the Mayo Alumni Association.

Dr. Irving S. Wright stated that the Committee on Public Information was encouraged by the high quality of performance by the Public Information Department with the help of Mr. Stephen T. Donohue, who was the Staff person responsible for the program. The Committee considered public information aspects of the Golden Anniversary Session. They were working with Merck, Sharp and Dohme to produce a film depicting the internist in practice which would be shown at the Golden Anniversary Session.

For the Committee on Educational Activities, Dr. Carleton Ernstene reported that in 1963-64, 19 postgraduate courses had been offered. Fourteen of these had already been held with five more scheduled before the end of June. The total number of registrants to date was 15,069.

The Board of Regents learned from the House Committee's report in November, 1963, that, after only two years, the need for additional private office space for the College Headquarters was apparent. An appropriation to the budget was approved, and $1,500 authorized to construct two offices at the north end of the first floor. The new facilities were serving the requirements of the administrative Staff, although there had been some minor problems with the heating and air conditioning systems.

An ad hoc committee for liaison between the ACP and the American Psychiatric Association had met in March, 1964. Dr. R. H. Kampmeier reported that both societies desired increased cooperation and submitted the following statement for approval:

> Having determined that there is need for closer association of the internist and psychiatrist in practice and the need for better understanding each other's problems and methods of diagnosis and treatment, the ad hoc committee recommends to the ACP and to the American Psychiatric Association the following:
>
> a. That a Task Force be appointed for a term of three years duration, goal limited, to implement the goals with three representatives of each organization.
> b. That Edward C. Rosenow, Jr. be recommended as Staff for the Task Force of the American College of Physicians and, Dr. William F. Sheeley be recommended as Staff for the Task Force of the American Psychiatric Association.
> c. That a National Institute of Mental Health [NIMH], grant application be recommended for submission by August, 1964 for implementing activities of this Task Force.

## Affiliate Members

Constitution and Bylaws changes ratified at the Atlantic City Annual Business Meeting created a special category of membership known as "Affiliate Membership." It was limited to members of the medical profession residing in Latin America and the Caribbean Basin area, whose qualifications had been approved by the International Medical Activities Committee. Affiliate Members were to be selected on the basis of their personal character, professional achievement, two years of training in the United States and demonstration of continued interest in scientific medicine. They would be endorsed by the program director in the United States who had been responsible for their training and the physician with whom they were working currently in their native country.

The candidates would be proposed for membership by the International Medical Activities Committee and subject to election by the Board of Regents. No dues were to be required of this group nor fees for attending College sessions. In addition, they were to receive the *ACP Bulletin* gratis and the *Annals* at the reduced rate.

The first 72 candidates proposed by the International Medical Activities Committee were the Kellogg Fellows, who were elected at the November Board of Regents meeting.

With the creation of this new category of membership, the Regents determined that a need existed to coordinate all international activities concerning both medical education and membership under the auspices of a single committee. The Bylaws were amended accordingly and approved at the Atlantic City Session, to change the name of the Committee on Latin American Fellows to the International Medical Activities Committee.

Another Bylaws provision changed the name of the Committee on Educational Program to the Educational Activities Committee. The new function of this Committee was to study and consider all educational programs of the ACP in their broadest aspects including the Annual Session, postgraduate courses, Regional Meetings, fellowships, *Annals,* and to recommend policy to the Board that would most effectively utilize the educational resources of the organization.

Coupled with these Constitution and Bylaws changes, plans were approved by the Board of Regents to develop postgraduate courses in South America. At the Interium Meeting in Detroit Dr. Phillip Lee, a Fellow of ACP, met with Dr. Pollard and me and suggested the College develop some educational programs for physicians in foreign countries. He was the administrative head of the government Aid for International Development. We thanked him for the offer but thought the College could do this without government support and we recommended this course of action to the Regents.

Three courses were scheduled; the first in Medellin, Columbia, in January, 1965; the second in Santiago, Chile in November of the same year and the third in Rio de Janeiro in January, 1966. The programs were to be conducted by professors in the medical schools of South America and patterned after ACP postgraduate courses given in the United States on general internal medicine subjects. The

"North American" (ACP) input was to be in the form of one professor per day to participate as guest lecturers.

Funds from the ACP, Kellogg Foundation, and Lilly Laboratories were to pay for simultaneous translation, projection equipment, and the expenses of the US speakers. Publication of any material and social activity would be financed from local resources. It was hoped that this activity would stimulate interest in holding other courses in South America and would strengthen the professional relationship between Latin American physicians and the College.

Congressional mail in 1964 reflected a decline in the activity of antivivisection groups. Bills before Congress were supported by only 11 Congressmen, compared with twice that many the previous year. This did not, however, deter activity already begun in the scientific community.

The AMA announced that a document concerning animal research was being prepared for presentation to public groups which included the principle of accreditation of animal care facilities. The National Society for Medical Research [NSMR], on the other hand, adopted the principle that instead of, or in addition to, combatting undesirable legislation proposed by the antivivisection group, the NSMR would adopt a more positive program and take the initiative in proposing legislation which would conform to its own goals and principles.

The College, being a constituent organization of NSMR, received a draft of a bill prepared by a committee of the Society's Board of Directors. This bill was adopted by the NSMR, although it was recognized that certain technical changes might be necessary before its introduction into Congress.

The Animal Facilities Accreditation Board [AFAB] of the Animal Care Panel of NSMR embarked on another effort, undertaking an impressive and ambitious program of personal visits to 25 institutions of various kinds which utilized animals for experimental work. The findings of the two-man visiting teams were reported, with the AFAB accrediting the animal facilities in 11 institutions, provisionally accrediting nine, and withholding accreditation pending recommended improvements and revisions in six.

These activities spoke loudly for the ability of those involved in the use of animals for scientific purposes to police their own houses and those of their peers. It constituted an effective answer to individuals and groups who would rather see government do the job. Although the inspections were carried out as a demonstration project and the techniques of evaluating and reporting the quality of facilities visited needed refinement, the AFAB expressed its intention to sustain this activity.

The College, with its large number of members engaged in research, had a duty to protect the interests of its constituents and ensure the establishment of a proper accrediting body. To facilitate this action, a NSMR communication to the Board of Regents stated that new financing would be required. The AFAB and its National Advisory Committee were contemplating a reorganization to make the AFAB more representative of the scientific community at large, placing it in a better position to attract financial as well as moral support. Action by the College was deferred until the Spring Meeting of the Board of Regents.

### Teaching and Research Scholars

The Fellowships and Scholarships Committee was asked by the Board of Regents in November, 1963, to consider the scope of the Research Fellowship Plan and suggest ways that it might be broadened or changed. Dr. Ray F. Farquharson, Chairman of the Committee, recommended to the Regents in Atlantic City in 1964 that a new Teaching and Research Scholarship Program be substituted for the existing ACP plan as follows:

1. The candidate be proposed and the application made on his behalf by the Chairman of the Department of Medicine and endorsed by the appropriate official of the university or college concerned.
2. Appointment of the scholar be for an initial term of three years; and that the scholarship may be awarded for an additional term of two years subject to request by the Department of Medicine and endorsement by the appropriate official of the university, and subject to the review of the scholar's accomplishments by the Committee early in the third year of the award. Should the scholar be appointed for a further two-year period his stipend would be $10,500 for each of those two years.
3. The university or college might supplement the stipend of the scholar, provided that such supplement did not entail any duties or activities not directly related to the purposes of the scholarship. It was understood that the ACP would be informed of any financial supplements.
4. The ACP should not accept financial responsibility for any ancillary benefits on behalf of the scholar. The new emphasis would focus on teaching and clinical research.

The Board concurred, and in November, 1964, the first two scholars were appointed for initial terms of three years for graduated yearly stipends of $7,500, $8,500 and $9,500. An extension of an additional two years could be obtained if the Chairman of the Department of Medicine and the appropriate university official petitioned the College. The stipend was then to be increased to $10,500 for the remaining two years.

The university or college would be allowed to supplement the scholar's stipend, provided that no additional duties or activities were imposed that were not directly related to the purpose of the award. (Appendix B)

The newly activated Medical Services Committee [MSC] met four times during the Atlantic City Annual Session to organize, review and interpret the directives of the Board of Regents. Among these directives, which included liaison with other medical organizations, such as the JCAH, the MSC was directed to conduct a continuing study of the implications of scientific advances in medicine to determine what effect new technology had on the quality of medical care and, in turn, on the economics of patient care. The MSC defined the following functions:

1. Provide liaison with ASIM, AMA, specialty groups and similar organizations to ACP members belong.

2. Expand activities by the College in the following areas: public relations and education; medico-legal concerns affecting internal medicine; hospital activities; maintenance of standards in internal medicine.
3. Conduct studies on the implications of scientific advances on quality of care and the effect of these advances on the economics of patient care.

Reporting to the Board of Regents on the Fourth National Congress on Voluntary Health Insurance and Prepayment, conducted by the AMA, the MSC noted how expensive the prolongation of life had become, even when it had lost its meaning. This capability to sustain ''life'' had come through a number of such techniques such as renal dialysis. The MSC indicated that this area deserved the thought and attention of the College and that the ACP should be aware of the social and economic implications of such scientific advances.

The inequality of charges to patients was also explored and the MSC pointed out that the technical aspects of medicine, procedures and laboratory tests, were paid by third parties, regardless of expense, whereas the cost of medical judgment, knowledge, and skill were not reimbursed realistically. The College was urged to study and suggest methods to place this inequity in proper perspective.

The MSC also recommended ACP attention to the quality of medical care in nursing and convalescent homes. The College should render what service it could to already existing agencies in order to foster improvements and better standards.

A subcommittee of the Residency Review Committee for Internal Medicine [RRC-IM] had been studying the one-year residency programs. Programs which conceivably could clearly be categorized as ''unique and highly specialized'' were only six in number. These were located at Roswell Park (Buffalo), Goldwater Memorial (New York), Hospital for Joint Diseases (New York), Highland View (Cleveland), City of Hope (Duarte), and the National Institutes of Health [NIH]. All except the NIH could affiliate with an existing three-year program. The NIH program should qualify without either review or special listing as a unique case of limited-category one-year training.

The ABIM Chairman, Dr. Thomas H. Brem, and Dr. Victor W. Logan, ABIM Librarian, made their report to the combined meeting of the Board of Regents and Board of Governors in April, 1964. They announced some major changes on the Board. Dr. William Werrell, who had been Secretary for the past 25 years, would soon be reaching retirement age, and a Search Committee had been appointed to find a replacement. In addition, it was likely that the headquarters would be moved from Madison, Wisconsin, and relocation in Philadelphia was a good possibility.

He presented some views on the problem of physicians who have difficulty with multiple choice question examinations. In the Board's opinion, it might be hard to devise an alternative examination for those who experience difficulty with this form of examination. The ABIM consulted several experts. In conclusion, they agreed that there were a few people who had real difficulty because of the examination format, but in most instances it seemed apparent that the candidate simply lacked knowledge and his own limitation was more likely culpable than the form of examination. They did not, therefore, plan to give any special examinations.

Slides were being used in the written examination, providing some advantages by offering practical visual material.

The problem of achieving breadth of observation in the oral examination was as always, considered difficult. Even though each examiner, for example, would like to observe a candidate palpate a spleen, it was obvious that there were not sufficient patients with palpable spleens in any given hospital where the examinations were being conducted, at the time of the examination, to observe each candidate in this procedure.

Dr. Logan presented some figures on the pass and fail rate for the different groups. The numbers of candidates examined had increased substantially over the previous four years, rising from 1,760 in 1960 to 1,792 in 1963. Of this group, there were 1,196 first takers in 1960 and 1,218 in 1963. Of the total candidates examined (11,114), 67 percent were certified, and of those who had passed the written examination, 88 percent were eventually certified.

Dr. Wallace Yater, the Secretary General and Chairman of the Membership Committee reported in April, 1964, that there were 32 Masters, 8,757 Fellows, and 4,172 Associates, for a total of 12,961.

In a report of the Publications Committee, Dr. Marshall N. Fulton, Chairman, stated that Dr. Thomas McMillen, *ACP Bulletin* Editor, had asked for retirement because he was moving from the Philadelphia area. It was agreed that the *ACP Bulletin* would continue essentially unchanged but editorial direction would be assigned to the office of the Executive Director. The Board approved my appointment as Editor of the *ACP Bulletin* and Miss Pearl Ott, who had been with the College since 1927 as Mr. Loveland's assistant, as editorial assistant.

In a report of the Military Affairs Committee, Dr. Theodore J. Abernethy, Chairman, made the following recommendations to the Board of Regents, which were approved.

1. That the ACP cooperate with the AMA Committee on Disaster Medical Care to the fullest possible extent by the following actions:

   a. Use of the *Annals* and *ACP Bulletin* for dissemination of appropriate educational materials relative to disaster medical care.
   b. Inclusion of papers and/or exhibits on disaster medical care on the program at the future Annual and Fall Sessions.

2. That the Chairman of the AMA Committee on Disaster Medical Care be informed by letter of the College's willingness to cooperate in this endeavor.

3. Finally, the Military Affairs Committee recommended that the Regents continue that Committee and that its name be changed to the Committee on Military Affairs and Disaster and Medical Care.

The Finance Committee, after discussion, agreed that the College had to begin planning for additional space. The present addition to the original building was inadequate even for the near future.

Immediately after the Atlantic City Session, an offset printing press and auxiliary equipment were acquired; a printing shop was constructed in the basement of the Headquarters Building. It was anticipated that this new facility would help the College economize on publication costs while increasing efficiency, flexibility and quality of material produced.

Another expenditure authorized by the Regents was for alterations to the heating and air conditioning equipment in the Headquarters Building. Efficiency had not been a hallmark of the system.

Encouraging results on the College's federal tax status were reported. The investigating revenue agent had advised the College by telephone that the claim had been approved in Washington and that our tax exempt status would continue.

Dr. Irving S. Wright, Chairman of the Ad Hoc Committee to Procure a Mace for the College, reported that the Committee was consulting with experts on the characteristics of wood for the purposes of artistic carving. He also reported on further communications from the silversmith firm of Garrard & Co. of London. The Committee, after review of alternative designs for the Mace, concluded that the shaft should be made of wood from the Plane Tree with a silver tip approximately six inches long. From this tip, proceeding toward the edge of the Mace, would be a narrow band of silver symbolic of the Serpent of Wisdom. The head of the Mace would be based on the design previously approved by the Board of Regents, which included the Book of Learning, the Lamp of Truth, and a medicinal herb. Garrard & Co. would be requested to submit more detailed designs for the head of the Mace and specific instructions for the size of the piece of wood required for the shaft. When the specifications were obtained, it was apparent that there probably would be enough additional wood to make gavels for presentation to various foreign professional colleges when ACP officials attended as representatives. It was anticipated that the Mace could be finished in time for use at the 50th Anniversary Annual Session of the ACP in Chicago.

Liberty Mutual, the carrier of the Professional Liability Program offered by Group Insurance Administrators [GIA] for the College, indicated disappointment in the number of College members participating in that plan. There were 2,008 members and 305 non-members associated with College insured members participating as of November, 1964. As of that date, there had been 455 notifications of professional liability claims or possible claims, with $276,284.35 paid in settlements. The reserve set aside for anticipated losses amounted to over $800,000.

Because of the disappointing response to this program, the carrier requested and received approval from the Board of Regents to set up a test area in a section of the country where Liberty Mutual agents could contact ACP members personally about the professional liability and optional premise plans. They wished to canvas the membership in one locality in order to better understand what limits, if any, were imposed by the coverage and how they could make it more attractive for College members.

Among young internists and investigators, increasing interest in the problems of cancer was developing. During a joint meeting of the Society of Clinical Investigation and the American Federation of Clinical Research in 1964, a Section on Cancer was established.

The ACP Committee on Cancer, I reported to the Board, believed that physicians were increasingly aware of the need for internists to participate in programs related to malignant disease. The College was an excellent body to promote the education of physicans about cancer and it could also usefully participate by acting as a conduit for important sources of current information about varied activities existing in this developing scientific field. The favorable progress in diagnosis and management of some varieties of cancer was reflected in the number and quality of scientific papers presented at the College's Annual Session and in the increasing participation of College members in cancer-related activities. Sixteen percent of the papers were directly related to cancer. The Committee made the following recommendations:

1. That an Annual Session section on cancer or neoplasm be created similar to sections on gastroenterology, metabolism, hematology, nephrology, etc.
2. That a major lecture or symposium be devoted to an aspect of cancer.
3. That programs at the Annual Session be directed to the public, emphasizing the health hazards of smoking.
4. That Dr. Michael Brennan be appointed as ACP representative to the Committee on Cancer.
5. That the College should provide representatives to the American College of Radiology's Committee on Cancer.

According to the Committee, the College had the reputation among many physicians of not being interested in cancer. Hence, a great number of quality papers were not being submitted for inclusion on the Annual Session program. The Committee on Cancer was established by the Regents for the specific purpose of encouraging participation of internists in activities relating to cancer and it urged the Board to take positive action to promote more College involvement.

The ACP had recently increased its participation in these activities by joining with other societies, specifically, the American College of Surgeons, the College of American Pathologists and the American College of Radiology, to develop interdisciplinary cooperative studies. Together they established the American Joint Committee on Cancer Staging and End-Results Reporting.

Chapter Two

# 50th Anniversary:
# Reflection and Self-Assessment

**1964-1969**

## II. 50th Anniversary:
## Reflection and Self-Assessment

### Part One (1964-1965)

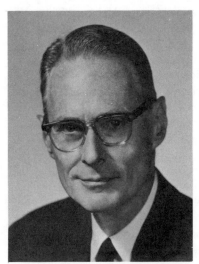

*Thomas M. Durant, MACP*

Thomas M. Durant was born in Evanston, Illinois, November 19, 1905. He attended public schools in Chicago and Washington, DC. His father was a business man. His grandfather started the first bank in Illinois at Shawnee Town, which reputedly turned down a request to lend money to Chicago after the great fire, considering the city a poor risk with a dubious future. One of his ancestors, related to Dr. Benjamin Rush, helped start the first library in Philadelphia. During his youth in Washington, DC, he was a contemporary and friend of Woodrow Wilson, and a member of the National Presbyterian Church, which fostered in Tom a life long interest in Bible studies.

Dr. Durant and his wife, Jean Margaret deVries, had two daughters, Carolyn and Catherine and one son, John, who is Professor of Medicine at the University of Alabama. Dr. Durant died in Philadelphia on June 21, 1977.

At the University of Michigan, he acquired a BS degree and finally an MD degree in 1930. After spending five years in graduate training at Michigan, where he was greatly influenced by the cardiologist, Frank Wilson, he moved to the Desert Sanitarium in Tucson, Arizona, where he became a close friend of John R. Paul, later the Professor of Preventive Medicine at Yale.

In 1936, Charles L. Brown appointed Tom as Assistant Professor of Medicine at Temple University. By 1946, he was a Full Professor and in 1956 he succeeded Richard A. Kern, also a former ACP President, as Chairman of Medicine. When he retired from Temple in 1966, he became the first full-time Chairman of Medicine at Albert Einstein Medical Center, an affiliate of Temple.

He served medicine in many official capacities, including: President of the American Federation for Clinical Research, 1945-46; Editorial Board of the *American Heart Journal,* 1950-1967; Associate Editor *American Journal of Medical Sciences,* 1951-1968; Chairman, *American Board of Internal Medicine,* 1957-1959; President of the College of Physicians of Philadelphia, 1961-1964; President of the American College of Physicians, 1964-65; founder of the Greater Philadelphia Committee for Pharmaceutical Sciences (a unique liaison organization between medical schools and top echelons of the pharmaceutical companies in Philadelphia); and Chairman of the Drug Research Board of the

National Academy of Sciences Research Council, 1968.

His numerous honors included the Strittmatter Award of the Philadelphia County Medical Society; The Shaffney Award of St. Joseph's College, Philadelphia, 1966; Distinguished Alumni Award, University of Michigan, 1970; Mastership in 1956 and Distinguished Teacher Award in 1972 by the American College of Physicians; and Doctor of Science from Franklin & Marshall College, Lancaster, PA in 1964. He was a member of Alpha Omega Alpha and Sigma Xi.

He was a member of the Association of American Physicians and gave the Plummer Judd Lecture at the Mayo Clinic in 1958. He was also a member of the American Clinical & Climatological Association, and a founding member of the American Osler Society, serving as its President in 1972-73.

Tom's professional attitude was patient-oriented. He urged his students to be "side of the bed" rather than "end of the bed" doctors.

In his Presidential Address at the Annual Session in 1965, he paid tribute to the newly inducted Fellows by describing them as "truly self-propelled learners." Presiding over the celebration of the 50th Anniversary of the College, Dr. Durant described, in detail, all of the significant happenings in the life of the College, and placed opposite each of these events some significant event that occurred in the general arena of medicine. The title of this talk was "The Days of Our Years". This historical vignette was later printed by the College in a booklet which still remains a popular reference work.

One personal anecdote illustrates the kind of influence Tom wielded. The wife of a new Fellow approached me in tears just after meeting Tom in a receiving line. She said, "All these years I've heard my husband talk about his wonderful professor, and now I have met him and I understand." The man had that kind of charisma.

At the convocation in Chicago, President Durant was particularly pleased to induct his son John into Fellowship.

In his presidential address, "Of Time, Talents and Purpose," he spoke very directly to the new Fellows.

> . . . you entered medical training with the blessing of a . . . background that made you superior persons from an intellectual standpoint; there can be no greater satisfaction in life than to have used the talents, not primarily for personal gain, but that which accrues to one's fellow man. . . . the key physician in this scheme is the expert generalist, a person involved with the idea that the whole person is more important than the individual parts. The physician's office is a detection center but also a health education center.

He outlined some very specific ways to use time efficiently, and quoted Albert Szent Gyorgi,

> . . . so I leave knowledge for safe keeping to books and libraries and go fishing, sometimes for fish and sometimes for knowledge. He urged all the Fellows to have time for work, recreation and love. It must be understood that the word "love" was used not in the sense of the Greek word "eros" but in the sense of "agape"- the Greek word meaning affection for and benevolence toward one's fellow man.

I first met Tom Durant in June, 1959 when as an aspirant I came East to meet with the Search Committee. Later I visited Mr. Loveland at Headquarters. At that time, I called on Tom to get advice about where my wife and I might wish to live. He gave me the name of a real estate man, good schools to consider for our 12-year-old son, and golf courses I might enjoy playing. In every way he was thoughtful, kind, and delightfully humorous. (He promised me he would never interrupt one of my stories if I would not interrupt his.)

Dr. Durant was the driving force in starting the Philadelphia Medical and Pharmaceutical group. This was made up of the Dean and Professors of Medicine of each school and the medical director and president of each of the large pharmaceutical companies in the Philadelphia area. Dinner meetings occur at frequent intervals and speakers are always ones who are interested in pharmaceuticals and relations to medicine. The director of the Food and Drug Administration, staff persons for congressmen, and leaders in medical education would be good examples of speakers. This group still meets at regular intervals.

In concluding this chapter it is fair to say that several very important things occurred besides the 50th Anniversary celebration of the College during Dr. Durant's year as president. I asked him what he thought was the most important event in his presidential year. He considered the founding the Tri-College Council which later evolved into the Council of Medical Specialty Societies to be the most important. I told him that I thought that even more important was the final solution to the long-standing problem of the term for Associate Members. With his strong urging, the College decided to make the Associate Membership a permanent membership, thus encouraging them to continue taking part in the College's educational programs. The name was thereafter changed to Member.

Dr. Durant was chairman of an ad hoc committee to set the criteria for the election of Associates (residents in training).

The committee recommended, among other things, that such a candidate should be proposed by three Fellows of the College and endorsed by the Governor. The reason was to make membership mean something. This seemed difficult and unnecessary when regular members needed only two Fellows to propose them. In addition, it was unlikely the Governor would know them and it would mean a lot of extra work for him to find out enough about the resident to make any kind of appraisal. At any rate, this was tried for one year (two Fellows to propose, Governor to endorse). The result was very poor. Only a few hundred responded. The following year the Regents authorized writing directly to the residents. The application would only need to be signed by the director of the training program. After all, this was a temporary form of membership and was intended to interest the resident in the College at an early age. This seemed to work and by 1977 there were about 14,000 such Associates.

He also was one of the founders of the Tri-College Council, which included the ACP, the American College of Surgeons, and the American College of Obstetrics and Gynecology. Later, the Council was expanded to include 21 specialty societies and became the Council of Medical Specialty Societies.

It was a very exciting year because of the celebration of our 50th anniversary but also for these rather substantial changes in the organization itself.

# 1964-1965

50th Anniversary, 46th Annual Session, March 22-26, 1965. College Mace first used in Convocation. Interim Sessions. Associates given unlimited term. Governors Club. South American postgraduate courses, Colombia. American Association for the Accreditation of Laboratory Animal Care. ACP/APA Task Force. Tri-College Council.

At the Fall Meeting of the Board of Regents in 1964, Dr. Thomas N. Durant, President, commented how favorably he viewed the activities at the Regional Meetings. He felt the meetings were of excellent quality and served a useful purpose. He remarked that during the few months that he had been in office, relations with American Society of Internal Medicine [ASIM] seemed to be very good. Dr. Durant discussed the idea that as an educational organization the College should become more active in studying the techniques of postgraduate education. It was not enough merely to schedule courses and meetings. The College was in a unique position to study the actual mechanics of effective teaching.

In the report of the Executive Director, I conveyed some information of interest about the proposed change in the Bylaws that would enable Associate Members to have unlimited terms. The matter of the length of term for Associate Members came to the Board of Governors from its Executive Committee. This problem had come up for discussion many times since the merger of the ACP and the Congress of Internal Medicine in 1926. At that time, members of the Congress were made "permanent" Associate Members unless they were advanced to Fellowship. Thereafter, new Associate Members were elected for three years before being eligible to advance to Fellow. If not advanced in that period their Associate Membership was terminated. Later, for a number of years, the term was extended to 10 years and then changed back to five years when it turned out that no more Associates advanced to Fellowship during the ten-year term than in the shorter period.

For several years before the Governors met in April, 1964, there was a growing number of Governors and Regents who felt that the College was losing some good internists, and it was obvious that most of the defecting Associates no longer participated in the educational programs of the College. It was recognized that some Associates would never complete the requirements for advancement to Fellowship, but the Governors thought it better to keep them associated with the College than to lose their interest entirely.

The recommendation to eliminate the time limit was presented to the membership at the 1964 Annual Business Meeting. The Regents had voted unanimously to delete from the Bylaws all reference to limit of term and to substitute the following: "An Associate should be eligible for advancement to Fellowship at the end of two years. Upon expiration of this two year period, the Associate shall be notified in writing by the Credentials Committee of his eligibility for advancement to Fellowship".

This action, however, was complicated by the fact that the motion was introduced at the Annual Business Meeting without prior publication, making a unanimous vote by the membership mandatory. There was vigorous discussion and a few negative votes on the motion were cast. The motion was remanded to the 1965 Annual Business Meeting and I was directed to publish the proposed amendment in the *ACP Bulletin* prior to the next meeting.

In November, having published the proposed Bylaws change, I reported to the Board that I had received only one letter and a few verbal communications in reaction. The general attitude was that some Associates would not care to advance to Fellowship if there was no fear of being dropped from membership. Some, however, suggested this might be an erroneous judgment. If it were the position of the Regents that Associates perform little service on behalf of the College, the same position might very well be taken about Fellows who behave in similar fashion. There was consensus that the College Fellows—as a class of membership—could be better structured.

An interesting side issue was raised by a staff person: If an Associate Member still received the *Annals of Internal Medicine,* there would be, at least, exposure to good educational material. Moreover, a non-member might not even subscribe to the *Annals.* Several Regents predicted that there would be just as many Associates advancing to Fellowship under the new system as under the old system. They expressed the opinion that many Associates would probably respond to the challenge even more vigorously, if advancement were not mandatory.

The matter was resolved at the 1965 Annual Business Meeting, when a simple majority vote finally settled this long-standing problem. From 1965, Associates were elected without limit of term.

Turning to other issues, I observed that the College probably had made a wise decision in establishing a Committee on Medical Services. I also felt that liaison with ASIM was improving. In addition to the usual report about headquarters, I described in some detail the trip I had taken to the Naval Hospital in Yokosuka, Japan, after the Annual Session. This was one of the programs at which the College provided representation at meetings in Japan sponsored by one of the three Armed Forces. It was a splendid meeting and several hundred Japanese physicians attending were received enthusiastically. In a final comment, I noted that I had participated in the centennial celebration of the Mayo Clinic in Rochester, Minnesota. I was also pleased to announce that at this meeting Dr. Dwight Wilbur, former President of the College and eight other Fellows, including myself received Distinguished Alumnus Awards from the University of Minnesota.

In addition to its deliberations in considering the membership questions, the Board of Governors expressed their interest in forming a Governors' Club for ex-Governors, organized along lines similar to the Regency Club, which was formed the previous year.

The financing of Regional Meetings was again subject for discussion in 1964; the Board of Regents deciding that Governors could charge a registration fee. The existing reimbursement system of up to $250 for non-social administrative costs of Regional Meetings with attendance under 200, and up to $500 for meetings with over 200 registrants, would continue. Statements of the disposition of all funds were to be submitted for review to the Committee on Finance and Budgets.

In another action related to the administration of the Regions, Governors were authorized to open local checking accounts in the name of the College for expenses associated with Regional Meetings.

A report by the Committee on Scientific Programs reviewed Annual Session attendance and the Interim Sessions attendance. Attendance at the Atlantic City meeting was compared with the previous Annual Session. It was the opinion of the Committee that bad weather was responsible for the decreased attendance. April weather was often bad in Atlantic City and could cut remarkably the attendance of physicians, who made a practice of driving to the meeting from surrounding metropolitan areas.

Attendance figures for the Los Angeles Interim Session compared with the first Interim Session in Detroit were very disappointing, particularly the response of physicians located in western states other than California. Originally the fall meetings were intended to be of a broad regional type, to accommodate many physicians who would prefer not to travel long distances to the Annual Session. If attendance at the Miami, Florida, meeting did not increase, the fall meetings would probably be discontinued.

The Finance Committee report also presented some data on the Annual Sessions. These compared costs from 1962-1964, showing gross costs of each meeting and gross costs per physician in attendance:

|      |              | Cost/Session | Cost/Physician |
|------|--------------|--------------|----------------|
| 1962 | Philadelphia | $109,377     | $19.75         |
| 1963 | Denver       | $126,868     | $42.19         |
| 1964 | Atlantic City| $115,246     | $31.75         |

The two Interim Sessions held during the same period showed the following costs:

|      |             |           |         |
|------|-------------|-----------|---------|
| 1963 | Detroit     | $ 27,642  | $26.62  |
| 1964 | Los Angeles | $ 42,577  | $50.33  |

It was apparent that meetings west of Chicago were higher in cost because of travel expenses, not only for the speakers on the program, but also for College Staff, Governors and Regents.

Expense allowances for program participants were reviewed at both the Atlantic City Session and the Fall Board of Regents Meeting. The Board decided that speakers who were invited (as opposed to those who applied) to appear on the basic science portion of the Annual Session program were to be presented an amount equal to first-class air transportation including ground transportation. For one appearance on the program they would receive $100 and $25 for each additional day necessitated by other appearances, excluding travel time.

Guest speakers who were full-time teachers or research workers in non-profit institutions, members of the medical corps of the Armed Forces, Public Health Service and Veterans Administration, were allowed first-class air transportation, ground transportation, plus $50 for one appearance and $25 each additional day.

Fellows and Associates of the ACP who were full-time teachers or research workers in non-profit institutions, members of the Medical Corps of the Armed Forces, Public Health Service and the Veterans Administration were allowed the transportation previously described, but reimbursement by the College would be limited to those who did not have travel funds available from other sources.

The Finance Committee also reported that the dues regulations currently in force were very difficult to administer and created a substantial volume of correspondence. Full time teachers at the rank of Associate Professor or below, researchers who received their salary from a medical school, and members out of medical school less than ten years were given varying preferential rates.

After considerable discussion, new regulations were adopted, predicated upon length of time out of medical school. The new schedule was as follows:

| Out of Medical School | Rate | No. of Members | Yield |
|---|---|---|---|
| 10 years or less | $15 | 530 | $ 7,950 |
| 11-15 years or less | 25 | 1,570 | 39,250 |
| 16 years and over | 40 | 7,125 | 285,000 |
| TOTALS | | 9,225 | $332,200 |

Of the total income from dues under the new schedule, $8 per member was credited to subscriptions, totalling $258,400. Prepaid Life Members (1,950) and those with dues waived (825) were an additional 2,775 members who would not be represented in the current dues income. Registration fees at the Annual Session for nonmember paying guests were brought into line with this new dues structure. Nonmember physicians out of medical school 10 years or less paid $20; 10 years or more, $40.

Dr. Ray Farquharson, Chairman of the Fellowships and Scholarships Committee, reported that the new category of Teaching and Research Scholars had awakened much interest. There were 20 outstanding applicants for this position, which caused difficulty for the Committee, as only two could be recommended for appointments.

Because of this favorable response, it was suggested that the College might add another position or a third Teaching and Research Scholarship. This did not seem practical, because the College was committed, for the time being, to a five-year scholarship for the early appointees. The brochure stated that if the scholar did well after three years, he could continue for another two years. For this reason no change was made in the number of positions at the November, 1964 meeting.

Plans for the 50th Anniversary celebration were progressing well. The design for the head of the new mace was selected early in 1964 and the Garrard & Company, Ltd., of London, silversmiths to Her Royal Majesty, Queen Elizabeth, completed work in September.

The wood from the plane tree on the Isle of Cos had been sent to the Forest Products Laboratory, Department of Agriculture, Madison, Wisconsin, where it was X-rayed for defects and studied under a variety of conditions. It was then treated with the preservative polyethylene glycol. The design for the shaft was carved figures and the opening words of the Hippocratic Oath in Greek. The work was being done at Williamsburg by Mr. Don Turano.

The Committee on Medical Services reported on a variety of subjects. In the opinion of members of the Committee, the relationship between ACP and ASIM had shown great improvement. There was little evidence of discord and a spirit of relaxed cooperation seemed to prevail. In conformity with the actions of the Committee, I had sent letters to many medical organizations in which College members were involved. Letters were also sent to major voluntary health agencies informing them of the existence and functions of this new Committee. These included a letter to the Director of the Food and Drug Administration, Dr. Joseph Sadusk. The Committee recommended, and the Board of Regents approved, that an appropriate committee be instructed to study what part the ACP and internists generally should play in "restorative medicine".

## Graduate Medical Education

In late June, representatives of the College met with the Citizen's Commission on Graduate Medical Education (the Millis Commission). Discussion centered around family practice and the role of the internist in that field. The Commission was considering 18 months as the required length of training in internal medicine for family practice programs. Although similar to the current requirements for Board certification by the American Board of Internal Medicine [ABIM], it was obvious that content and emphasis might be different.

Since training for such practice, no matter what it was to be called, would be based fundamentally on internal medicine, the Board of Regents, had, in November, 1963, adopted the following statement as the official policy of the College on family practice:

> The American College of Physicians recognizes there is a shortage in the number of physicians engaged in family practice. In view of the fact that family practice comprises a substantial portion of the work of many internists, the College has a strong interest and responsibility in the supply, quality, training and continuing education of physicians engaged in the family practice of medicine at its highest level. In order to promote this interest and responsibility, the Board of Regents will exert every effort to make effective the College's influence in the solution of these pressing problems including representation on all appropriate bodies and committees considering these problems.

Some apparent friction had developed between the principal national societies engaged in physical medicine. Quite naturally, the College's interest was in the complete care of the patient, with rehabilitation an integral part of such care. It was with this in mind that the Board of Regents, through the issuance of the following statement, encouraged its members—particularly internists—to take an increased interest in the rehabilitation of the patient:

> The American College of Physicians is committed to the principle that internists must be responsible for the complete care of the patient. The teaching and practice of internal medicine encompasses four aspects as it relates to a person whose func-

tion is threatened or limited by disease, illness or injury. These aspects are: Prevention, Diagnosis, Therapy and Rehabilitation.

Any one or all of these areas may require the skills and cooperation of allied specialists, health personnel and community services. Rehabilitation includes the restoration of function in the following areas: Physical, Mental, Vocational and Social.

By virtue of his broad training the internist is the logical coordinator of and participant in the long-term care and rehabilitation of the chronically ill or handicapped person. Consistent with its long-standing interest in all fields of medical education and research, the ACP will promote and encourage medical education and research in rehabilitation. This educational program should be emphasized at the undergraduate, graduate and postgraduate levels.

## Golden Anniversary Session 1965

The city of Chicago hosted the Golden Anniversary Session which celebrated the ACP's 50th year. Letters of congratulation were received from the Chicago Society of Internal Medicine and the Institute of Medicine of Chicago, both of which were celebrating their own 50th anniversaries. The American Medical Association, the Royal College of Physicians of London and the President of the United States, Lyndon Johnson, among many others, sent their congratulations.

The National Board of Medical Examiners had also been founded in 1915. This Board presented the College a beautiful scroll of congratulations and good wishes. The Board of Regents in turn presented them a similar congratulatory certificate.

For the first time, the Marshall of the Convocation led the academic procession into the auditorium carrying the new College Ceremonial Mace. It stood four feet two inches in length; the head was made of silver and gold. At its center, designed in a modern spirit, were the twin serpents of Aesculapius and the Lamp of Wisdom, the Book of Knowledge and the Poppy, all symbolic of medicine and its practice. The rough texture of this central feature contrasted with the extremely fine surface of the Mace head proper and the silver gilt finial atop the spire represented the flames of the Torch of Progress. Around the base of the head, the words from the first aphorism of Hippocrates were engraved: "Life is short and Art is long".

The shaft of the Mace was made of wood from the Great Plane Tree of Cos. Carved at the top of the shaft were two plane trees and beneath one of these, the bearded figure of Hippocrates holding a skull with several students sitting at his feet. Twin serpents were carved at the base together with the first words of the Hippocratic Oath in Greek: "I swear by Apollo, . . . "

Gavels were made from those portions of the limb that remained and these were presented to the Royal College of Physicians of London and the Royal Australasian College of Physicians, as mementos of the occasion.

Several interesting projects were described by the Committee on Public Information. Dr. Irving S. Wright, Chairman, described the operation of the press headquarters for the Golden Anniversary Session and cited the very good attendance by press representatives. At the invitation of the College, the National Association of Science Writers was scheduled to have one of their regional meetings at the Conrad Hilton Hotel. There were three Golden Anniversary projects initiated by the Public Information Committee which had been completed:

1) An anniversary medallion, commemorating the Golden Anniversary of the founding of the College would be given gratis to all Fellows who registered. Those not registered at the meeting could purchase these medallions for $3.50. These were made available by the generosity of Lilly Company.

2) A very attractive historical booklet was printed based on Dr. Durant's opening address, entitled, "The Days of Our Years . . . A Short History of the ACP from 1915-1955". This booklet was made possible through the courtesy of Wyeth Laboratories. This would also be given to all registrants at the time Dr. Durant made his presentation.

3) Finally, the Committee was pleased to announce the completion of a motion picture entitled, "Portrait of An Internist". This depicted the typical activities of a typical internist. Following the Annual Session, this would be made available for presentations at College meetings and to the general public via television and screenings to clubs. This film was financed by Merck, Sharp & Dohme. As an interesting sidelight, the movie was made at the Hartford Hospital; the movie producers had the extreme good fortune of filming a staff physician and a Fellow of the College who combined good acting ability with a fine demonstration of the kind of work internists do.

The report of the Executive Director at the April session noted that the number of members as of the April session totaled 34 Masters, 8,666 Fellows and 3,521 Associates, for a total of 12,221. I mentioned also that 20 percent of candidates were then elected directly to Fellowship.

I announced that a printing department had been established at the Headquarters, improving the Staff's ability to get things printed on time and in an attractive manner.

Total physician registration at the Annual Session in Chicago was 3,863, only 200 more than in Atlantic City the year before. Average physician registration between the years 1956-1960 was 3,928, but in the past five years, it had dropped to 3,768. A more marked decline was offset by the attendance of over 5,000 physicians at the Philadelphia Annual Session in 1962.

The weather, in large part, was responsible for the relatively poor showing in both Atlantic City and Chicago. These attendance figures were not exactly consoling to a growing organization, and pointed to the importance of constantly seeking excellent programs with innovative teaching methods.

In matters of membership, the "Manual of Rules, Policies, and Procedures of the American College of Physicians" read in part:

> While it is not officially stated in the Constitution and Bylaws of the College that only citizens of North America shall be admitted to full membership in the College, it is the policy of the Board of Regents and of the Committee on Credentials to discourage the admission to the College, physicians who are not citizens of this continent.

Since citizenship was no longer a criterion for the American Board of Internal Medicine examination, provided the training was taken in US or Canada, and this policy did not involve a change in either the ACP Constitution or Bylaws, the following statement was substituted in the "Manual" by the Board of Regents, on the recommendation of the Credentials Committee: "The Board of Regents approves the election of non-citizens to full Fellowship in the College when such a candidate meets all other requirements except residence and citizenship." In the future, when an outstanding physician from another country was proposed who fulfilled all the requirements, citizenship and residence would not prohibit his or her election to regular membership.

The administrative Staff felt strongly that one further step needed to be taken regarding dues which had been revised the year before. Numerous letters were received at College Headquarters asking how to define "basic science." There were members who were primarily basic scientists who worked part time in clinical departments, some with the title, for example, of Associate Professor of Physiology and Internal Medicine; others who were primarily clinicians worked part time in basic science departments. The Board of Regents decided to bill the basic scientists on the same basis as other members (length of time out of medical school).

The Board of Regents authorized the Editor of the *Annals* to spend up to $6,000 for color plates to illustrate papers where color was more effective than black and white. The Board also authorized publication of the *ACP Bulletin* on a monthly basis.

The high caliber of applicants for the new Teaching and Research Scholarships impressed the Board of Regents. Reversing its decision at the 1964 Fall Meeting, the Board approved a recommendation that two additional scholarships be made available for a three-year period beginning in 1967. This was made possible by discontinuing the five-year term for all scholars.

In March, 1964, an ad hoc committee of the College had met with representatives of the American Psychiatric Association [APA] in Chicago, for the purpose of exploring the integration of certain aspects of internal medicine and psychiatry. It was generally agreed that the interests of each of the groups had much to contribute to the other in the practice of their respective specialties. To accrue a better understanding of psychiatric objectives and techniques, the committee examined prevailing educational methods— undergraduate, graduate, and those for physicians in practice. Frankly recognizing the antipathy of many undergraduates to the psychiatric approach, and the limitations of postgraduate or continuing education in terms of the few practicing physicians it reached, College representatives concluded that the best means for the integration of psychiatry with internal medicine was through consultation at the bedside.

Having determined that there was a need for closer association of internist and psychiatrist in practice, and for better understanding by each of the other's problems and methods of diagnosis and treatment, the Regents appointed a Task Force to serve for three years. Areas of common concern between the organizations were to be explored and methods of effective collaboration developed.

One of the first activities of the Task Force was the filing of a grant application, late in 1964, in the name of the College to the National Institutes of Health, entitled, "General Hospital Psychiatric Education Project". The College proposed, in conjunction with the APA, to demonstrate how state and local ACP and APA component units and members could best collaborate with key hospital staff to establish continuing psychiatric education programs for practicing physicians in the community. This was a direct attempt to develop and expand, among ACP members, skills required for the care and management of emotional disturbances associated with somatic illness.

In a status report at the 1965 Annual Session, Dr. R.H. Kampmeier, Chairman of the ACP/APA Task Force, informed the Board that the joint grant application to the National Institute of Mental Health [NIMH] for the study of psychiatric teaching at the community hospital level had been denied. The ACP/APA Task Force was to meet again to discuss a new grant proposal which would respond to the NIMH objections. In the meantime, some pilot programs were started.

At the 1964 Board of Governors meeting, there was a fair amount of discussion about the Interim Sessions. With a final vote of 31-25, the Governors recommended to the Board of Regents that the fall meetings be discontinued after the Miami Interim Session, in deference to Regional Meetings. The Governors expressed the opinion that attendance at Regional Meetings was discouraged in those years when the fall meeting occurred in the same geographic area. Yet many local physicians had not attended the last two Interim Sessions. However, the Board of Governors decided that they would not make elimination of fall meetings an official request to the Regents until after the attendance report of the Miami meeting was obtained.

The Board of Governors affirmed the decision to impose no limitation on the term of Associates and agreed with the principle that periodically Associates should provide evidence of continued participation in the educational activities of the College. They also voted to establish a Governors' Club along the following lines:

a. to be an organization primarily for former Governors, although current Governors were to be invited to meetings.
b. during the Annual Session that there be a Governors' Reception.
c. that it be "no host".
d. that wives be included.
e. that the first meeting be held in 1966 at the New York Annual Session.
f. that the Executive Director and his wife be invited.
g. that the current Chairman of the Board of Governors be the Chairman of the Governors' Club for ease of coordination of this activity with other activities of the College through the Executive Director's office.

For the ABIM, Thomas H. Brem, Chairman, reported that 1,206 physicians took the oral examination in 1964. Of the number of candidates examined, the passing rate was 61.7 percent of first time takers; of all candidates 65 percent passed the examination. Eventually 80 percent of candidates passed their oral examinations and became certified. For some candidates, this process took two or three years. In October, 1964, 2,116 took the written examination. Of this group 1,291 were first time takers and 60 percent of these passed. Of the 825 repeaters, 20 percent passed.

The examination, according to Dr. Brem, was remarkable in its validity, based on a test of discriminatory power. The Board analyzed every item for its discriminatory power on the basis of how the top 25 percent taking the examination did on these items compared to the bottom 25 percent of all takers. The test yielded a number called a Bi-Serial r Index of discretionary power. The perfect question would have an index value of 1.0, meaning that all the top takers got it right and all the bottom takers got it wrong. Fifty percent of the questions in the test had a Bi-Serial r Index greater than four-tenths (0.4), 85 percent of the questions had an Index greater than three-tenths (0.3) and only 10 percent of the questions were below two-tenths (0.2).

Dr. Brem announced that since the death of ABIM Executive Director, Dr. William Werrell, the Board had appointed Dr. Victor Logan, a Fellow of the College to take over the operation of the ABIM. The Board had also decided to move the headquarters to Philadelphia. There were several reasons for this move, including the establishment of closer communication with the ACP and proximity to the National Board of Medical Examiners [NBME]. All the mechanics of ABIM examinations including printing, distribution, collection, storage, and analysis were being accomplished for them by the NBME. ABIM continued to make up the questions, but the NBME had the machinery, including data processing, and the capacity to assist the ABIM in its task of processing examinations.

The Residency Review Committee in Internal Medicine [RRC-IM] accepted several recommendations from the ACP/APA Task Force, and these were incorporated in the new edition of the *Essentials of Approved Residencies*. It was obvious to the ACP/APA group that general hospitals were going to have the first influx of Medicare patients with psychiatric disorders. Probably, residents in medicine would receive the main brunt of this caseload because psychiatric residencies were relatively scarce in community hospitals.

The Animal Facilities Accreditation Board [AFAB] was set up in 1963 by the Animal Care Panel to undertake voluntary inspection of various institutions and organizations throughout the country in which experimental animals were being utilized. This activity was a countermeasure to repeated threats of federal legislation designed to regulate experiments on animals. Teams of voluntary inspectors made visits to 26 institutions during 1964, and deficiencies were reported to the AFAB. This pilot program demonstrated the feasibility of voluntary inspection and ''policing'' entirely free from federal interference.

The pilot project was purposely limited as to duration and financing, but it indicated a permanent, privately supported body could be set up to carry on accrediting procedures. Representation on the Animal Care Panel at that time was constituted of commercial as well as professional members. The Board of Directors reflected the thinking of both groups. The scientific community felt that it must be represented by scientists only, if such a voluntary accrediting body were to command respect and have the authority of persuasion.

The panel proposed, therefore, to the ACP Board of Regents, as well as to 14 other national scientific organizations, that a new corporation be established. It was to be known as the American Association for the Accreditation of Laboratory Animal Care [AAALAC]. Membership was to consist of scientific and educational organizations; each would appoint one representative to the Board of Trustees. The Trustees were then to appoint a Council on Accreditation.

Institutions visited would be charged a fee, but this would not be sufficient to meet the budget. Member organizations were, therefore, asked to make voluntary contributions and the College decided to contribute $1,000 annually to this operation.

### South American Educational Activities

Concerning the Latin American Fellowship Program, the College learned that the Rockefeller Foundation was terminating its yearly contribution of $25,000. This grant had been used to fund a course at Cornell, "Methods of Internal Medicine", instruction in the English language, and medical orientation for the Fellows upon their arrival in the United States. The Kellogg Foundation, which had subsidized travel and employment through grants, reported to the Board of Regents that it would be too expensive for them to finance this course, inasmuch as it cost $1,000 per person, plus the stipend to Fellows.

Some modifications were made in the schedule of the incoming Fellows and, at least for the following year, English language instruction was to be given in a tutorial program and run concurrently with the course in internal medicine at Cornell. Other means of obtaining financial support would continue to be explored.

There were 140 registrants for the first ACP postgraduate course held in Medellin, Colombia, in March. Over two-thirds were from Colombian medical schools outside Medellin and the remaining one-third were from Medellin and its surrounding areas. A registration fee of 300 pesos for the non-academic registrants was charged and 150 pesos for those connected with a medical school.

Both the College representatives and the faculty from the seven medical schools in Colombia were pleased with the turnout. The pediatricians had held a three-day course in 1960 and a brief course in endocrinology was presented in 1961. This postgraduate course was a first rate internal medicine experience. In response to enthusiastic support and the recommendations from the visiting professors, the Regents decided to authorize another course, tentatively scheduled for the Fall 1966.

The Committee on Cancer reported to the Board of Regents on two important studies concluded recently. The first was a New York State Department of Health study on the routine use of vaginal cytology during the three years 1958, 1962, and 1963. It revealed that vaginal cytology performed on 17,698 adult women hospitalized regardless of the reason for admission, had detected four unsuspected carcinomas of the cervix per 1,000 patients. The Committee proposed, therefore, that an explicit statement be issued urging that a vaginal cytology examination should be as much a part of the routine work-up of female patients as urine examination or hemoglobin determination. The Committee also welcomed the suggestion to send a notice to the membership recommending this policy.

The Committee also reported on a recent survey which alleged that only 52.5 percent of internists advised patients not to smoke. On the basis of the overwhelming evidence on the health hazard of cigarettes in the genesis of emphysema as well as lung cancer, the Committee proposed that the College lend its influence to the prevention of these diseases by recommending to ACP members that they inform their patients about the health hazards from smoking.

After extensive discussion, the Board of Regents passed a motion which, in effect, authorized dissemination of information concerning both of these suggestions through normal College channels, including the publication of editorials and scientific papers in the *Annals,* presentation of papers at the Annual Session, and making the ACP mailing list available to the US Public Health Department (as it had done with a mammography brochure) for dissemination of authoritative statements. It, however, did not wish to promote the routine use of any one procedure in clinical medicine as College policy.

The College representatives to the American Joint Committee for Cancer Staging and End Results Reporting reported that they were taking an active part in the difficult task of developing classifications for all sites of anatomical cancer and field testing of the proposed classifications. The program would extend over many years, and "even when adequate staging has been accomplished for a particular site, it would require a great deal of educational effort to get it accepted and used by the medical profession." It was hoped that a classification would be completed in 1965 for an acceptable field trial on disseminated carcinoma of the breast.

### Tri-College Council

During his presidential year, Dr. Durant had attended an informal meeting with representatives of the American College of Obstetricians and Gynecologists and some British guests. Discussion was about the possible need for an interdisciplinary council in the United States. Such a council existed in England and was very useful as a meeting ground for the various specialties. Its main function in England was to establish grounds of agreement on issues related to licensing and certifying specialists. The Regents authorized Dr. Durant and me to explore it further; a meeting was held in January, 1965, with representatives from the American College of Surgeons, the American College of Obstetricians and

Gynecologists and the ACP. As a result, a Tri-College Council was proposed and approved by all three Colleges.

The new Council held an early meeting with the AMA Board of Trustees to explore how specialty societies might be more active in AMA. Projected plans included expansion of the Tri-College Council to include the major society which represented each specialty for which a certifying board existed. The AMA representatives were reluctant to proceed with specialty societies representation in the AMA House of Delegates. But shortly after this they formed a permanent committee to be known as the AMA Interspecialty Committee, whose function was to advise its Board of Trustees about organizational problems relating to AMA's scientific programs and other matters.

It soon followed that the Tri-College Council was renamed the Interspecialty Council as the American Academy of Pediatrics and the APA joined. Within a few years all the major specialty societies for which there was an official certifying board became members, and the name was changed to the Council of Medical Specialty Societies [CMSS]. Its purposes were to be:

1. To promote communication among the specialty organizations concerned with principal divisions of medicine.
2. To share administrative experiences and to seek mutually advantageous solutions to administrative problems.
3. To promote advances in medical education through joint programming and to provide broader perspectives on patient care.

Other details of the Council's membership and administration were presented. The Board of Regents approved the recommendation that the three immediate past presidents of ACP serve as the College representatives to the Council. Thus, each year one new appointment would be made. Current members would include Drs. Franklin M. Hanger, Wesley Spink, and Thomas Durant.

At one early meeting, CMSS met with representatives of the American Association of Medical Colleges [AAMC] to explore possible formal association. It was decided that informal communication would be helpful, but the CMSS desired to be an independent body.

At about this time there was another multi-organizational body known as the Medical Intersociety Council. It was composed of representatives of the AAMC, the AMA, American Hospital Association [AHA], a number of academic societies and a number of clinical specialty societies (mostly the same as those in CMSS). Its purpose was to be a listening body in Washington for various legislative matters of interest to medical bodies. This group met for several years but performed no function not already covered by some of the other groups mentioned above.

Dr. Durant thought that the beginning of the Tri-College Council and its development into the CMSS was the most important event of his year as President. He agreed that the final establishment of the Associate Membership without limit of term was most important for the ACP, but the CMSS would be most important to medicine generally.

The Joint Commission on Accreditation of Hospitals [JCAH] announced the appointment of Dr. John D. Porterfield, III (FACP), of the University of California, Berkeley, as Director to replace Dr. Kenneth Babcock.

The first signs of cramped physical conditions began appearing at the College Headquarters. The printing department needed room to expand, but at that time there was no solution to the question of space. The Board of Regents was told that within a few years, consideration would have to be given to providing additional facilities.

## Part Two (1965-1966)

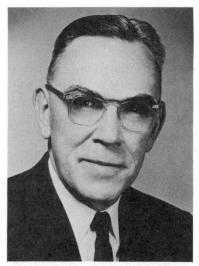

*A. Carlton Ernstene, MACP*

Arthur Carlton Ernstene was born in Parker, South Dakota, on August 4, 1901. He died on March 12, 1971 in Cleveland. He is survived by his son, Marshall.

He was graduated from the State University of Iowa, where he received both his Bachelor of Arts and Doctor of Medicine degrees. His graduate training included internship at Henry Ford Hospital, a residency at the Thorndike Memorial Laboratory, Boston City Hospital, and research experience at Beth Israel Hospital in Boston, where he was Assistant in Medicine from 1928 to 1932. He also served as Assistant in Medicine (1927 to 1930), Instructor in Medicine (1930-31), then Faculty Instructor (1931-32) at Harvard Medical School. He became Head of the Department of Cardiovascular Disease at the Cleveland Clinic, and in 1948 became Chairman of the Division of Medicine at the Clinic. He continued in that position until his retirement in 1966.

During World War II he served as a Lieutenant Commander, USNR, completing his tour of duty as Chief of Medicine at the U S Naval Base Hospital No. 3 in the New Hebrides Islands.

Dr. Ernstene was a member of numerous medical societies, including the AMA in which he served as Chairman of the Section on Internal Medicine (1956-57), American Heart Association (President 1959-60), and American College of Physicians (President 1965-66, Master 1970). He was also a member of the Association of American Physicians, the American Society for Clinical Investigation, Central Society for Clinical Research, and the Interurban Club.

In 1950 he was elected Vice President of the American Clinical and Climatological Association and maintained active interest in that society until his death. He was a Diplomate of the American Board of Internal Medicine and the Subspecialty Board of Cardiovascular Disease.

He was awarded the Gold Heart of the American Heart Association and Honorary degrees of ScD from John Carroll University and Baldwin-Wallace College. He was a member of Phi Beta Kappa and Alpha Omega Alpha. During his professional career he maintained an active interest in clinical investigation, as evidenced by the publication of about 100 papers dealing with a wide spectrum of cardiovascular diseases and a monograph, *Coronary Heart Disease.* He was, however, primarily a first-rate clinician.

Dr. Irving Wright, President-Elect of the College, said of Dr. Ernstene, "Throughout his very active and productive life he maintained a modest, soft-spoken, quiet mien. He engendered a spirit of warm friendship and a close relationship with a host of fellow physicians. He was a gentleman in the best sense of this term."

In characteristic fashion, Dr. Ernstene was very specific in his interpretation of the "responsibilities of Fellowship". He understood Fellowship as being more than a testimonial of qualification. Fellowship represented the mark of the true internist, carrying with it a number of lifelong responsibilities: dedication to a self-imposed program of continuing education, continuing education of colleagues, leadership in residency training programs and humane sensitivity in patient care. The true internist, in his view, recognized the patient's need to know, explaining to the patient the nature of his problem, the mechanisms and significance of symptoms, the rationale of treatment and the characteristics of the course of illness. He emphasized the importance of instruction to the patient, given unhurriedly and in understandable and convincing terms, and of adequate explanation of the problems to the patient's family.

The first suggestion that the College should create an educational self-assessment program occurred during Dr. Ernstene's presidential year. Although not all the Regents were enthusiastic about this project, Dr. Ernstene gave this movement his vigorous support, which was very helpful during its incipient stage.

Reflecting on the events of the 50th Anniversary celebration, Dr. Ernstene told the Regents at their meeting in November, 1965,

The achievements of the College during its first half-century comprise a record of which we can rightfully be proud and for which we are indebted to those who have gone before us. We must recognize, however, that times are changing rapidly and that these changes are confronting us with new challenges and greater opportunities. One of the most important of these, it seems to me, is a task for the Committee on Educational Activities which is now charged with overall planning and evaluation. The indispensable need for continuing education for the physician was one of the basic reasons for the founding of the College, and the need today is greater than ever before. The number of new graduates from our medical schools is not keeping pace with the increase in our population, and it is imperative, therefore, that all possible means be employed to prevent deterioration of the skills and competence of physicians in practice.

I had personal cause to remember Dr. Ernstene's sensitivity as physician and friend. At the Sunday night dinner for Officers and Regents during the 1966 Annual Session in New York City my wife, Esther, fainted and fell, cutting her lip. Dr. Barondess called one of his colleagues, a plastic surgeon, who gave her immediate attention. (Several weeks later, I discovered she had had occurrences of atrial fibrillation which continued thereafter, resulting in a hemiplegia in 1973.) During this 1966 Annual Session, we shared our suite with Dr. Ernstene; he was most considerate throughout and in every way a pleasure to be with.

Dr. Ernstene invited the Right Reverend Bishop Fulton Sheen to give the Convocation Address. Bishop Sheen's topic, "There Are No Diseases, Only Sick People", noted the importance of the sense of touch. After the ceremony Bishop Sheen complimented us on one of the best ceremonials of this type he had ever attended.

I met Carl Ernstene on two occasions before becoming Executive Vice President of ACP. The first meeting occurred during a vacation at Grand Lake, Colorado. He invited me to go trout fishing with him. His father, who was vacationing with him, advised us against going because it wasn't the kind of day trout would be apt to take the fly. We went anyway and climbed to an elevation of 11,000 feet. We saw hundreds of cutthroat trout, but didn't get a nibble. The next day his father went to the same place and caught his limit.

I next met Dr. Ernstene at an AMA meeting; I was asked to discuss a paper he had given.

During Dr. Ernstene's term, his wife became progressively more disabled and needed much care at home. Carl's dedication to his wife was made manifest to me when he called one day in early autumn and offered to resign, because he would not be able to travel very often for the College. I told him that if he came to the Board of Regents meeting in November and attended the Annual Session in New York, we could exempt him from representing the College at Regional or other meetings. I suggested that he would have to refuse all other meetings, or we would have difficulty explaining his absences at College meetings to our Board of Governors and other College members. We were able to work out arrangements that enabled Carl both to work satisfactorily for the College and provide adequate attention to Mrs. Ernstene.

He portrayed an even-handed patience in his presidential duties under these trying conditions that fall, when he had to choose a new Chairman of Local Arrangements for the Annual Session. The incumbent Dr. Stanley Bradley, professor at the Columbia College of Physicians and Surgeons, was unable to spare the necessary time. Dr. Ernstene asked Dr. Jeremiah Barondess to take over this job. Dr. Barondess later became a College Governor, then a Regent, and finally President.

# 1965-1966

Self Assessment. Headquarters fire. Affiliate Members. Dr. Edward Huth made Associate Editor, *Annals*. Millis Commission. Family Practice. RRC-IM *Guide for Residency Training Programs*.

In his report to the November meeting of the Board of Regents, Dr. A. Carlton Ernstene, President, announced with deep regret the sudden and unexpected death of Dr. Ray Farquharson. He described Dr. Farquharson as "A devoted Fellow, Governor and Regent and member of many College committees, on several of which he served as chairman. He will long be remembered as one of our most loved and admired members. The College can ill-afford the loss of such a wise and gracious counselor."

Dr. Ernstene then commented on the Interim Session in Miami on October 7, 8 and 9. From the standpoint of those who had attended, it seemed very successful. Meeting facilities were excellent, and the program was very good. Attendance, however, was disappointing. Apparently, physicians beyond the immediate Miami area did not attend in any considerable numbers. Dr. Ernstene raised the question, "Is there a need for the fall meetings, and do these meetings accomplish more than the Regional Meetings?" In his opinion, the answer was negative, and he was in agreement with the recommendation of the Executive Committee and the Committee on Educational Activity that the project be discontinued.

He indicated that, in addition to a meeting of the Millis Commission, he had also attended the Conference for Medical Specialty Groups on the Medicare Law at the AMA and the White House Conference on Health.

His most important charge to the Board, as previously noted, was to the Educational Activities Committee, and reflected his strong committment to the idea of self-assessment in continuing education.

Dr. Ernstene also emphasized the ever growing role in the College epitomized by the expanding activities of the Committee on Medical Services.

In the report of the Executive Director, I mentioned that the two buildings which were owned by the College had been designated historically important by the Philadelphia Historical Commission. This body has legal authority to preserve certain structures in the city. The only disadvantage to the College was that it would not be able to demolish the buildings, or change their external appearance without the consent of the Historical Commission. I reported that through my efforts with the West Philadelphia Corporation, the Historical Commission had given the College permission to demolish the adjoining building if we agreed to make any future additions to the present building conform to the present architecture. Of incidental interest I reminded the Board of Regents that the adjoining building, occupied by the Group Insurance Administrators, had been a farmhouse during the Civil War.

During the evaluation of Interim Sessions, I confirmed that the fall meetings had had adequate publicity, and I felt that the Governors in the southern states had done everything possible to publicize the meeting. In spite of this, it was obvious that physicians outside the Miami area did not attend in sufficient numbers. In summary, I commented,

In many ways, the year 1965 will be considered historically important for medicine generally. With the enormous changes in our government programs to help solve health needs in this country, there has never been a time when leadership by our profession is more needed. The College seems to me to be an ideal organization to develop such leadership as no other large medical association has such solid support from the best men in practice, education and research.

At the AMA conference on the pending Medicare Law, the essential features of the law were presented by AMA staff, and it was pointed out that if physicians, through medical organizations, refused to participate in the Medicare program, such action might expose the organization to the application of the Sherman Antitrust Act. Furthermore, a physician's right to practice in a hospital was not vested. He was obligated to abide by reasonable rules and regulations imposed by the hospital administration, and such rules might rightly require the cooperation of the physician in assisting the hospital to participate in the Medicare Law.

In order to keep the College well informed on developments in rules and regulations, a representative was appointed to an AMA sponsored committee.

There was a prevalent feeling among the memberships of the American College of Surgeons [ACS], the American College of Obstetricians and Gynecologists [ACOG] and the ACP that specialty groups were not well represented in the AMA House of Delegates. Representatives of the three organizations had met late in 1964 to discuss the possibility of forming an interspecialty council. Guidelines were drawn up and approved by the sponsoring societies, delineating the purposes of the new council as described in the previous chapter.

At the first meeting held in September, 1963, the name, Tri-College Council [TCC], was adopted. This meeting, although lengthy, was not very productive. Several more sessions were required before the value of the project could be properly assessed.

The Executive Committee's report included the suggestion that Associates of the College be required to attend certain educational functions of the College. Past discussions had raised the question of the purposes of such a requirement: If the purpose was to indicate continued interest in the College, then the requirements would only need to include attendance at College functions. If, on the other hand, the requirements were to indicate an interest in continuing postgraduate education, then a much broader interpretation of acceptable attendance at educational functions of many types might be adopted. It seemed to be the consensus that only attendance requirements of Associates should be considered at that time and that these should be limited to College functions. After study, the Board of Regents postponed decision pending a survey by questionnaire which would be sent to all Associates to determine their current attendance at College or other educational activities.

The survey of the Associate members showed that well over 90 percent of the members did participate in significant continuing medical education programs. Dr. Phil Corr, Regional Governor of California, thought that such a mandatory requirement would necessitate making exceptions to the rule, and he did not think all the Governors could interpret the need for exceptions evenhandedly. I suggested to the Board of Regents that if this were to become a requirement for members it should also include Fellows. This seemed to turn the tide toward no attendance requirement for anyone.

The Executive Committee announced that the College had received $125,000 from the estate of Dr. James D. Bruce, President of the College in 1941. A memorial award in his honor had been established in 1946 following his death. The income from the legacy was $5,000 a year. A decision by the Board of Regents on how this fund was to be used was required. While attending another meeting in Ann Arbor, I had sought out Miss Mabel Kelly, Dr. Bruce's secretary and the only surviving executor of his estate. Because of Dr. Bruce's long-time interest in postgraduate education, Miss Kelly respectfully requested that the Board of Regents consider the Department of Postgraduate Education in Medicine, University of Michigan, as a possible place where all or part of this money might be allocated. I pointed out to her that it would seem that if Dr. Bruce had intended the University of Michigan to be the only recipient of the money, he would have put it in his will. Dr. Bruce had provided for a similar amount to be bequeathed to the University of Michigan as well as to the Michigan State Medical Society for the same purpose.

A committee was appointed to consider the disposition of this bequest.

Approximately $4,000 from the first year's income in 1965 was forwarded to the Department of Postgraduate Education at the University of Michigan to provide a suitable memorial from the College for Sheldon Auditorium in their new continuing education building. The University of Michigan used the gift to purchased sound equipment for the auditorium. The Ad Hoc Committee recommended that because of Dr. Bruce's interest in postgraduate education, the income after the first year be used for much needed research in education. In 1967, this fund was put to good use in the scholarships program and to support postgraduate courses in South America.

The Educational Activities Committee, in its report, suggested that the following be considered by the Committee on Scientific Programs:

a. That an experiment in teaching be tried at the forthcoming 1966 or 1967 Annual Session. This would consist of inviting 12 professors, each representing a specific field of internal medicine.

b. That each be invited to meet with no more than 15 Associates for one hour at lunch or some other time to provide an occasion to ask questions of the professor, in the belief that through this intimate contact, the Associates would enjoy a valuable learning experience.

Finally scheduled at the 1968 Annual Session in Boston, the ''Meet the Professor'' sessions were very successful and have become a regular part of the Annual Session program, open to all attendees.

The Committee discussed the continuing education of the internist at great length and identified the following problems areas:

a. Education at the community hospital level.

b. Requests that educational filmstrips be made available for members.

c. Development of educational films in conjunction with other scientific organizations.
d. Definition of the responsibility of the ACP in the field of continuing education for the internist.

The Committee concluded that it was evident that continuing education was the most important factor affecting medical care in the future. If that premise were correct, then the College should lead in this field. At a recent White House Conference on Medical Health and Education, it had been pointed out that proper mechanisms to foster continuing education were poorly developed and in many areas, completely lacking. The Committee believed that the area of continuing education should occupy the Committee's attention for the next several months.

The Publications Committee announced that Dr. Edward Huth had begun full time service to the College in his capacity as Associate Editor of the *Annals* in July of 1965. Dr. J. Russell Elkinton expressed gratitude for this increased help. He noted that in the face of the present explosion of scientific activity and information, editors and publishers of medical journals had to be alert if they expected to fulfill their function adequately. He quoted Sir Theodore Fox, recently retired editor of *The Lancet*, who had lectured on the problem of the future of medical journals. In "Crisis in Communication", Dr. Fox divided the functions of the medical journal into that of a repository of new information, and, secondly, of a medical newspaper. Dr. Elkinton believed that the *Annals* should continue to function in both capacities and had discussed this matter in an editorial entitled, "Too Much To Read", which appeared in the October issue, 1965.

## Headquarters Fire

In the early morning hours of Thursday, February 17, 1966, fire destroyed a considerable portion of the new wing of the Headquarters building. A defective electric motor in one of the air conditioning units was presumed to be the cause of the blaze. The new addition built in 1961, would have to be rebuilt.

Fortunately, all membership records, proposals for new membership, postgraduate courses registration and files, and all pre-registration for the 1966 New York Annual Session were intact. Two *Annals* manuscripts on a desk in the process of being edited were lost, but the rest were in a steel filing cabinet and were only scorched around the edges.

The Addressograph plates in the Circulation Department were relatively untouched and were it not for the fact that all advertising records were destroyed, the *Annals* would have been delivered on time. Despite these problems, the April, 1966 *Annals* was mailed to subscribers only a few days late.

The long walnut table in the Loveland Board Room sustained considerable water and smoke damage, but it was possible to refinish it. The new College Mace, used for the first time the previous year at the 50th Anniversary celebration in Chicago, as well as the Caduceus, the President's Badge, and other memorabilia, survived the fire intact. An oil painting of Mr. Edward R.

Loveland, the former Executive Secretary of the College, that hung in the Board Room was completely covered with soot, but fortunately was restored to virtually perfect condition.

By good fortune, the pre-Civil War farm house adjacent to the Headquarters structure, which the College owned was, at the time, occupied by the Group Insurance Administrators. With the cooperation of the Claypooles, administrators of the insurance programs, most of the College Administrative Staff along with the Editorial Department of the *Annals* were crowded into the building until the damaged wing could be rebuilt. By reopening a third floor of the house and using the basement in an undamaged part of the Headquarters building, the College Staff was able to operate at near normal capacity during the rebuilding.

The R. M. Shoemaker Co., which had erected the burned out wing five years earlier, estimated that it would cost approximately $325,000 to rebuild. In April, 1966, the Finance Committee stated that it seemed prudent, in restoring the structure, to incorporate some improvements over the previous building. The following November, the Board appropriated $70,000 in the 1967 budget to cover estimated costs. Among the items approved for installation were (1) a more sophisticated heating/air conditioning system, replacing the electronic controls with pneumatically operated controls to eliminate most of the fire hazards present in the old control system; (2) a sprinkler system; (3) completion of the third floor for offices, and (4) carpeting. While these improvements cost more than could be realized from the settlement with the insurance companies, funds were available in the Operating Fund Surplus and could be utilized without dipping into the Building Fund, the Endowment Fund or solicitation of special assessment from membership.

Reconstruction began in June, 1966, and it was hoped that reoccupancy could begin shortly after Christmas.

## Annual Session 1966

In spite of the hardships imposed by the fire, the 1966 New York meeting, which occurred only two months after the fire, recorded the largest attendance at an ACP Annual Session to that date. A total of 5,224 physicians registered, of whom 3,373 were members. Together with spouses, exhibitors, and medical students, a total of 7,804 attended.

The traditional hospital clinics were not held. Instead, several hospitals kept "open house" for physicians interested in visiting particular institutions. The TV sessions were highly successful, though there were some anxious moments over a lost signal which was found just minutes before the first session was to begin. In view of the success of the televised sessions, it was decided that the hospital clinics would not be presented at the Annual Session scheduled for San Francisco.

In his out-going Presidential report in April, 1966, Dr. Ernstene offered the following assessment of the year's work. He believed the removal of restrictions on the length of Associateship adopted the previous year was a great step forward. He thought it would sustain the continued interest of many members who might be lost to the College had we retained the old mandatory rule (advance to Fellow or be dropped). More importantly he felt that the new rule would encourage the retained members to avail themselves of the educational opportunities of the College. Dr. Ernstene felt that the change would increase the stature of Fellowship and would not reduce the traditional standards of excellence that the College expected of its members.

During the past year, he said, the College's new interest in the socioeconomic problems of medicine had become known among other professional groups. The statement approved by the Board of Regents in November, 1965, was well timed to publicize the College's desire to help solve problems in the area which the Millis Commission had been studying. Inasmuch as a great majority of internists were already doing a significant amount of primary care, the proportion who chose general internal medicine might be increased by making a broad intern year an integral part of residency training and reducing the requirements for admission to the examination of the American Board of Internal Medicine [ABIM] to two years beyond internship.

The development of the Tri-College Council had stirred a great deal of interest among specialty societies. In fact, the formation of the TCC stimulated the AMA to set up its own interspecialty committee.

I reported that the total membership as of April, 1966, was 12,987: 34 Masters, 9,266 Fellows, and 3,687 Associates.

In my update on the rebuilding of the Headquarters offices, I informed the Board that the contractor's final estimate was $325,000. This quotation included some additional essential changes: A duct type of air conditioning would be installed as planned originally, eliminating individual units in each room. Also, a modern sprinkler system and smoke detection devices would be placed in the original building.

The report of the Committee on Medical Services recommended that the College adopt ethical guidelines for clinical investigation. Dr. J. Russell Elkinton had represented the College at a meeting in Chicago on this subject. He observed that, to his knowledge, the statement presented to the conference was considerably more detailed than all previous codes of ethics. After extensive discussion the representatives of the three societies for clinical research and the ACP presented the point of view that this code was much too specific and rigid. They, proposed to replace it with the general statement of principles adopted by the World Medical Association in 1964, known as the Helsinki Declaration, and urged its endorsement by these several medical associations. Everyone agreed it would be desirable to write a short introductory paragraph indicating this endorsement. In addition to this action, it was recommended that the ACS, the Society of University Surgeons and perhaps the two corresponding bodies of pediatricians be approached to see if they also would endorse the statement. The proposed preamble was as follows:

We the undersigned medical organizations wish to reaffirm the principles of medical ethics of the American Medical Association which have governed the actions of

American physicians. In addition, with respect to human experimentation we endorse the principles set forth in the Declaration of Helsinki by the World Medical Association.

Following a long discussion about the principles of medical ethics of the AMA, and in view of the fact that only a few of the principles had anything to do with medicine and physicians, and because there are other ethical principles which physicians embrace, Dr. Elkinton recommended the following preamble to the Board.

We the undersigned medical organization endorse the ethical principles set forth in the Declaration of Helsinki by the World Medical Association concerning human experimentation. These principles supplement the principles of medical ethics to which the American physicians already subscribe.

At the Annual Business Meeting, a motion was presented which sought to prevent the acceptance of a bill before the US House of Representatives relative to laboratory animals. The following telegram was dispatched:

In formal action at its 47th Annual Session, the 13,000-member American College of Physicians took a strong stand against this or any other bill or amendment which places control of any aspect of medical research, including animal laboratories associated with hospitals or research facilities, under control of the Secretary of Agriculture. This would introduce a grave threat to medical research. We urge you to take immediate, urgent steps to defeat any such proposals.

During the year, the interest of the ACP in socioeconomic problems in health care increased. Representatives of the College had met with the Ad Hoc Committee on Family Practice of the AMA's Council on Education and presented a statement approved by the Board of Regents in November, 1965. The document emphasized the ACP commitment to help solve problems in this area.

## Millis Commission

At another meeting with the Millis Commission (The Citizen's Committee on Graduate Medical Education), the College expressed awareness of the need for more physicians in family practice, but emphasized that "family practice" and "general practice" were not synonymous terms. A great majority of general internists performed "family practice" limited to adult patients.

It again became apparent that the College should state its views on general medical care, family practice, and the movement to establish a certifying board of family practice. In order that the Board of Trustees of the AMA might become more familiar with the internist's viewpoint before the matter was referred to the House of Delegates, the ACP Board of Regents in April, 1966, approved the following statement prepared by the Committee on Medical Services:

In recognition of the manifold efforts being made to resolve the many problems pertaining to the declining number of physicians in the field of family practice; and cognizant of the fact that physicians of widely varying background, training and specialty orientation currently function as family or personal medical advisers; and in view of its own stated interest in these problems; and while supporting the efforts of the American Academy of General Practice to elevate educational standards by prolonging the period of training for those wishing to qualify as family practitioners, the American College of Physicians feels a responsibility to express its opinion that family practice is not a separate discipline; and that current efforts to upgrade the status of general practitioners by means of board certification will not be successful in solving the problems in this field.

Physicians offer knowledge and availability. Society appears to wish the greatly expanded medical knowledge of today to be more readily available on a personalized basis. Two basic questions exist. First, how can more physicians be interested in the problems of family practice, and second, how can we make more effective use of all the physicians in this field? A number of devices are available by which physicians' services may be made available more readily. Among these are group practice (multidisciplinary), associations of physicians trained in one specialty, clinics and other affiliations of physicians, to mention but a few. Perhaps a more practical method of increasing the availability of physicians with skills oriented toward family practice would be to broaden their training in the behavioral sciences and other appropriate disciplines, so that a physician in any branch of medical practice would be equipped to perform as a family practitioner or medical adviser, in accordance with the dictates of his own preference. The College urges that more study of this matter be made by all interested parties.

Dr. Ernstene proposed an additional solution:

The number of internists performing family practice might be increased by making the internship year an integral part of residency training and reducing the requirements for admission to the examination of the American Board of Internal Medicine to two years of residency training beyond the internship. A third year of residency training might then be credited toward eligibility for the examinations of the Subspecialty Boards in Medicine. It remains to be seen whether the American Board of Internal Medicine will look favorably on such a change.

Discussion on this matter did not cease with the publication of the Regent's statement in the *ACP Bulletin* in April, 1966. Activity, in fact, intensified when the reports of the Citizen's Committee on Graduate Medical Education (the Millis Commission) and the AMA Council on Medical Education's Ad Hoc Committee on Education for Family Practice (Willard Committee) were published. In the following year, the Board would consider its position again at great length.

A White House Conference on Health and Education emphasized that mechanisms for the continuing education of physicians were poorly developed and completely lacking in many areas. It also became apparent that there was an attitude in official health circles that if physicians did not develop a plan of continuing education, one would be developed for them.

The Educational Activities Committee reported to the Board of Regents in April, 1966, that a program of continuing medical education for the internist should be a major concern of the College. They indicated that there was evidence that some physicians' study efforts were ineffective and unproductive, not directed toward better patient care.

While ACP postgraduate courses, Regional Meetings and Annual Sessions were helpful, many members declared they had no way of knowing which areas of medical knowledge were inadequate in their intellectual data base. They could not keep up with the flood of new information. This was demonstrated each year when a number of residents exposed to good residency and fellowship training did poorly on written ABIM examinations. It was difficult for these physicians to identify their deficiencies, because neither the Board exams, nor any other programs, were structured to provide clues to areas of weakness.

Dr. Hugh R. Butt, Chairman, then outlined what his Committee had done and made several recommendations. The following were pertinent:

He had spent considerable time at the National Institutes of Health [NIH], where he encountered a strong feeling that the ACP was an ideal organization to develop new techniques in continuing medical education. The NIH expressed readiness to be helpful in implementation.

The use of TV programs was explored, but the Committee did not feel that this alone could fill the total educational needs.

### Self-Assessment Plan

Dr. Butt described the feeling of many members that current ACP programs were simply not enough. His conversations with members revealed that their biggest concern was that they lacked guidance about what the practicing physician should study. Obviously the single most important problem was that the physician could not identify his areas of deficient knowledge.

Advancement in electronic and computer techniques directed attention to the development of self-examinations for the physician. He could assess his own knowledge. These new techniques made it possible to set up a voluntary self-assessment program in a nonthreatening, confidential manner. *Life, Time* and General Electric were forming a General Learning Corporation. Through Dr. Hayes Caldwell, ACP Governor for Arizona and physician to Henry Luce, head of *Life* and *Time*, this group offered financial support. The Committee, believing that the program, if possible, should be self-supporting, did not accept the offer.

At the Board of Regents meeting in April, 1966, the Committee concluded the College and the profession generally must develop a plan for continuing medical education, or it would be developed for the profession. The College should develop a plan for voluntary self-assessment of educational needs, and this should be done in a helpful and nonthreatening manner.

The Committee requested that the President appoint a small ad hoc subcommittee to study this matter and present a formal recommendation at the November, 1966 Board meeting.

Representatives of the TCC met with the AMA Board of Trustees early in 1966 and expressed the desire of the specialty societies for closer liaison and more direct communication with the AMA. As a result of this conference, the AMA Board of Trustees formed the AMA Interspecialty Committee. Its members were to be comprised of one representative from each of the dozen or more boarded specialty groups.

The functions of the TCC were reviewed, and it was decided that the Council could be more effective with the addition of representatives from other specialties. The American Academy of Pediatrics [AAP] and the American Psychiatric Association [APA] would be included and other specialty societies considered.

The Medical Intersociety Council, representing a number of professional organizations, was formed to provide a forum to those in the medical community. At its first meeting, representatives of the ACP, ACS, ACOG, AMA, AAP, Association of Professors of Medicine [APM], American Hospital Association [AHA], American Surgical Association [ASA], and the Association of American Medical Colleges [AAMC] met with various government experts from Health, Education and Welfare [HEW], NIH, the Food and Drug Administration [FDA] and Medicare.

The government representatives expressed the need to establish open lines of communication with the entire medical profession and not exclusively through the AMA. The AMA was represented in the group in proper perspective to the total aspect of medicine; patently it was not the only organization capable of speaking for medicine. College participation in this body provided an excellent opportunity to offer expertise on medical legislative matters at a high governmental level.

Results of the three ACP-APA pilot programs in community hospitals in Houston, Nashville, and Boston encouraged the College to reapply to the National Institute of Mental Health for a five-year grant. This was designed to explore and promote the education of internists and other practicing physicians in psychiatric techniques along with the integration of psychiatric services into the hospital setting. The ACP-APA Task Force concluded that the three pilot study prototypes were applicable to hospitals in a variety of settings.

The Methodist Hospital in Houston appointed a psychiatrist to the staff and a service in psychosomatic medicine was in the planning stage.

In Boston, at the Faulkner Hospital, a psychiatric service was integrated with the medical and surgical services. Psychoneurotic patients were cared for on an outpatient basis and a staff of six psychiatrists were appointed to contribute consulting and supervising services. Psychiatrists made weekly visits to physicians' offices where the psychiatrist observed the practicing physician examine a selected patient. Every third week the six psychiatrists and the practicing physician would meet together for exchange of information.

Another approach to the problem was developed by the St. Thomas and Baptist Hospitals in Nashville. The two institutions were located one street apart and the combined 800-bed complex had an attending staff largely common to each. They jointly presented two-hour evening seminars, led by a psychiatrist, twice monthly, for eight to ten internists who were representative of the teaching committees of the hospitals. A four-day postgraduate course was planned for 12 internists who had completed residency and were practicing in the hospitals.

It was hoped that these three programs would provide prototypes of continuing education for ACP Members in psychiatry and psychosomatic medicine, as "open" clinics developed in community hospitals. Residents moving into practice from such hospitals would profit from these programs.

Experience with the program showed that those who participated found the exercise worthwhile, but were reluctant to add new members to the group. This one factor, excluding those who had not "suffered together", determined its failure as an expanding program.

It had long been the policy of the College to have an active program for visiting spouses at the Annual Sessions. Because the Chairperson of the Ladies' Entertainment Committee was responsible for the Ladies' Program, the Board of Regents allocated funds to permit the Committee Chairperson to attend the preceding Annual Session.

In order to provide for future expansion of College Headquarters, the Board of Regents empowered the Executive Director to acquire real estate in the immediate vicinity of the headquarters as properties were placed on the market. Total expenditure for that purpose was not to exceed $75,000 during 1967.

During the ensuing few years, nine houses were purchased, seven on Osage Street and two on Pine Street. Although only one house was immediately adjacent to ACP property, in no place on Osage Street were there more than two consecutive houses not owned by the College. Our intention was to refurbish the houses and negotiate trades in order to obtain houses which could be demolished, providing land on which to build as the College's need for office space continued to expand.

The Board also appropriated $25,000 to the Residency Revolving Loan Fund to ensure that sufficient funds were available to meet requests anticipated during the coming year. An appropriation of $3,000 was approved for 1967 to provide Teaching and Research Scholars travel allowances to attend Annual Sessions.

The ACP film, "Portrait of an Internist," now two years old, continued its popularity and was solidly booked through 1966. Over five million had viewed the film on television and 1,258 groups with a total audience of 65,139 had seen the presentation. It was made available for showings through another calendar year.

In 1966 a new pamphlet entitled, "What is the American College of Physicians", was distributed for dispensing in members' waiting rooms; this was another effort to increase public awareness about internal medicine and the ACP. It was also mailed to those who inquired about the ACP and distributed at various College functions.

The incoming president, Dr. Irving S. Wright, had been searching for some means of strengthening ties with the Royal College of Physicians of London. He was exploring the possibility of a jointly sponsored convention in 1968, when the ACP Annual Session was to be held in Boston. He received enthusiastic support from the Regents. The idea was presented to the Royal College and the President and his Board approved. This promised to be an inspiring scientific event as well as an important step in international relations. Representatives of all the Royal Colleges were contacted and invited to attend as guests of the College.

The Commission on Professional and Hospital Activities [CPHA] experienced a tremendous growth in its computerized programs (PAS and MAP). This success was attributed largely to the services these programs offered to hospitals, which were attempting to meet the utilization review requirements of Medicare. CPHA purchased 35 acres of land in Ann Arbor, near the North Campus of the University of Michigan, as site for a headquarters building. Preliminary plans called for an initial building of about 65,000 square feet. Meanwhile, CPHA installed a second large computer. The Commission paid a monthly rental for data processing equipment that approximated $24,000.

A wholly-owned subsidiary, MedicaData, Inc., was created to provide a mechanism for protecting its tax-exempt status. The new corporation would be permitted to perform research for profit-making organizations and certain other agencies. The 1966 budget of CPHA exceeded $2 million and growth projections indicated a 1968 budget approaching $5 million.

The fruits of the work by the American Joint Committee for Cancer Staging and End Results Reporting were finally realized when the first six fascicles on the staging and reporting of cancer were published and made available for purchase. They included clinical staging systems for cancer of the breast, larynx, cervix, corpus uteri, pharynx, nasopharynx, oropharynx, and hypopharynx. The sixth fascicle included methods for reporting cancer survival and end results.

It had been apparent for a number of years that Joint Commission on Accreditation of Hospitals [JCAH] accreditation activities should be extended beyond the acute care hospital to other health care facilities. The most pressing need in the early to mid-1960s had been the area of nursing homes and homes for the aged. After many years of hard work to bring together many separate organizations, a plan finally emerged to provide a mechanism for accrediting health care facilities and services under the aegis of the JCAH. The National Council for the Accreditation of Nursing Homes, with support from the AMA and the American Nursing Home Association, volunteered to turn over its files to the JCAH.

Problems were introduced by this newly enlarged program, including the necessity to secure a sufficient number of well-qualified surveyors to establish fair and acceptable standards for certification satisfactory to the Commission and comprehensible to the institutions. It was necessary to increase the JCAH headquarters personnel budget.

Difficulties were encountered from the beginning. Approximately 50 percent of the extended-care facilities surveyed were denied accreditation during the six months after the JCAH initiated the program. In striking contrast, only four percent of acute care hospitals were refused accreditation during the same period. Another 20 percent of extended-care facilities were accredited for only one year.

The third Interim Session of the ACP was held in Miami Beach on October 7-9. The opinion of the few attending was that the program was excellent and the facilities left little to be desired. Attendance, however, was so disappointing that the Board of Regents decided no future fall meetings would be scheduled.

Late in 1966, the membership of the College mourned the passing of one of its most distinguished members, Dr. George Morris Piersol. Dr. Piersol made more extensive contributions to the College than almost any other member.

He was an Officer of the College for more than half of his 44 years as a member. He served as President in 1933-34 and Secretary General from 1926 to 1932 and 1937 to 1951. As Chairman of the Committee on Credentials, he was largely responsible for the College's exacting requirements for membership, but recognized the importance of reasonable flexibility in applying the standards based on the applicant's talents, opportunities and objectives.

In his later years, as College Historian, he traced the founding, developments and accomplishments of ACP in the history, *Gateway of Honor*. To recognize his devoted service to the ACP, he received the highest awards that the College could bestow: a Mastership in 1948 and the Alfred Stengel Award in 1951.

# Part Three (1966-1967)

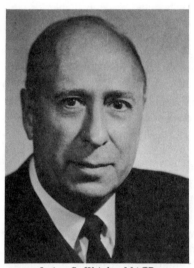

*Irving S. Wright, MACP*

Dr. Irving S. Wright was born in New York City in 1901. With his first wife Grace M. Demarest, he had two children, Barbara and Alison. He married Lois Elliman Findlay in 1953. A lifelong resident of New York City, Dr. Wright received his baccalaureate (1923) and medical (1926) degrees from Cornell University. Following graduate experience at the New York Postgraduate Hospital and Medical School, he was appointed Professor of Clinical Medicine and Head of the Department in 1938. He held this position until 1946. In 1952 he became Professor of Clinical Medicine at Cornell University Medical College, reaching emeritus status in 1968. He served his alma mater as president of the alumni association for one year and later as a trustee of Cornell University from 1960 to 1965. Concomitant with his professorship at Cornell, he was Physician to the New York Hospital, Consulting Physician in eight other New York and New Jersey hospitals, and Physician to the Metropolitan Opera from 1935-1962. During World War II, he was Consultant in Medicine to the Surgeon General of the Army.

The author of more than 350 scientific papers, contributor to several medical textbooks, and author and/or co-author of other scientific texts, Dr. Wright achieved international recognition for his studies of peripheral vascular disease. Long interested in thrombosis and embolism, he pioneered the use of anticoagulants as a form of therapy.

He was president of the New York Heart Association in 1949 and of the American Heart Association in 1952; in both organizations he also served in other capacities. Elected to Fellowship in the American College of Physicians in 1934, he was Governor for New York for eight years, Regent for six years and was elected President in 1966. He served on many committees of the College and frequently gave papers at Annual Sessions. He lectured in numerous medical centers abroad, and such visits brought him honorary memberships in distinguished societies in Argentina, Chile, Colombia, Cuba, Peru, Sweden, Switzerland, and the USSR. He is a Fellow of the Royal College of Physicians of London and an Honorary Member of the Royal Society of Medicine of London.

Numerous United States agencies sought his advice and counsel. He gave his talents generously to the National Research Council, National Advisory Heart Council, National Heart Institute, and President's Commission on Heart Disease and Stroke. In 1960 he received the Albert and Mary Lasker Foundation Award and served on its jury from 1962 to 1975. In recognition of his meritorious and devoted service to the College over a span of nearly 40 years, and for his outstanding achievements in medicine, the College awarded him a Mastership and the Alfred Stengel Memorial Award.

At 77, he founded the American Foundation for Aging Research and in 1982 served as its President. The objective of this organization is to raise funds to support young investigators in the study of mechanisms of illness and disability involving elderly patients.

When the President's Commission on Cancer, Heart Disease and Stroke made its report, Dr. Wright was assiduous about implementing its recommendations. He was instrumental in actions which established centers for study of these diseases in all parts of the country. He contended that places like New York City would have little need for such centers, because adequate facilities already existed for treating stroke victims, whereas, in places like Fargo, North Dakota services might be meager. I advised him to travel more to places like Fargo, because in that city there was an excellent hospital and a very good multidisciplinary clinic, in addition to the fact that transport of stroke victims was far simpler in a small town such as Fargo than it was in larger cities like New York. He laughed and agreed that he had used a poor example.

Dr. Wright suggested that the Nominating Committee of the College should always consider candidates for the positions of Regent who showed potential for assuming the Presidency. He was always concerned about high quality leadership, as this suggestion exemplified.

He enjoyed meeting and hosting distinguished guests. On one occasion he invited Esther and me to New York to have dinner with Dr. and Mrs. Brian Pringle, who was then president of the Royal College of Physicians of Ireland. During cocktails I proposed a toast in Gaelic (given to me by Miss Joan Murphy, my assistant). It was apparent that they understood not one word, and when I conjectured that perhaps my Gaelic was deficient, Mrs. Pringle commented "Oh, we are not Irish, we're British".

Irving was always an enthusiastic individual with many visionary ideas. He was anxious to establish agreeable relationships with most people, and he was tireless in pursuing his objectives. Working with him was easy, for he always wanted full support for his ideas and wanted to be informed when he was wrong.

During my early years at the College, Dr. Wright, who was past president of the American Heart Association [AHA], was very interested in public relations. (When Dr. Dwight Wilbur was President in 1958-59, the College had employed a full time public relations officer, but it did not work out.) In 1961, Dr. Wright asked me to dinner in New York to discuss with him and the man who had started the AHA's public relations program the possibility of creating a similar division in the College. In a letter Dr. Wright suggested we establish such a department; its officer would be responsible to the Public Relations Committee and administratively responsible to me. This was unacceptable to me because I felt that all Staff had to be directly responsible to me and secondarily to a committee upon assignment. I felt so strongly about this that I told Irving that if the Board of Regents adopted this suggestion I would resign and return to California. He recognized that the College was different from the AHA, and we worked out a successful plan to employ a part-time public information officer who would work with the media to report on the Annual Sessions and all other educational activities of the College.

Dr. Wright was the force that brought the official mace of the College into being. On a trip to London with his wife, Irving talked with A.G. Styles at Garrard's of London about the mace. Styles designed the head and heel of the mace. Dr. and Mrs. Wright then traveled to the Isle of Cos. When Lois Wright saw the famous plane tree she exclaimed, "Why don't you get a branch and make the shaft of the mace from that?" Irving tried to get permission to obtain a piece of wood from the tree through one of his former colleagues, who had become a professor in Cos. This effort failed, and he feared that the mace would have to be made of metal. However, the Board approved obtaining more information and asked for a later report. During this time Dr. Theodore Abernathy, a Regent from Washington, DC, prevailed upon a patient, Henry R. Labouisse, the Greek Ambassador to the United States, to intercede. The request went through channels, including the Ambassador, to the King of Greece, to the Mayor of Cos, who later attested to the wood's authenticity.

The course of negotiations also involved Mr. Henry A. Baehr, Agricultural Attache at the US Embassy, who received the wood from the Honorable John Zigdri, Parliamentary Deputy for Cos. When the branch from Hippocrates' tree arrived, it was inspected and seasoned by Dr. Ray N. Seaborg at the University of Wisconsin's Forest Product Laboratory. Don Turano, a sculptor in Washington, DC, designed the shaft, which was carved by a wood sculptor in Williamsburg, Virginia. Dr. Wright was surprised and pleased at this outcome. His plan to have Garrards of London make the head of the mace was accepted.

Dr. Wright's flexibility and facility in helping the Board reach a consensus brought many of his ideas to fruition, as in this instance. After the completion of the mace, he proposed that a suitable College necktie be designed. Incorporated in the tie, designed by Brooks Brothers, was a replica of the head of the mace.

He may be given credit for establishing the Regency Club in 1964. He also initiated the idea of having the President and Executive Director speak at the Regency Club luncheon. This proved to be informationally valuable, both for me and for the older Regents.

Reviewing his presidential year, Dr. Wright recalled that he was representing the College at a Regional Meeting when we called him about the fire in the west wing of the College. He had looked forward to presiding in the Loveland Board Room, but the fire and subsequent reconstruction frustrated this hope. Indeed, he never presided at a meeting at College Headquarters, since all Board meetings were held elsewhere throughout the period of reconstruction.

Dr. Wright was proud of the colloquium: "The Changing Mores of Biomedical Research". He picked all the speakers and felt that had he been as astute in selecting stocks, he would have become a millionaire.

An amusing incident occurred at the colloquium. Mr. Elmer Jones, the convention manager, had not set up the limit timers. He felt speakers at the colloquium were so distinguished that it might bother them to see the red light come on when their time was up. When Dr. Wright learned of this, he jokingly told Mr. Jones that distinguished speakers needed the timer the most. Our Secretary General, Dr. Wallace Yater, suggested that Mr. Jones run a red carpet up to the stage. Since this would have cost several hundred dollars, I would not approve. Mr. Jones asked me what to tell Dr. Yater, and I said, "Tell him you can't find me." Later I explained the cost to Dr. Yater and told him I was sure he didn't want to pay for it. He laughed and agreed with me.

## 1966-1967

Primary care and family practice. Tri-College Council renamed Council of Medical Specialty Societies. AMA Interspecialty Committee. AAMC Council of Academic Societies. JCAH Extended Care Facility Accreditation. Regional Medical Programs for Heart, Cancer and Stroke.

Eleven months after fire destroyed the west wing, the Administrative Staff of the American College of Physicians moved into the reconstructed building. The claim for damage to the structure was settled for $341,079.29. The final cost of several improvements not covered by insurance, but approved by the Board of Regents in November, 1966 totaled approximately $66,000; the addition of offices on the third floor cost $10,000. The cost of the fire protection system was $44,000. The sprinkler system was absolutely essential because putting cement instead of wood floors in the rebuilt wing would have meant constructing a completely new building. The system was installed throughout the new addition and in those parts of the old section where practical. The front reception lobby and the committee rooms on the second floor were excluded because the ceilings did not permit installation of four-inch pipes. These rooms, however, were equipped with smoke detection devices.

The approved carpeting for the entire building and rearrangement of some of the executive office space involved no great additional cost. The air conditioning system cost $12,000. Though an entire air duct system could not be installed, it was possible to introduce a very sophisticated system of controls which would operate pneumatically rather than electronically, minimizing fire hazards which were present in the old building.

At the Fall meeting of the Board of Regents in November, 1966, a change was made in the Fellowship Pledge. The first motion was to rescind the second sentence in the first paragraph, "I have voluntarily accepted membership in this College", and the complete third paragraph, "Further I will avoid commercialism in all my professional activities. I will refrain from seeking the public eye for purposes of seeking self-advancement and I will ask fees commensurate with my services and adjust to the circumstances of the patient"; and the first sentence of the last paragraph, "Finally, I condemn and will avoid all debasing money trades with brother practitioners". These were all deleted. The Fellowship Pledge then read as follows:

> I appreciate that the American College of Physicians has been created to foster the best principles and traditions of our calling. I solemnly pledge to the utmost of my ability I will live in conformity with its ideals and regulations. Now, therefore, I dedicate myself to practice medicine following the Golden Rule and the precepts of the Oath of Hippocrates; to place the welfare of my patients ever before my own; to respect the reputation of my College; to supplement, as occasion requires, my own judgment with the wisdom and counsel of competent medical specialists; to render assistance willingly to my colleagues; to extend freely my professional aid to the unfortunate; to seek increase in medical knowledge by continuing study, by attendance at important gatherings of my professional brethren, by association with physicians of eminence and by free exchange of experience with my colleagues.
>
> I will strive constantly to spread among all physicians the noble ethics of practice set forth in the Constitution and Bylaws of the College.

Dr. Wright, presented an interesting idea for strengthening the ties of the ACP with the Royal College of Physicians of London [RCP(L)]. He woke me at an early hour one morning and proposed that the ACP jointly sponsor an Annual Session with the RCP(L). He called Dr. R.M. Kampmeier, ACP President-Elect, and Sir Max Rosenheim, President of RCP(L), in London. Coincidentally, Sir Rosenheim was to be in New York the following week, and he and Dr. Wright met. Sir Rosenheim was enthusiastic about the idea. They agreed on Boston for such a meeting because it would be less costly for the British traveling to our country, and that 1968 would be the ideal year because it would be the 450th anniversary of the Royal College of Physicians.

Following an ACP sponsored trip to the 1966 International Society of Internal Medicine meeting in Copenhagen, a entire group of ACP Members spent a few days in London, where Sir Rosenheim and the Royal College of Physicians scheduled an afternoon scientific program for the visiting Americans and sponsored a reception at their impressive new headquarters building. Sir Rosenheim and some of his colleagues invited Dr. Philip Corr and me to dinner and displayed obvious enthusiasm about the proposed joint meeting in Boston. I reported this to Dr. Wright, who happily transmitted it to the Board of Regents to support approval of his plan.

## Primary Care

This year was crucial for issues related to the training of internists. On the one hand, though the Millis Commission and the Willard Report had brought the issue of "primary care" to the attention of ACP, AMA, and the American Academy of Family Practice, the College position had opposed the trend toward new training and certifying programs for family practice, espousing internal medicine as a "primary care" specialty. On the other hand, more and more residents in internal medicine were choosing to go into subspecialty training. Both the American Board of Internal Medicine [ABIM] and the Residency Review Committee for Internal Medicine had defined a minimum of 24 months of general internal medicine training, stating that graded patient responsibility must be an absolute minimum core requirement. They insisted that the training and supervision of treatment in these programs must be done by qualified internists.

At this time, ABIM required four years of training in internal medicine, two of which were general, before taking the ABIM examination. Previously, only two years of practice were required before the candidate could be admitted for examination. Another plan to encourage primary care was proposed, which would require a candidate to take two years in pediatrics and two years in internal medicine, and then be certified in both.

The November report of the Executive Director called attention to the 1965 Board of Regents resolution regarding family practice, which was revised at the Board of Regents meeting in April, 1966. I concluded that without these statements the College probably would have been unable to influence either the Citizens Commission (Millis Commission) or the AMA Ad Hoc Committee on Education for Family Practice (Willard Committee) since few members of these bodies seemed to recognize that internists provided a good deal of primary care. Internists in practice commonly work in conjunction with pediatricians, and such patterns should be recognized as a team practice that provides excellent family health care.

I also attended a meeting on continuing education at the AMA, which was called to reconsider the AMA position and role in this area. The House of Delegates had turned down a "national plan" idea. This plan had been the result of a joint effort by nine professional societies, including AMA and ACP. The AMA House of Delegates rejected, rather peremptorily, all recommendations set forth in *Lifetime Learning for Physicians*. The concept of a "university without walls" was imaginative and original. After further discussions in Chicago, the AMA decided to continue exploring and implementing parts of the program. I emphasize this as a good example of the College's influence at various society meetings.

I then described the 9th International Congress on Internal Medicine in Amsterdam, which 130 ACP Members and wives attended. Following the Congress, part of the group went to Copenhagen, Stockholm, and Oslo. In Stockholm, we were guests of Drs. Jorpes and Biorck, at the Karolinska Hospital. Both were Honorary Fellows of the ACP. Following a luncheon, Dr. Biorck spoke to the group on "Sweden - Past and Present."

Closing my report to the Regents, I announced that I had been elected president of the Carleton College Alumni Association. Wesley Spink, Past President, was also an alumnus of this midwestern college.

The Board of Regents was impressed with the caliber of applicants for the new Teaching and Research Scholars, and approved a recommendation from the Committee on Fellowships and Scholarships that one additional scholarship be made available for a three-year period beginning in 1967. Inasmuch as the first two scholars had been promised that they could have the fourth and fifth year, the Regents concluded they could add one scholar starting with the period of July 1967 to 1968.

The House Committee concluded that the College Staff was adequately supervising property maintenance and oversight by busy physicians was no longer necessary. The Committee was discharged with thanks.

The Educational Activities Committee proposed a voluntary educational program designed to provide members with an opportunity for self-evaluation of their current factual knowledge of internal medicine. The exam could be taken privately, in the home or office, and only the participant need know the results. The questions were to be prepared by specifically designated ACP committees and a special firm engaged to send the test questions to subscribers, computer grade the examinations, and return results to participants. The entire project would be handled outside the College administration; complete confidentiality would be guaranteed.

While there was no way to know how the membership would receive this plan, we believed that the College must lead the way in self-assessment and be the first to offer its members such an opportunity to participate in a voluntary program. Considering the ACP's leadership in continuing education, such a step presented opportunities for future development, even if only several hundred participants enrolled in the first program. Despite the recognition of the uncertainties and difficulties of a self-assessment project, the Educational Activities Committee recommended that the project be pursued. The Board of Regents concurred and initiated the first task by selecting nine subspecialty chairmen to write the questions.

Dr. R. H. Kampmeier, Chairman, described the current activities of the ACP/APA Task Force. The pilot projects to develop several prototypical educational models for training practicing internists in the emotional aspects of disease was the basis for reapplication for a National Institutes of Mental Health [NIMH] grant. The three programs were in progress at Methodist Hospital in Houston, Texas, St. Thomas and Baptist Hospitals in Nashville, Tennessee, and in Faulkner Hospital in Boston, Massachusetts. Dr. John Graham, College Governor for Massachusetts and Chief of the Medical Services at Faulkner Hospital was directing the project in the latter hospital.

The Board of Regents accepted a recommendation by the International Medical Activities Committee to rescind that portion of the Bylaws which waived dues for the category of Affiliate Membership. A dues fee of $6.00 per year was established, which included the *ACP Bulletin* and *Annals.* The Regents also approved a new application form for Affiliate Members. Finding it difficult to obtain letters of endorsement from Latin American Fellows, the Committee recommended that the applicant furnish the name of his preceptor during training in the US and the name of the chief of service under whom the candidate was working presently.

## Council of Medical Specialty Societies

Dr. Thomas M. Durant described a meeting of the Tri-College Council held on May 7, 1966. The newly formed Interspecialty Advisory Committee to the Board of Trustees of AMA was discussed, as well as the existing Medical Intersociety Council, which was partly sponsored by the AMA and the Association of American Medical College [AAMC]. The consensus being that the Tri-College Council would be more effective with representation from additional specialties, the constituent bodies decided to support the inclusion of the AAP and the APA. The Tri-College Council was renamed the Council on Medical Specialty Societies [CMSS].

Three interspecialty organizations have been established in the United States since the formation of the CMSS in 1966. The first of these was the previously mentioned AMA Interspecialty Committee. This was developed in the hope that specialty societies could gain representation in the House of Delegates. Unhappily, it was treated simply as an advisory body to the AMA Board of Trustees with little clout.

## Council of Academic Societies

The second interspecialty organization was established when the AAMC formed a Council of Academic Societies [CAS] early in 1967, consisting of academic groups and those with limited membership such as the Association of American Physicians and the American Surgical Association. Later, colleges such as the ACP were invited to join.

The third, the Medical Intersociety Council, was made up of a great number of clinical and academic societies and while active, its major concern was the exchange of information with various agencies of government. After a few meetings this organization was discontinued.

A principal objective of the CMSS was to achieve adequate specialty society representation in the House of Delegates of the AMA. When the AMA Interspecialty Council was created, need for the CMSS was questioned. The representative societies responded that a definite need existed for an interspecialty organization independent of the AMA.

The AMA, the ACS, the AHA, and the ACP had established the Joint Commission on Accreditation of Hospitals [JCAH] in 1951. In the 14 years of its existence, the hospital accreditation standards had been amended several times. A new administration in 1966 introduced several additional accrediting activities and a general expansion of services. A review was initiated in 1967 to determine if standards were current and enforceable in the light of prevailing medical knowledge, hospital administration, organization and practice, and the capability to evaluate the level of quality of patient care.

The procedure of the JCAH was to consult, examine, grade (and accredit or not accredit) a candidate hospital. While the administrator of a hospital was result oriented, the JCAH was more concerned about the capability of the institution to deliver quality care and the dialogue stimulated between the physician and administrative members of the hospital staff and the JCAH physician surveyors.

In 1966, the JCAH expanded to include review of extended care facilities. Most of 1967 was spent revising definitions, JCAH standards and possible interpretations, and the survey procedures for this new activity. Three classes of non-hospital institutions were identified: post-hospital extended care facilities or convalescent hospitals; long-term care facilities, not necessarily post-hospital, but providing continuous service in nursing homes; and domiciliary homes, which presented mainly supportive care with regular and intermittent nursing and medical service. Any other institution which did not fit one of those categories would be offered a "non-accreditation" service to review its operation and help it decide if it wished to become identified with one of these categories.

The JCAH also expanded into the accreditation of rehabilitation facilities. A contract was signed to provide administrative, executive, and field survey accreditation services for the Commission on Accreditation of Rehabilitation Facilities. This commission, which included rehabilitation centers, sheltered workshops and homebound programs, wanted to be involved in integrated programs concerned with health care. The JCAH studied and reorganized the structure, distributing responsibilities of setting standards and making decisions within the categories of expertise and competence. In addition, this relationship with the JCAH provided an integrating influence on the philosophy of accreditation of health services. It was not easy, but the JCAH hoped to develop a central umbrella under which all accreditation services in the field of health care could be accommodated.

The ACP Board of Regents was asked by the JCAH for an opinion about a stipulation that a member of the medical staff be on the governing body of a hospital. A motion was passed in April, 1967, approving, in principle, official representation of the professional medical staff on governing bodies of hospitals. However, this was revised in November to state:

> The Board of Regents wishes to clarify its previous approval in principle on requiring official representation of medical staff on governing bodies of hospitals. It is clear that in many hospitals, whether government, religious, university, or other, it would be impossible for the hospital to adopt such a rule, it being prohibited either by law or fundamentals of organization. There is evidence to show that on some occasions such an arrangement actually has interfered with good policy procedures. In many hospitals, close liaison between the governing body and the medical staff is accomplished by an effective joint conference committee which has regularly scheduled meetings (these should be at least four or more times a year). Another method of involving medical staff in policy making is to appoint individuals to governing body committees. For these reasons, the Board of Regents continues to

approve medical staff representation on governing bodies of hospitals, but on a voluntary, rather than on an obligatory or mandatory basis.

Interest in animal experimentation reached a fever pitch in 1966 with 25 to 30 pieces of legislation introduced into Congress. Anticipating a rapid expansion of activities in view of actual and contemplated federal legislation, the American Association for Accreditation of Laboratory Animal Care [AAALAC] submitted a request for financial support to the National Institutes of Health [NIH]. In April, 1967, it was reported to the ACP Board of Regents that the NIH was unable to act on the request for funds until definitive legislation was passed.

There was unanimity in the AAALAC Board of Trustees that it should continue with its original program of inspection and certification of laboratory animal facilities on the basis of voluntary application from various kinds of institutions. Requests for accreditation continued, although at a slower rate. Uncertainties emerged concerning the internal stability of the AAALAC when the administrative head of the association took a leave of absence due to illness, and the Chairman of the Board resigned. The search for a full-time executive director, with staff support, was begun late in 1967, and a schedule of inspections was set up for early 1968. Financing continued as in the past, with expenses of site visits covered by fees charged for inspection. In view of the uncertainty of both the nature and timing of congressional action, the AAALAC Trustees considered it more important than ever that a non-governmental agency maintain its surveillance of facilities. This was considered important from the aspect of animal care and the public interest in animals. The ACP continued its support.

The ABIM was faced continuously with the problems of examining an increasing number of applicants and, at the same time, improving the written and oral examinations, in an effort to continue their efforts to distinguish between qualified and unqualified candidates with efficiency and fairness. Two major projects planned for 1966 involved a critical reevaluation of both the oral and written examinations.

The objectives of the reevaluation of the oral examination were threefold:

1. Standardization of the environment of the examination was sought, to eliminate many variables inherent in the use of different patient populations in many different hospitals with dissimilar physical and ancillary facilities. The ABIM achieved its objectives in part by increasing the Board from 12 to 15 members and by developing a cadre of experienced examiners.

2. Within the framework of a practical bedside examination based on the management of the patient at hand, the format of the examination was scrutinized to eliminate unnecessary variables affecting the fairness of the examination. This was a difficult task and was unlikely to be entirely achieved.

3. The grading procedure was observed critically in order to increase discrimination in the criteria for success or failure. The Board was aware unhappily that the majority of candidates fell into a grey area between those who had clearly passed and those who had clearly failed, and the

ABIM was determined to refine its capability to discriminate. An experimental grading system under trial in the first two examinations in 1966 promised to be useful.

Of serious concern to the ABIM, and worthy of College attention, was the six percent increase in the oral examination failure rate during recent years as compared to a stable rate for many years previously. It was possible that this phenomenon paralleled the 26 percent increase in candidates who had failed previously one or more oral examinations. But the possibility that residency programs were not training candidates adequately could not be dismissed; a large number of failures were due to deficiencies in history-taking, physical examination, and synthesis of a diagnosis.

Although there seemed to be widespread agreement that the written examination accomplished its purpose effectively, new techniques and formats were being studied by a review committee.

The ABIM announced that it had leased half a floor at the National Board of Medical Examiners' new headquarters in Philadelphia and that Dr. Palmer Futcher, FACP, would succeed Dr. Victor Logan, FACP, as Executive Director of the Board. Dr. Futcher was an Associate Professor of Medicine at Johns Hopkins and was to assume his new position on January 1, 1967.

Considerable discussion in 1966 revolved around the problems faced by those who operated training programs in large charity hospitals. With the advent of Medicare implementation, there was little doubt that strong efforts would be exerted to make these hospitals open-staff community hospitals. The Residency Review Committee in Internal Medicine [RRC-IM] and the ACP was concerned lest the teaching and supervision of such programs fall into the hands of unqualified physicians. For that reason they presented to the Board of Regents the following statement which was adopted as ACP policy:

1. In the training of Residents in Internal Medicine, the primary responsibility for the teaching must be held by qualified internists.
2. The ultimate responsibility for patient care on graduate teaching medical services must be the responsibility of qualified internists.

The National Institutes of Health introduced new regulations in training programs which affected International Fellowships. In April, 1966, the International Medical Activities Committee reported that new legislation excluded any person not a citizen of the US from all NIH traineeship programs. The Committee interceded and expressed its concern to officials of the NIH.

Dr. Pollard, a Committee member, subsequently learned from Dr. Karl Mason, an NIH official, that any traineeship program would be allowed by special request to have 10 percent of their program positions filled by foreign trainees. Unfortunately, very few programs in existence had even ten trainees in one division of a department of medicine and most programs had only two to four, eliminating them from consideration. Individual approvals were extremely rare. The International Medical Activities Committee was directed to convey the College's concern in person to proper officials of the NIH, and specific members of government, to urge a more far-sighted and flexible regulatory policy with respect to foreign trainees.

The College's Kellogg Fellowship Program was directly affected. Most Kellogg Fellows compiled marvelous records of achievement in their medical schools upon their return to Central and South America. Since the training took place in the United States, there was no dollar drain and no significant "brain drain" from those countries. Figures showed that almost 200 such trainees had returned to their homelands. Only one returned permanently to the USA.

## Annual Session 1967

The 48th Annual Session of the College held in San Francisco in April, 1967, was by all standards a great success. With over 5,000 physicians registered, including 2,991 members, this Session took its place among the larger ACP meetings in recent history.

In an endeavor to focus the attention of other learned professional groups on the importance of the ACP, President Wright conceived the idea of a public colloquium on the "Changing Mores of Biomedical Research". This was presented as a regular part of the Annual Session program; its success exceeded all expectations. Panelists invited by Dr. Wright were: Judge Warren Burger, United States Court of Appeals, Washington, DC, later Chief Justice of US Supreme Court (Law); Professor Joshua Lederberg, PhD, Stanford University (Genetics); Sir Peter Medawar, FACP (Hon.), National Institute for Medical Research, London (Genetics); Thomas Starzl, MD, Chief, Surgical Services, VA Hospital, University of Colorado Medical School (Transplant Surgery); Professor Samuel Stumpf, PhD, Vanderbilt University (Philosophy); Professor David Krech, PhD, University of California, Berkeley (Psychology). Each presented his views on the subject as it related to his discipline. Two "challengers," Dr. Rene Dubos of Rockefeller University, and Dr. Chauncey Leake of the University of California, San Francisco, then questioned the expressed views of the panelist, and encouraged cross-examination of opinions by members of the colloquium. Faculties and students from the San Francisco schools of medicine, philosophy, law, religion and psychology were invited. Through such interdisciplinary presentations, the Board hoped to strengthen the role of the College in matters of current public concern.

The Convocation Oration was given by Dr. Lee A. DuBridge, PhD, President, California Institute of Technology, on "Exploring the Solar System."

While the San Francisco Annual Session program was a fine one, major changes were anticipated for the 49th meeting to be held in Boston in 1968. It had become clear in recent years that division of original papers into clinical sessions, clinical investigation, and basic science had served its purpose. In the future, original papers, whether clinical or research in nature, were to be scheduled in subspecialty areas of interest: cardiology, pulmonary diseases, allergy and immunology, gastroenterology. The Board of Regents felt that this change would make it possible to present basic science and clinical papers relating to the same subjects during the same session.

Another innovation to be inaugurated in Boston was the "Meet the Professor" sessions. Attendance at these informal sessions would be limited to 15 participants to facilitate dialogue with the professor and provide ample opportunity to discuss subjects within his/her realm of expertise. Initially, 12 were scheduled to run throughout the week; each would last one and a half hours.

Increased interest by the profession in the Annual Session of the College was reflected in the record-breaking number of 650 abstracts submitted for the 1967 meeting. Custom at this time required the President to rate and set all submitted abstracts in priority. So many submissions necessitated that this labor, henceforth, would be divided among members of the Committee on Scientific Program. The Board of Regents designated a Cochairman of the Committee, who would serve for a number of years and provide continuity to the work of the Committee. The President continued to invite all guest speakers, remained in charge of the Convocation and bore responsibility for general supervision of the entire scientific program. The cochairman presided at the meetings of the Committee and with the approval of the President, implemented decisions of the Committee.

Amendments to the Constitution and Bylaws ratified at the San Francisco Session outlined the qualifications for Fellows, Associates and Affiliate Members, including methods of proposal and privileges of Fellows, Associates, and Affiliate Members. These newly adopted Bylaws facilitated the admission of qualified candidates to membership in the ACP.

Under the new rules, the Governors were given more latitude in proposing candidates for Associateship. Though an individual may have been dropped previously and failed the Boards, now he might be again eligible for membership. It was up to the Governor to decide on those who had failed the ABIM examination and would never take it again. However, if the ABIM examination had never been taken, nor scheduled, the candidate was not eligible. Age ceased to be a criterion. Instead, time out of school was the new guide and published material was no longer an absolute requirement for advancement, except among candidates who failed to show other evidence of professional growth.

At the Board of Governors meeting in April, 1967, the Executive Committee proposed for the first time, that the name "Associate" be changed to "Member". This was taken under advisement for further study. The Executive Committee of the Board of Governors, with the Board's support, also suggested that a new category of membership be defined to include young physicians still in training in order to interest them in the College at an early stage.

The Board of Governors received the results of the questionnaire sent to Associates, which yielded a 64 percent return. Of this group, 96 percent of the total showed adequate activity in ACP and other continuing medical education programs. The Governors reported to the Board of Regents that these results satisfied the Committee that the Associates were indeed taking an active part in continuing medical education activities.

Another recommendation was forwarded to the Board of Regents relating to the number of annually awarded Masterships, based on a motion made by W. Philip Corr, Chairman of the Board of Governors' Executive Committee. Since there were so many members of the College deserving of this honor, it was recommended that number of Masters be increased gradually over a period of years, emphasizing the maintenance of present standards. Dr. Corr pointed out that the College was electing exactly the same number of Masters each year, virtually unchanged despite the doubling of membership. The Governors felt that it would be advantageous to have at least one Master from each region of the College. It would be stimulating and helpful to the new members of the College to meet and get to know physicians who set such fine examples of loyalty to the College, and to medicine generally.

The Executive Committee also conveyed to the Board of Governors my analysis of physician practice among the College members: 8,532 of these were in private practice and 2,767 were engaged in other activities. Of the latter, 1,125 were on medical school faculties, 815 worked full time on hospital staffs and 220 were in military services. The primary specialty of internal medicine was indicated by 7,030 members, 693 of whom were over 65 years of age. Other specialties cited included cardiology, allergy, gastroenterology, psychiatry, dermatology, neurology, pathology and radiology.

At the April meeting of the Board of Regents, I reported that total membership had reached 13,650, of which 32 were Masters, 9,673 were Fellows, 3,839 were Associates and 106 were Affiliates.

In relation to family practice issues, I noted that the position of the College was hard to explain because there simply were not enough internists to fill the gap left by the disappearance of general practitioners. By stating that it did not think the proposed "new" family physician concept would attract many, the College was placing itself in a reactionary and negative position. I urged that the College assume a more positive position of leadership by demanding more internists and, in fact, demanding more physicians of all types.

In matters of government relationships, I advised that the College use care not to bite off more than it could swallow. It was easy to go to Washington and be "for" something. It was much harder to make the College's position heard effectively when it was "against" something. The College could very easily be maneuvered into being almost always against AMA positions. This would be harmful to both and would be exactly what the social planners would like. The College could operate best in this area by working closely with those associated with the government who were at least friendly to the College, such as Philip Lee, Ivan Bennett, John Layne, Dwight Wilbur, and James Cain.

The Committee on Cancer reported that since its April, 1966 meeting it had conducted a systematic examination of the relationships of internal medicine to cancer care. The study was organized into three main sections:

1. The role of the internist in cancer.
2. Needs of internists concerned with the cancer problem.
3. The role of the Cancer Committee of the ACP.

Conclusions of the study were summarized:

The contributions of the physician in practice to the large clinical problem of neoplastic disease are conceived to be in the area of knowledge and use of new diagnostic procedures, such as cytology, radioisotopes and radiologic examinations; sophisticated triage which requires contemporary information on the indications and limitations of radiotherapy and surgery for specific tumor entities, and medical management of disseminated neoplastic disease which at the present time includes approximately two-thirds of all patients.

The physician in a teaching institution has responsibilities for student, house officer, fellow and practicing physician training in the natural history of the varieties of neoplastic disease, the mechanisms of distorted physiology in the tumor-bearing human host, and in medical therapy. In cancer research institutes, the internist plays a central role in the conception and conduct of clinical research. In the regional programs the internist will have major functions in training, representation on tumor boards, dissemination and interpretation of current research information, as well as direction of the medical management of patients with neoplastic disease.

Conclusions of the second section, "The Needs of Internists Concerned with the Cancer Problem," premised that

> . . . If it is accepted that the internist has important and diverse roles to play in the clinical problems of cancer, he is in a position to accept the responsibilities of clinical research and complex patient care. Although internists increasingly recognize their enlarged obligations in neoplastic disease, additional emphasis is still required.

One important need identified was recognition by the ABIM of one year of training on an approved medical oncology service toward fulfilling requirements to take the ABIM examination. Additionally, the Committee concluded that more questions on ABIM examination in the field of neoplastic disease might well stimulate the internist's interest and facilitate recognition of deficiencies in knowledge of neoplastic disease.

Finally, the Committee discussed its relationship to the overall function of the College, noting its potential and actual areas of usefulness:

1. A forum for interdisciplinary association.
2. Availability of the Committee members to the Board of Regents as consultants in the area of cancer.
3. Committee services to aid the Scientific Program Committee of the College in screening abstracts for the Annual Session in order to select the best quality papers for presentation.
4. Organization of postgraduate courses on cancer under College auspices, initiated by individual members of the Committee.
5. The Committee report emphasized to the Board of Regents that the very existence of a Cancer Committee within the structure of the ACP constituted significant and necessary recognition by the nation's leading physicians that the problem of neoplastic disease is an area of importance to internists.

The national office of the Regional Programs on Heart Disease, Cancer and Stroke, had entered into a contract with the American College of Surgeons [ACS] to establish standards and evaluate institutions to determine their competence and qualifications as cancer centers. To this end, the ACS Cancer Commission consisted of representatives of all medical specialties, selected professional and non-professional organizations, and consultants from allied medical and professional services.

The Cancer Commission was formed to assist the Division of Regional Medical Programs of the US Public Health Service in implementing the provisions of Section 907 of Public Law 89-239:

> The Surgeon General shall establish, and maintain on a current basis, a list or lists of facilities in the United States equipped and staffed to provide the most advanced methods and techniques in the diagnosis and treatment of heart disease, cancer, or stroke, together with such related information, including the availability of advanced specialty training in such facilities, as he deems useful, and shall make such list or lists and related information readily available to licensed practitioners and other persons requiring such information. To the end of making such list or lists and other information most useful, the Surgeon General shall from time to time consult with interested national professional organizations.

Physicians would have an important role in the Regional Centers Program on Cancer; the ACP Committee on Cancer considered it a matter of importance that the College participate actively in this national effort to improve the quality of medical care. The Board of Regents voted to continue the Committee and authorized it to propose an outline of standards for internal medicine which could be utilized by ACP representatives to the Cancer Commission.

The activities of the AMA Advisory Committee on Occupational Therapy, American Registry of Physical Therapists' Advisory Board, and American Physical Therapy Association were all concerned about the existing and increasing shortage of professional paramedical personnel. There were only 13 schools for the allied medical professions, and these were fashioned along the lines of the first one at the University of Pennsylvania, established in 1950. It was estimated that within the next few years 60 more institutions would build paramedical programs around existing physical therapy and occupational therapy schools, in addition to those being developed. Both the Veterans' Administration and the Department of Health, Education and Welfare [HEW] estimated a potential shortage of one million individuals in the paramedical professions. The heart, cancer, and stroke programs being organized across the nation also confirmed this projected shortfall. The College, aware of immediate and increasing demands, decided to maintain active lines of communication in these burgeoning fields.

The National Research Council's [NRC] Division of Medical Sciences continued to be active in advising agencies of government and studying medical problems of interest to the scientific societies represented in the Council, including the College. One activity that commanded attention during 1967 was an Efficacy Study of Drugs for the Food and Drug Administration [FDA]. The FDA had entered into a contract with the National Academy of Sciences [NAS] through the NRC and its Drug Research Board [DRB], on which the College was represented. The DRB was charged to review all drugs approved by the FDA from 1938-1962 for proof of clinical effectiveness. Confronting the group was the enormous task of evaluating more than 4,000 drugs.

The DRB fulfilled an important mission of the NRC by commenting upon the various regulations issued by the FDA which affected every doctor in the United States, whether active practitioner, clinical investigator, or scientist. The College, through its postgraduate education programs and the Annual Session, had taken an active part as a national society in bringing to the attention of the membership such important problems as the issue of informed consent.

A survey of the College membership determined that a significant number of members was interested in a "Group Plan for High Limit Accidental Death and Dismemberment Insurance." The Group Insurance Administrators [GIA] for the ACP were authorized to secure a master policy and proposals from several insurance companies were reviewed. Bankers Life and Casualty Company of Chicago made the best offer and was selected.

The Board of Regents took under advisement a policy statement on the matter of "Smoking and Health" and approved the following resolution: "The Board of Regents of the American College of Physicians endorses the warning issued by the Surgeon General of the dangers of the use of tobacco."

In November, 1967, the Regents completed deliberations on the funds from the James D. Bruce estate, and approved the award of five traveling scholarships in the amount of $500 each, for a period of three years beginning in 1968. The balance of income from the legacy was made available to the International Medical Activities Committee and was used to support South American postgraduate courses sponsored in conjunction with the College.

Two memorials were established by the Board of Regents in 1967 in recognition of Dr. George Morris Piersol, Past President, Past Secretary General, and Master of the College, and Dr. William C. Menninger, FACP, both of whom had died in 1966. One ACP teaching and research scholar a year was to be designated the George Morris Piersol Teaching and Research Scholar. To recognize his distinguished contributions to the science of mental health, the William C. Menninger Award was established. Dr. Menninger had been a College Governor for Kansas, 1949-1958; a member of the Board of Regents, 1958-1963; and the First Vice President of the ACP, 1964-65. The award was supported by the Menninger Foundation.

Because of uncertainty concerning the number of copies of the College history, *Gateway of Honor,* needed at the time of initial printing, 1,000 fewer copies were bound than had been printed. While this saved a considerable amount of money at the time the book was made available, all of the 3,000 bound copies had been distributed. For this reason the additional 1,000 copies were bound and made available.

The College received a fortunate offer from the W.B. Saunders Company to index the *Gateway of Honor,* including composition and preparation of negatives for offset printing without cost and the College assumed the cost of printing.

Everyone who purchased a copy of the *Gateway of Honor* was sent a free index.

For many years, Surgeon Generals of the Army, Navy, Air Force, and Public Health Services had been automatically appointed Governors of the ACP during their term of service. The Committee on Military Affairs and Disaster Medical Care thought that a modification was needed; that the Governors for the respective services should be internists and members of the College. In actual practice, when the Surgeon General had not been an internist or Fellow, most College liaison was conducted by a deputy who was usually a Fellow. The Committee opinion was that if the deputy were made Governor, liaison between College Headquarters and Washington would be enhanced and greater interest in ACP affairs among the military would follow. The Committee recommended therefore, that the Surgeon General of a military service should become, automatically, College Governor, provided he was a Fellow and he wished to assume the duties himself. If the appointee was an internist but not a Fellow, he was to be elected directly to Fellowship and subsequently receive an appointment as ACP Governor. If he was of another discipline, he was to be asked to nominate a Fellow of the College within his office who could then be appointed.

Now that Associates were granted membership without limit of term, Life Membership in the College was available for them, at identical dues rates as for Fellows.

Membership cards had been distributed annually upon receipt of the member's dues. This expense was mitigated by the decision to issue a permanent membership card, similar to the laminated Life Membership card, at the time a member was elected to ACP.

A bill was introduced in Congress by Senator Lister Hill (North Carolina) which called for the creation of the post of Under Secretary of Health. There existed no office for the overall coordination of federal health programs, and since further reorganization of HEW in the field of health was being contemplated, the President of the College wrote to the HEW Secretary emphasizing that,

> The American College of Physicians, representing 15,000 internists in this country, would appreciate the opportunity for its President and certain other officers to meet with the Secretary or his designated representative, to express our views in favor of Senator Hill's bill. We are in agreement with the proposal that the Under Secretary of Health should be the senior policy adviser on all health programs in the Department. We recognize that while it is not possible to place all programs, for example, Medicare, under the direct administrative control of this Secretary, we believe that he should be able to speak for the Secretary in all health policy matters.

The American Society of Internal Medicine [ASIM] Liaison Committee was informed of the action and invited to use its "grass roots" organization to work with the College in a cooperative venture to help implement the intention of Senator Hill's bill.

In related action, the Board of Regents approved a recommendation that the College's Committee on Comprehensive Health Services replace the Subcommittee on Governmental Activities in Medicine and report directly to the Medical Services Committee. This new committee would relate to the Public Health Service by serving as a consultant to the Bureau of Health Services, to assist in the development of government financed programs in personal health care.

## "Forces Reshaping Medicine"

With the great variety of laws, regulations, projects, studies and the like, which seem to be spawning utter confusion in the minds of most of us, [wrote Dr. James W. Haviland, Chairman of ACP Medical Services Committee, in the June 1967 *Bulletin*] it may be worthwhile to review and summarize some of the activities presently in progress which will reshape the delivery of health care as we know it today. Some are frightening, some are irritating, some are interesting, but all of them deserve understanding, so that the medical profession can maintain the quality of medical care even in the face of the almost inevitable erosion occasioned by bureaucracy.

Certainly the federal legislation of recent years is the best known of any of these factors. Medicare and Medicaid (P.L. 89-97) need no further discussion. The Regional Medical Planning Program (P.L. 89-239 or the "DeBakey Program"), likewise, is well known and is being actively pursued in many areas. Less well known is the recently enacted comprehensive health planning legislation (PL. 89-749) which provides money for each of the states to establish comprehensive health planning groups, with at least half the advisory council composed of "representatives of the consumers of health care".

This feature of strong representation by the consumer public is becoming popular in all sorts of federal health activities at the present time. The Office of Economic Opportunity programs (OEO or antipoverty programs) have just begun to be recognized for what they are, that is, easily identified by their stressing the development of the concept of "neighborhood health centers", in which the federal agency brings in complete medical care teams to community areas where the local resources are felt to be either inadequate or improperly placed.

Medicine's activities in this field, [Dr. Haviland continued] have come in for a good deal of recent discussion. The Millis Commission Report (Graduate Education of Physicians) with its emphasis among other items, on the development of large numbers of "primary physicians", and the Willard Committee Report (The Ad Hoc Committee on Education for Family Practice) with its emphasis on a similarly trained and functioning physician entitled, "The Family Physician", have given strength to the recently published plans and suggestions of the American Academy of General Practice for training the family practitioner of the future. The AMA, through its Board of Trustees and Council on Medical Education, has been active in sponsoring these reports.

The Association of American Medical Colleges published its report, (the so-called Coggeshall Report), giving still another approach to the way in which physicians should be educated in the future. It is also well known that curriculum revisions are under active consideration in a great many medical schools around the country. Some revisions are actually in operation or about to be activated. In many instances, however, they are still in the discussion phase, but all of them seem to be looking toward the requirements of training physicians functioning in a day of great increases in scientific knowledge, specialization, computerization, and yet coincidentally trying to meet demands for large amounts of personal physician care.

[Dr. Haviland concluded his *ACP Bulletin* article by saying] Medicine has as one of its key responsibilities in the immediate future, the maintenance of quality of the product it delivers.

Clearly, there were many questions facing the medical community concerning the delivery of health care. The ACP was active either formally or informally through its own committee system and representation on a number of committees and commissions of other organizations.

## Emergency Care

Yet another area of increasing concern to the medical community, emergency first aid and medical care, was the topic of a report by the Committee on Trauma and the Committee on Shock of the National Academy of Sciences and the National Research Council. Outlining the basics of the report in my January, 1967 Executive Director's Page in the *ACP Bulletin*, I noted,

Transportation of the injured to the place where expert care can be given will become increasingly important. Committees could learn much from studies of how this was done by the Armed Services. In World War I, 8 percent died before getting to the medical facility. This figure dropped to 4.5 per cent in WW II, to 2.5 percent in Korea, and is less than 2 percent in Vietnam. . . . There are fewer patients today who get any of their medical service at home. In the past few years, the total percentage of a physician's service involved in making home visits has dropped from nine percent to less than five percent. The injured person has learned that the place to go is the emergency room in the nearby community hospital. It would seem a primary responsibility of all physicians to make sure that competent and expert professional service is available at the hospital. This cannot be adequately solved by having foreign graduates staff such facilities without supervision.

I also wondered why,

In our country known for its technical know-how, . . . we can communicate with astronauts in space, but can't get a communication system operating so an ambulance can be in voice contact with the emergency room it is approaching. . . . All kinds of improvements in communications are essential. Emergency departments need to be categorized by depth of service and some system of accreditation should be developed.

I noted in conclusion:

Some other general directions should be considered. We should develop trauma registries to develop material for long-term studies of the natural history of various injuries. Hospital Trauma Committees should be active. Convalescence, disability and rehabilitation should be studied and programs developed for rehabilitation of all injured and not reserved only for the permanently disabled. Medico-legal problems deserve emphasis and lay coroners should be replaced everywhere by medical examiners who are not only physicians but highly qualified forensic pathologists. Autopsies should be a routine procedure on all accident victims. Finally, much research in trauma should be encouraged.

The members of the College should join their surgical colleagues on these trauma and emergency committees. There is too much at stake, [I cautioned] to presume that accidents are primarily the concern of surgeons. For example, internists have much greater responsibilities in prevention of accidents and, because of their knowledge of shock, heart disease and the effects of drugs, they should take an active part in this pressing problem.

The Board of Regents, having gone on record in both November, 1965, and in April, 1966, concerning the family practice situation, directed the Medical Practice Committee to study The Millis Commission Report and the Willard Report in detail.

## Family Practice

On September 30, 1966, the ACP sponsored a meeting of the MPC Ad Hoc Subcommittee on Family Practice with the (AMA) Willard Committee in Chicago. The previous policy statements of the College concerning family practice and factors affecting medical manpower problems were reviewed in detail, thereafter, by the Medical Practice Committee. The resulting Board resolution in November, 1966, responded to the Willard Report and endorsed the Millis Commissions' statement of educational and organizational goals set forth in Chapter 4 of the Millis Commission report entitled, "The Graduate Education of Physicians," and embodied in its four principal goals:

a) The preparation of more physicians with the desire and the qualifications to render comprehensive continuing health services.
b) The development of programs of graduate medical education which give greater emphasis to the training of physicians for cooperative effort among all members of the health professions in order that each patient may be provided with the combination of skills and knowledge best adapted to his particular needs.
c) The development of better procedures and agencies for systematic continuing review and improvement of graduate medical education.
d) To increase the attention given to the needs of medicine as an integrated scientific and professional whole.

The Regents were, however, unable to endorse the "Intent" of the Report of the AMA's Ad Hoc Committee on Education for Family Practice entitled, "Meeting the Challenge of Family Practice". That report recommended, among other things, the establishment of a certifying board and separate autonomous departments in medical schools with full-time faculty.

The Willard Committee report had defined a family physician as one who:

1. serves as the physician of first contact with the patient and provides a means of entry into the health care system;
2. evaluates the patient's total health needs, provides personal medical care within one or more fields of medicine, and refers the patient when indicated to appropriate sources of care while preserving the continuity of his care;
3. assumes responsibility for the patient's comprehensive and continuous health care and acts as a leader or coordinator of the team that provides health services; and
4. accepts responsibility for the patient's total health care within the context of his environment, including the community and the family or comparable social unit.

The AMA Ad Hoc Committee also contended that family practice was a specialty because the composite body of knowledge utilized by the family practitioner is significantly different from that of other specialists.

The Regents were of the opinion that family practice was a type of service or a function, and, therefore, not so different from the function of existing specialties as to warrant a completely new type of training. It was pointed out that the "Essentials for Approval of Examining Boards in Medical Specialties" contained the statement:

> A specialty board (primary, subsidiary or affiliate) in a medical specialty should represent a distinct and well-defined field of medicine. It should reflect advancement in medical knowledge and practice. It should be concerned primarily with organs or systems or broadly useful methods of diagnosis and treatment.

The Board of Regents reemphasized its previous policy set forth in resolutions on family practice adopted in November, 1965, and April, 1966, and averred that policy already adopted adequately indicated directions in which solutions to these problems could be achieved. The Board urged increased support from all available sources for the development of more and better trained physicians, particularly internists and pediatricians, to meet the comprehensive health needs of the American people.

The final conclusion to the study of these issues was presented by the ACP Medical Services Committee in a point by point analysis of the Millis Commission report to the Board of Regents for its approval at their November, 1967 meeting.

Through its representatives, ACP was active on several other fronts. The improvement of standards of residency training, while the immediate responsibility of the RRC-IM, was a matter of deep concern to the ABIM. According to the Board, it was apparent to all who assisted in the oral examinations that an appalling number of candidates were poorly grounded in fundamental clinical procedures used by qualified internists. A statistical study was undertaken to define accurately these deficiencies and this knowledge was to be made available to directors of residency programs. Further, grading of training programs on the basis of success of candidates in ABIM examinations was also undertaken. Training program directors and the RRC-IM were to be notified, but since the ABIM was aware that many failures were due to too early or too heavy exposure to subspecialties without adequate responsibility for patients, it was resolved that a minimum of two years of general medical training with adequate patient responsibility—including experience during the internship—was the minimum core requirement for training in internal medicine. Training in subspecialties could make up the remainder of required residency training.

A resolution which had been adopted by the RRC-IM was approved by the Board of Regents. All members of the RRC-IM were concerned lest the teaching and supervision of some programs in large charity hospitals fall into the hands of unqualified physicians. For that reason they recommended the following policy statement which was approved by the Board of Regents in November, 1966.

1. In the training of residents in internal medicine the primary responsibility for the teaching must be by qualified internists.
2. The direction of care of patients on graduate teaching medical services must be the responsibility of qualified internists.

The RRC-IM was also active during this year formulating a definition of what constituted broad field training for internal medicine, and adopted the following statement:

Since the ability to study and care for the whole patient is one of the distinguishing characteristics of the internist, the Committee believes that ample opportunity for broad training should be provided in every approved program. During this time the resident should have direct responsibility for patients who are not preselected for subspecialized consideration or treatment. In this situation the resident will encounter an unselected spectrum of diseases in patients, and in so doing learns to study and work with them in the broadest sense. Indeed, the opportunity to see in consultation occasional problems from the surgical, pediatric, obstetrical and psychiatric fields is considered entirely appropriate.

At the conclusion of his program, the resident's total graduate medical educational experience should have included not less than two years of graded, direct patient-care responsibility in the broad field of internal medicine.

Subspecialty training adds depth of knowledge and skill in the areas of major organ systems, and is a vital part of the education of an internist. The residency program should include a well-organized experience in many of the special disciplines, such as cardiovascular disease, gastroenterology, pulmonary disease, endocrinology, hematology, and rehabilitation, among others. Such experience may be provided by the ready availability to the resident of qualified consultants and teaching in the subspecialities for patients on an unselected general medical service, as well as or in addition to rotations through a series of subspecialties. Such rotations for a period shorter than two months ordinarily are not advisable. These rotations should ensure appropriate and continuing resident responsibility for patient care.

Since the medical resident's later experience in practice will include a large number of patients with neurological and psychiatric problems, it is advisable that adequate opportunity for familiarization with these fields be included in the program.

A similar requirement was written into the RRC-IM *Guide for Residency Programs in Internal Medicine* which required that

. . . at the conclusion of this program, the resident's total graduate medical educational experience should have included not less than two years of graded direct patient care responsibility in the broad field of internal medicine.

Primary patient responsibility was defined as,

. . . when, during a period of training in internal medicine predominantly devoted to clinical experience, the applicant directs the total care of the majority of the patients for whom he has responsibility, under supervision of the attending staff.

The Board of Regents approved the new *Guide* at its meeting in April, 1967.
The Millis Commission recommended that if internship was eliminated, one year less should be required for Board certification. In opposition, the ABIM

stated "We believe a man needs four years of formal training beyond graduation from medical school".

The ABIM changed its eligibility requirements for the certification examination, establishing a principle that anyone qualifying should have two years of training in the broad field of internal medicine with primary patient responsibility. This would include a straight medical internship. Although the Board preferred the straight medical internship, rotating internship under a new definition would also qualify a candidate if it included eight months of internal medicine. Rotation through subspecialties would count as broad basic internal medicine training provided the person on that subspecialty rotation was not working in a consultant capacity but was actually taking care of patients on that service.

The written examination would be given at the end of four years of formal training instead of at the end of two additional years of practice. This would enable candidates who found themselves deficient in certain areas of internal medicine to be in a better position to take further specific remedial training over the next two years. It also appealed to foreign applicants who found it difficult, because of expiration of their visas, to take the written examination after two years of experience just following the period of formal training.

The ABIM was deeply interested in the proposed programs for education of the "primary care" internists. Since it was acknowledged that a large number of internists functioned in this role, the Board studied what steps might be taken to ensure excellent training and maintenance of high standards for physicians who wished to pursue this mode of practice. In collaboration with the American Board of Pediatrics [ABP], the possibility of joint training programs, which might include other specialties, was investigated early in 1967. While it appeared probable that such joint programs could be established, the maintenance of high standards for each specialty might make the training of large numbers of qualified primary care "pediatrician-internists" difficult.

The ABIM decided late in 1967 that it did not wish to set up a separate examination for this purpose. The matter was discussed with the ABP. The two Boards jointly proposed that a combined program in medicine and pediatrics be offered so that in four years a person could be certified by both Boards. Any plan of training for family physicians, the Board stated, should be experimental for the moment.

The workload of the ABIM increased in response to new educational challenges in internal medicine and examining increasing numbers of candidates for certification. While the number of candidates taking the written examination remained stable at approximately 2,200 per year, the number of candidates eligible for the oral multiplied due to the backlog of candidates who had failed previously. Since only about 1,300 could be examined in the five oral examinations given each year by the ABIM, steps were taken to increase the number of cities where the examination would be offered and to make the oral examinations more fair and efficient.

An expansion of the Board from 16 members to 20 was planned and a technique of "mini orals" devised, whereby each Board member would conduct one-half to one day examinations. Examinations consisted of four to eight candidates reviewed at the designated institution by a Board member and one of his faculty or associates as coexaminer.

The failure rate in both written and oral examinations had remained at a high level for three years, the ABIM reported, and this disturbing statistic could be attributed either to improper examination techniques or poor preparation of candidates in residency training programs. Since a large number of failures in the oral examination were "laid at the door of inadequate or discriminating history taking and incorrect performance of the physical examination," the ABIM took steps to rectify the situation. Questions were introduced into the written examination emphasizing these aspects and illustrated material in the form of photographs, X-ray films, microscopic slides, and electrocardiograms were incorporated into the testing format.

The oral examination had received careful scrutiny in the previous two years by a committee headed by Dr. Craig Borden. In most participating hospitals, the physical setting of the examination and the selection of patients for candidates had been improved in such a fashion as to reduce the importance of extraneous factors detracting from the candidate's performance. By using Emeritus Board Members and enlisting a corps of experienced Senior Guest Examiners who participated for a full examination, after a preliminary training period, the quality of examiners had been maximally assured. The technique of oral examination was standarized as much as possible by limiting questions to various facets of the problems presented by the patient at hand. The grading technique and means of deciding on success or failure, likewise, was standarized to a considerable degree and was under study for further refinement.

In a meeting of the ACP Committee on Medical Services, Dr. John Layne, one of the members, reported on the work of the Subcommittee on Governmental Activities in Medicine:

> The report to . . . President [Johnson] by HEW, "Medical Care Prices" (February 1967) was reviewed in some detail . . . It involves not only items of economic import, but also many other far-ranging recommendations which well represent the platform from which may be launched the present Administration's future plans and activities in the health care field. ("Comprehensive community health care systems should be developed, demonstrated and evaluated"; "Cost-reducing methods of reorganizing the delivery of services in hospitals and other providers of health services should be developed, demonstrated and implemented"; "Federally supported health care programs should be used to train physician assistants, evaluate their performance, and disseminate the results"; and "HEW should undertake an intensive examination of frequently prescribed drugs to assess the therapeutic effectiveness of brand name products and their supposed generic equivalents", are but a few of the recommendations.) Dr. James Cain talked of the deliberations of the President's Health Manpower Commission. He mentioned two problems in particular that are plaguing the Commission: 1) The health manpower shortage, to which the requirements of the military contribute significantly, and 2) The absence in the Federal government of any coordinating body in the field of health services. He made a strong plea for the establishment of an objective advisory group (similar to

the Economic Advisory Council) which could study and effectively advise the President and Congress in matters relating to health legislation.

Another important report was submitted by Dr. Thomas M. Durant, from the CMSS, which met in special session in Chicago on January 14, 1967. In addition to representatives from the three originally represented Colleges (ACP, ACS, and American College of Obstetricians and Gynecologists [ACOG]), also present was Dr. Robert G. Frazier, Secretary of the Association of American Physicians [AAP], Dr. Raymond Waggoner of the American Psychiatric Association [APA], Dr. Walter E. Barton, Executive Director of the APA, and Dr. Roger C. Berson, Executive Director of the AAMC.

Dr. Berson, presented a interesting and instructive report of the activities of the AAMC in the implementation of the Coggeshall Report; summarized as follows:

1. A Washington office was established by the AAMC.
2. An organization of administrators of teaching hospitals was formed within the AAMC.
3. Regional meetings of the AAMC were being encouraged.
4. The objectives of the AAMC were being restudied and would be restated.
5. A Council of Academic Societies representing clinical and preclinical fields was being formed as a part of the Association.
6. An attempt had been made to develop a part of the organization concerned with allied health professions.
7. An ad hoc committee was appointed to review the Millis report.

Following Dr. Berson's report, the Council discussed again in some detail its objectives as an organization. The Board of Regents approved the suggestion of Dr. A. Carlton Ernstene that the representatives to this Council be the President, President-Elect and the Chairman of the Committee on Medical Services.

## Part Four (1967-1968)

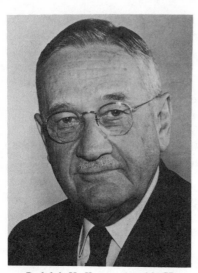

Born January 15, 1898, in Clarksville, Iowa, Dr. Rudolph H. Kampmeier married Blanche Davis in 1922. They had one daughter, named Joan. He obtained his AB degree at the State University of Iowa College of Liberal Arts, in 1920. He continued at the University, earning his MD in 1923. Following an internship at St. Mark's Hospital in Salt Lake City, Utah, in 1923-24, he entered private practice for a year in Utah, then accepted appointment as Instructor in Medicine at the University of Michigan Medical School from 1925-1929. He was Instructor of Medicine at the University of Indiana School of Medicine in 1929-30, then returned to private prac-

*Rudolph H. Kampmeier, MACP*    tice for three years in Castle Rock, Colorado. In 1932, he was appointed Assistant Professor of Medicine at Louisiana State University School of Medicine, advancing to Clinical Professor in 1935. He served as Visiting Physician at Charity Hospital in New Orleans from 1932-1936.

In 1936, Dr. Kampmeier began his lifetime association with Vanderbilt University School of Medicine in Nashville, Tennessee. Appointed Assistant Professor of Medicine in 1936, he became Associate Professor of Medicine in 1938 and advanced to Professor of Medicine in 1953. In 1963, he was made Emeritus Professor of Medicine. During his faculty tenure, Dr. Kampmeier served in numerous positions including that of Director of the Department of Medicine during World War II, while Dr. Hugh Morgan was away in military service. From 1946-1966 he was Director of Postgraduate Continuing Education. He also served as Visiting Physician at Vanderbilt University Hospital.

His leadership in both local and national medical societies included membership in the American Medical Association, Association of American Physicians, American Clinical and Climatological Association, and Southern Medical Association [SMA]. He was President of the SMA in 1964-65, He was a Diplomate of the American Board of Internal Medicine, and served as Guest Examiner from 1955-1958 and in 1961-62. He was also Associate Chief Examiner for the National Board of Medical Examiners from 1948-1954.

His long association with the AMA included membership in the Section on Internal Medicine, of which he was Secretary from 1956-1959 and Chairman in 1959-60. He was an AMA Representative to the Residency Review Committee for Internal Medicine, 1963-1969, and served on the Awards Committee and Scientific Exhibits Committee from 1963-1970. He was Chairman of the Department of Continuing Education in 1971, Site Surveyor from 1968-1978, and participant on the Committee on Preparation for General Practice from 1957-1959, the Joint Study Committee on Continuing Education, 1961-62, and made field trips for the Section on Nutrition Information in 1966-67.

Dr. Kampmeier served on a great number of governmental committees, among which were the Advisory Committee on Cancer Control, 1963-1967 and the Mid-South Regional Medical Program, 1967-1971; the Committee on Medical Research of the Office of Scientific Research and Development, 1943-1949, serving as responsible investigator for that agency's "Study on Penicillin in Syphilis". He was involved in wartime studies in nutrition for the Surgeon-General's Office of the Army, 1944-45, and participated in studies for the Interdepartmental Committee on Nutrition for National Defense, in surveys in Ecuador (1960), Lebanon (1961), and Jordan (1962). He was a participant in numerous government sponsored conferences and other seminars from 1958-1965, being called upon particularly as an authority in venereal disease control. Also clinically well versed in problems of mental health and in geriatrics, he participated in White House Conferences and on commissions and committees in these areas from 1955-1971.

Among his numerous awards were the AMA's Rodman E. Sheen Award, 1975; Thomas A. Parran Award, American Venereal Disease Association Award, 1975; William Freeman Snow Award, American Social Health Association Award, and the Founders Medal of the Southern Society for Clinical Investigation. He is also a Fellow of the Royal College of Physicians of London and of Ireland, and a member of Sigma Xi and Alpha Omega Alpha.

A prolific writer, Dr. Kampmeier was author of many articles, chapters, and several books, most notably: *Essentials of Syphilology,* 1943; *Physical Examination in Health and Disease* (4 editions), 1950-1970; *History of the Vanderbilt Department of Medicine,* 1925-1959, c1981; and *History of Tennessee Medical Association,* 1930-1980, c1981.

At various times, he edited the *Southern Medical Journal, Southern Medical Bulletin* and the *Journal of the Tennessee Medical Association.* He was President of the Southern Medical Association in 1965, the Nashville Academy of Medicine and Davidson County Medical Society in 1951, and of the Tennessee Medical Association.

A Fellow of the ACP since 1928, Dr. Kampmeier was Governor for Tennessee from 1954-1961; a Regent from 1961-1966; President-Elect and President in 1966-67 and 1967-68 respectively. He returned to the Board of Regents as Past President from 1968-1970. In 1972 he became a Master, was recipient of the Alfred Stengel Award in 1973, and the first recipient (1981) of the Ralph Claypoole Award, established in 1979 for distinguished achievements in the clinical practice of internal medicine.

Dr. Kampmeier was a hard worker who believed in very high standards, yet never took a judgmental approach in advising other physicians. As a member of the Residency Review Committee, he was especially adept at communicating his decisions in language designed to support and help program directors who were trying to improve their residency training activities.

At Vanderbilt he was popular with all doctors, but he especially tried to make the practitioners feel welcome in the academic centers. His success was remarkable.

He told me once that most of the indigent people in the clinic referred to him as "Dr. Camp Fire", which they could pronounce more easily.

Upon his retirement from Vanderbilt, he continued as a clinician, acting as a regular consultant and visiting physician to the Southeastern Tennessee Psychiatric Institute. His participation on a joint committee between the American Psychiatric Association [APA] and the ACP was most helpful. For a time, the language of the two groups was not mutually understood and Dr. Kampmeier, widely conversant in both disciplines, could explain the College position in a way that made the Committee work effectively and smoothly.

### "The Doctor as A Scholar"

Dr. Kampmeier reflected his devotion to his profession in his Presidential address, which be began by quoting Sir William Osler.

Thucydides it was who said of the Greeks, that they possess the power of thinking before they acted and acting too.

Dr. Kampmeier asked,

Does it not characterize the physician as he practices his profession? Is this not implied in *The Doctor as a Scholar*!

. . . I wish to speak of [the physician today] as a scholar, a *Man Thinking*, as defined by Ralph Waldo Emerson . . . and the pressures that beset him . . . technology, society, law and government. These are forces which in the future conceivably may transform the life of a scholar into that of a skilled technician. I have no worry about the first attribute of the scholar, *curiosity* . . . For most physicians I have little concern about a second attribute of the scholar. *Perserverance* in the continued and steadfast pursuit of knowledge . . . is shown by his growth in professional competence acknowledged by his peers . . . It is the remaining three attributes . . . with which I am concerned today: *initiative, originality,* and *integrity.* How to withstand the oppressive forces of technology, society and government is the medical scholar's dilemma today . . ."

He observed that the younger physician, who lacking the leavening of accumulated clinical experience . . . tends to cling to the objective data obtained by a "machine" or in the laboratory . . . Erroneous deductions drawn from laboratory findings take their toll both in morbidity and mortality. How best to bend today's technologic tools to their controlled use is one of the dilemmas of the medical scholar . . . Meeting . . . the demands of society tax[es] the scholar sorely, . . . and may immobilize and even paralyze his scholarly assets. [In the patient's expectations] lies the paradox: the promise of health or cure and the inability to provide it. This is a major dilemma.

Although he believed that the medical scholar might still have freedom to pursue a course of action, nevertheless as a scholar he or she encountered the force of government and law, whose constraints are almost immutable. He held that the only way to cope with the government was for the profession to try to influence its decisions by offering advice. Although professional input frequently would be ignored, making the effort was mandatory, since it was essential to a scholarly, rather than a political solution, to health problems.

Another dilemma which each physician must face is whether or not to continue treating end-stage disease and allow the patient to die with dignity. [Quoting again Emerson's characterization of the scholar's relation to society, Dr. Kampmeier concluded,] In the right state he is *Man Thinking*.

In an interview in April, 1982, Dr. Kampmeier recounted to me the details of a postconvention tour in 1967 on which he and Mrs. Kampmeier traveled with 50 ACP Members and their spouses. In Hawaii, the group was hosted by ACP Governor, Dr. Morton Berk, and the Staff at Tripler Army Hospital. In Tokyo they spent an educational day with Professor Hideo Ueda, Chief of the Second Department of Internal Medicine of the Tokyo University Hospital and his Staff; in Hong Kong, Professor Alexander J. S. Fadzean, Chairman of the Department of Medicine at the University of Hong Kong and his staff conducted a splendid educational program. Professor Fadzean was a Fellow of the Royal College of Physicians of London [RCP(L)] and also a Corresponding Fellow of the ACP. He was obviously delighted to entertain the touring group. The Kampmeiers gave a cocktail party for the group and Professor Fadzean and his staff at the Mandarin Hotel.

Rudie and Blanche then left the group and traveled via New Delhi, Teheran and Cairo to Dublin, to represent the College at the Tercentenary Celebration of the Irish College [RCP(I)]. President of Ireland Eamon de Valera and Dr. Kampmeier, among others, were made Honorary Fellows. At the reception, after learning that Dr. Kampmeier was from Nashville, President de Valera recalled that many years before, his plane had been grounded at Nashville. At a tea, Dr. Kampmeier presented to Dr. Brian Pringle, RCP(I) Immediate Past President, a silver Philadelphia Bowl for the Royal Irish College on behalf of the ACP.

In 1968, Rudie and I traveled to England where we were inducted as Fellows of the RCP(L) on June 6. Dr. Elkinton, Editor of the *Annals*, was also made a Fellow on July 25 in London. Later in 1968, during Dr. Pollard's ACP presidency, the Kampmeiers, the Pollards and the Rosenows spent nine days in London, attending the 450th Anniversary Celebration of the Royal College of Physicians, then traveled to Dublin, where Rudie was made an Honorary Fellow of the RCP(I).

Dr. Kampmeier, Dr. Chester Keefer and I met with people at the National Broadcasting Corporation, who were hoping to set up a medical information broadcast service to be used in doctors' offices. The medical information would be interspersed with background music, with the scientific information channeled into the physician's office and the background music into the waiting room. We concluded it was unrealistic to expect that a doctor would take time in a busy office to listen to medical information, but this did not dissuade radio experts from efforts to sell the program. Pharmaceutical manufacturers were to provide the financing, contingent upon a sufficient number of subscriptions to support it after its introduction. Since physicians were unable to ascertain what they could expect to receive in such a package, the venture failed from lack of popular support.

Mrs. Kampmeier, always a pleasant but objective observer of her husband's activities, told me on many occasions that she thought her husband talked too long. I reassured her and advised her to watch the audience during his speeches. Dr. Kampmeier was a captivating speaker, and his audiences were always attentive. An indefatigable companion on his travels, Mrs. Kampmeier had one colorful habit at which Dr. Kampmeier sometimes balked. She loved flowers and could not leave behind gifts of flowers in hotel rooms. She insisted on taking them home or to their next destination. Dr. Kampmeier did not like to do this and on one occasion, I remember, he refused to take them along.

The success of the *Medical Knowledge Self-Assessment Program,* launched in 1967, exceeded all expectations, even in its first modest publication. Subscription projections were the subject of the usual office guessing games. I won, not by accurate prediction, but by "nearest" guess, 2500 subscriptions, which turned out to be only 50 percent of the actual response: The first edition drew 5000 physicians in response to the initial mailing.

Incidentally, at an early planning meeting, one professor had questioned the usefulness of the program, stating that any physician could tell what he needed to know by looking at the table of contents of an up-to-date textbook of medicine.

The title of the program had an interesting origin. Our bookkeeper, Miss Hannah Tyndall, one day asked me if I wanted a particular expense item charged against the "medical knowledge self-assessment program"; she had to give it some name to identify it for accounting purposes. That name was exactly appropriate, and following *MKSAP's* success, Miss Tyndall was rather proud of the fact that she had named it.

When the College and the American Society of Internal Medicine [ASIM] were planning their first joint meeting, Dr. Kampmeier told me that the ASIM President did not consider it wise for the Executive Directors of the two organizations to be present. Mr. William Ramsey had been recently appointed to the ASIM position, and it might not have been a matter of concern to him. However, I was opposed to such an exclusion, noting that one of my agreements with the Board of Regents was that there would be no executive sessions of the Board or of most committees which would exclude my presence, except when the subject related to the terms of my income or performance of my duties.

More pertinently, being excluded from such a meeting with the ASIM officers would make my job very difficult. I was prepared to resign my position if the ASIM officers were adamant on the point. Dr. Kampmeier agreed with me and so informed the President of ASIM, who withdrew the suggestion. My attendance had an important effect on my capacity to carry out the Regents' policies in this important matter.

# 1967-1968

*MKSAP-I.* Phoenix meeting-ACP/ASIM. Millis Commission report. RCP(L) 450th Anniversary. ACP/RCP(L) Joint Meeting, Annual Session, Boston. ACP Distinguished Teacher Award.

At the November Board of Regents meeting, Dr. Rudolph H. Kampmeier, President, reported that he, the President-Elect, the Executive Director, the Treasurer and a Regent-At-Large had represented the College at an invitational meeting with the AMA Board of Trustees in October. The meeting was convened to provide "for a general discussion of current socioeconomic problems that affect physicians" and to review "the question of representation by the specialty groups within the AMA structure".

The ACP representatives anticipated an unstructured conference for tentative exploration of these and related topics, but at the meeting an agenda was presented to the participants, listing: 1) Specialty group representation within the AMA structure; 2) Establishment of a Board of Family Practice; 3) Reorganization of the Department of Health, Education and Welfare [HEW] and establishment of a position of Under Secretary of Health; and 4) Health care, medical and hospital costs, manpower shortages and increasing public demands.

The ACP representatives were invited to comment on each topic. Discussion of the proposed AMA Interspecialty Council was the most significant subject of the meeting. The AMA Board's position was quite bluntly and clearly stated: The American Society of Internal Medicine [ASIM], because of its interest in socioeconomic aspects of medical practice, was more sympathetic and more helpful to the AMA than was the College. Since the ACP, until recently, had expressed no interest in this aspect of medicine, the AMA implied to those present that the choice of the ACP or the ASIM for internal medicine representation on the Council was the prerogative of the AMA Board of Trustees. The Trustees' position was that members of the Interspecialty Council should represent practicing internists rather than the academic segment and that if an ACP Fellow were nominated, the candidate should also be acceptable to the ASIM. Dr. Dwight Wilbur, then President of the AMA, appointed Drs. James Haviland and W. Philip Corr as ACP representatives to the Council.

The ACP reiterated its stand on the establishment of a Board of Family Practice. Although questioning the efficacy of such a move to meet current problems in health care delivery, the ACP did not oppose it and was ready to advise the American Academy of Family Physicians on graduate programs in internal medicine if a certification program was established.

There was general agreement on a resolution to create a position of Under Secretary of Health in the reorganization of HEW.

The final agenda item, review of health care and manpower issues, however, was "obviously too large for even a bow" at this meeting.

Continuing his report, Dr. Kampmeier proposed to the Board of Regents that they provide for better continuity in Annual Session planning by appointing a Chairman for the Program Committee who would serve three years, with the

President acting as Cochairman. The Board concurred, and Dr. Walter Frommeyer was appointed as the first Chairman to serve the longer term.

Dr. H. Marvin Pollard, President-Elect, proposed that the offices of Second and Third Vice President be abolished. Notwithstanding Bylaws definitions, in recent practice the Nominations Committees had used these offices simply to hold over qualified Governors for nomination to the Board of Regents in the succeeding year. Having no meaningful committee functions, the offices were extraneous. Dr. Pollard proposed that the offices be replaced by the addition of three new Regent positions, and the Board concurred.

In my report, I reviewed the status of the National Institutes of Mental Health [NIMH] Grant for community hospital pilot programs to educate internists in psychiatric and emotional aspects of disease. Dr. Kampmeier was cochairman of this ACP/APA Task Force Project. The success of the project was uncertain and outcomes might be dependent on whether the College was really in a good position to implement educational programs at the community hospital level.

I emphasized the need for continuing Board review of the increasingly expressed desire of specialty organizations for a voice in representing their interests in government, the AMA and other bodies affecting their status. Currently, the College was involved in three specialty-oriented efforts, the Interspecialty Society Council (later known as the Council on Medical Specialty Societies), the Medical Intersociety Council and the AMA Specialty Society Advisory Committee. I was Secretary for both the ISC and the MIC To date, these had offered intersocietal social and mutual educational opportunities but had little impact on the need for united action.

## MKSAP I

Work on the first ACP *Medical Knowledge Self-Assessment Program, [MKSAP]*, progressed rapidly in 1967. Nine subspecialty chairmen were appointed in the areas of neurology, cardiovascular disease, gastroenterology, pulmonary disease, infectious disease and immunology, hematology, rheumatology, endocrinology and metabolism, and renal disease. Each chairman then selected a committee of five members with one representative from general internal medicine on each committee to emphasize clinical practice.

The chairmen of the *MKSAP* committees met in Philadelphia late in 1966 and were briefed by the staff of the National Board of Medical Examiners and the Educational Activities Committee of the College, concerning the type of questions desired and the purpose of the self-assessment program.

Test questions were prepared and in October, a prospectus outlining the program and a registration form were mailed to all College members. The cost was $10 for College members. Distribution was scheduled in January, 1968. By December, 1967, 4,500 applications were received.

The Board of Regents agreed that following the completion of the program for ACP members in January, the College should repeat the program for members who did not sign up initially and for nonmember physicians, at fees of $15 for members and $25 for nonmembers. A coded answer sheet and the bibliography were included in the subsequent subscribers' package for self-scoring. In further action, the Board reversed a previous decision to make group scores available to the College. It had assumed that group information would support more effective planning of postgraduate courses and the scientific programs of the Annual Session. After further study, the Regents concluded that knowledge of the scores might not only be minimally helpful but, in fact, foster improper interpretation and make many physicians reluctant to subscribe. The scores would therefore be destroyed immediately, without construction of group scores. To guarantee confidentiality, the score would be known only to the participant.

The Ad Hoc Committee on Continuing Education, which planned the *MKSAP,* was directed to continue its work to further develop and refine the program.

The result of the first program was a resounding success. Approximately 5,000 College members ordered it, and over 4,000 returned it in time for machine scoring. A total of 10,500 were distributed during the next three years and an additional 1,000 were printed.

In a follow-up survey, participants complimented the program and most considered it "a challenging, humbling, and educational tool." Nearly all responders were interested in having the program repeated in two or three years, and many expressed a desire to know how they stood in comparison to peers. The President reported great enthusiasm for *MKSAP* at Regional Meetings. The bibliography was well received as it allowed easy access to answering questions and stimulated additional study in weak areas of knowledge.

Many directors of residency programs and chairmen of departments of medicine purchased the program for use in undergraduate and graduate teaching. Several national specialty groups contacted ACP headquarters indicating that they were planning similar programs in their particular fields. The favorable publicity the College received indicated that internists were conscientious about continued education, tried hard to "keep up", and would engage in self-appraisal without coercion.

The Board of Regents moved to repeat the *MKSAP* every three years and authorized the President to appoint an ad hoc committee to plan another program.

In light of this success, the Educational Activities Committee was encouraged to pursue other modes of continuing education. The Committee was studying the use of large screen television, which was popular at the Annual Sessions, and believed that, as the audio-visual medium improved, it would become a major conduit to disseminate information. For this reason, the Committee was investigating the possiblity of producing television and audio tapes on specialized subjects to be made available to members. The Committee would report the findings of its feasibility study to the Regents in 1969.

In November, 1967, the relationship with the ASIM was considered to be satisfactory, but it was quite clear that many issues would emerge in the future on which the College and the Society would experience divided interests. Development of clearly understood policy positions for both organizations was essential to adequate representation of internal medicine at many levels.

Reflecting on that period in a recent conversation with me, Dr. Kampmeier wondered why there had been increasing tensions between the two organizations. We agreed that much of this was due to differences in goals, organization and individual perspective. When the College decided against addressing issues of prepaid health insurance in 1956, the ASIM leaders believed that the Board of Regents was enthusiastically supportive of the emerging new organization. This was not the case. A number of Regents had been enthusiastic, but most felt that an organization formed on the basis of socioeconomics alone would surely fail. The role of addressing these fields of interest in internal medicine would then inevitably revert to the College. This was reported to me by Mr. Loveland, who had been in attendance at all the discussions pertaining to these matters in 1956.

As ASIM became more active, the differences became more apparent to the leadership of both organizations. The Board's attention to ASIM relations and their respective roles consumed much of their meeting time. During 1963-64, these matters were fraught with much friction and misunderstanding. Dr. Wesley Spink urged that the College go its own way and ignore the ASIM. The Regents then approved the establishment of a Medical Services Committee, which only exacerbated the situation. It quickly became apparent that something had to be done to restore a cooperative atmosphere that would nevertheless allow each society relative independence.

During the early part of 1967-68, Dr. James J. Feffer, President of the ASIM, was extremely upset on many occasions, sometimes with reason and sometimes because of misunderstanding. The ACP then initiated a proposal for a joint conference where cooperative efforts could be formulated. The top leadership of ACP and ASIM met in Phoenix, Arizona, and a much better relationship resulted.

President Kampmeier sent a memorandum to the members of the Executive Committee of the Board of Regents outlining both the causes of the strained situation and the outcome of the ACP meeting with the ASIM Board of Trustees. The Executive Committee recommended that the Regents consider having consultations between both organizations leading to a top level conference with both Boards, or appropriate representatives of each, to discuss the present position and possible future directions the ACP-ASIM relationship might take. A similar memo was circulated to the Regents by the President prior to the November meeting. He felt he had inherited ill feeling and controversy. Dr. Kampmeier said,

> The growth in strength and prominence of the ASIM as a spokesman for the internist in the socioeconomic field is without question and is easily documented . . . The "know-how" of ASIM in the socioeconomic field has made it the logical consultant or advisor for internal medicine in the current climate of governmental regimentation of medical practice and care. In grappling with these everyday problems of the internist's livelihood and his status as a practicing specialist, the ASIM had filled a vacuum left by the ACP . . . In addition to the contributions which daily met the eye of the internist "in the field" the ASIM offered the opportunity for many physicians to play a role in an attempt to direct trends in providing medical and health care . . . [In contrast to the ACP] the ASIM offers

numerous activities to its membership in which they could be officers on the board of the state arm of the ASIM, in a well organized "grass roots" cadre of "contact men" with congressional members of the respective states; as representation of internal medicine on committees or commissions to state medical societies dealing with matters of third party contacts, insurance, etc.; and upon advisory committees or commissions to state government.

It was Dr. Kampmeier's belief that there were three courses open to the College to solve this growing problem. The ACP could:

1. make the decision that each organization go its own way with an understanding that it would be foolish for the College to attempt competition with the well organized machine of ASIM in the socioeconomic sphere;

2. attempt to maneuver an amalgamation, or an assimilation of the ASIM at the top or national level, with the development of a plan to maintain and foster activities at a state level. This would permit a unified voice for internal medicine at the national level; or

3. [develop] a true liaison with the Society at a top policy level, with a committee composed of representatives of the Board of Regents and their Board of Trustees respectively.

At the November Regents meeting, Dr. Kampmeier called upon me to comment on this matter.

. . . This Board, [I said] could be making decisions at this time which will affect the very future of the College. Many attempts have been made to improve liaison with this very worthy organization, many of whom are College members.

There are several reasons I believe liaison is difficult and to a degree ineffective. The difference in goals has made communications seem somewhat less than urgent. The difference in age and maturity of our respective leadership hasn't helped smooth out differences. Organizational differences are striking—the ASIM being a federation of similar, though not identical state organizations, whereas the College is not very much a locally oriented organization.

Before trying to solve any more present problems in our relationship with ASIM, it is my hope that all of you will give careful thought to this question. What course should be taken now which would be best for the public, internal medicine and the American College of Physicians and its members twenty years from now? I have tried to do this and I firmly believe the members of both organizations would be best served by one organization. I believe the time for us to make this decision is upon us for the following reasons:

1. ASIM is increasingly active and more effective in seeking positions which would make it the spokesman for internal medicine—[in its words]—"The only large organization made up of internists only."

2. Financially, ASIM will need to find other sources of money.

3. ASIM has a limiting field of activity unless it expands into the scientific and educational field. There are already many signs this will be an inevitable trend.

4. Times have changed in the past 11 years. It is no longer possible for the College to avoid action in the socioeconomics of health care, if it is to continue its position of leadership.

5. In order to implement effectively some of the programs now in an early stage of development, we will need help in many local areas.
6. More opportunities for our members to be active. This is, I think, the most important of all. In the past the College has in general reacted to requests and actions of the ASIM. Now I think we should be prepared to meet with their top policy body and explore mutual problems and solutions . . . I urge you to come to some such decision at this time. It seems to me if we sidestep this issue it is quite possible that twenty years from now ASIM and not the ACP will lead the internist.

I outlined a possible method of merging these two societies. Although these ideas were not accepted, when a possible merger was considered again in 1972, these old suggestions were very much like the ones that were finally agreed on by the Board of Trustees of ASIM and the Board of Regents of ACP.

The Board of Regents approved a motion that a committee be appointed by the President to initiate negotiations or serious discussions with the Board of Trustees of the ASIM at the top level.

## ACP and ASIM Meet in Phoenix

The first meeting of the ACP-ASIM Liaison Committee was held in Phoenix, Arizona in early February, 1968. The Committee consisted of the Immediate Past Presidents, Dr. Wendell B. Gordon, ASIM and Dr. Irving S. Wright, ACP; the Presidents, Dr. James J. Feffer, ASIM and Dr. R. H. Kampmeier, ACP; the Presidents-Elect, Dr. Robert S. Long, ASIM and Dr. Marvin H. Pollard, ACP; Dr. Blain Z. Hibbard and Dr. Joseph T. Painter, members of the Board of Trustees, ASIM; Dr. Carter Smith and Dr. James G. Haviland, members of the Board of Regents, ACP; and the Executive Directors, Mr. William R. Ramsey of ASIM, and myself. The activities of the two organizations were reviewed and the respective objectives and areas of overlapping interest in which communication and liaison between the two societies might be essential to the good of the community of internists and to American medicine were identified.

Those present reaffirmed that the ACP had clear responsibilities for the ongoing or continuing education of internists, for representing internal medicine in undergraduate and graduate education, for the certification of competency as a specialist, as well as responsibility for the hospital environment in which the physician practiced.

The ASIM's responsibility was directed toward the socioeconomic aspects of practice, third party contracts, fees and reimbursements, and personal standards of providing medical care in the office and hospital.

Dr. Kampmeier reported that all the participants generally agreed that,

The broad area of delivery of medical care was an area in which it was essential that excellent liaison be established, one in which forces external to the two organizations might become devisive to the detriment of the practice of medicine and the nation's health. This area includes so-called family practice or primary physicians, relationships of the internist to other medical associations (AMA, AAGP, possibly . . . specialty societies), and of paramount importance the voice of the internist if called upon to advise with, or testify before governmental agencies and/or committees of the executive and legislative branches of our federal government . . . It was apparent that by proper liaison, the better representation of internal medicine might be selected for a given assignment, but that upon occasion and dependent upon attending circumstances, strength might be lent by joint representation of the two organizations as a demonstration of a unified front in internal medicine.

A joint statement for information to the membership of both organizations was drafted at the conclusion of the meeting to be circulated over the signatures of both Presidents. The statement read:

> In recognition of the desirability of closer liaison between the American College of Physicians and the American Society of Internal Medicine, a new liaison committee has been established to represent the top policy level of both organizations. This committee consists of the President, President-Elect, and immediate Past President of each, and two members of the Board of Trustees. The first meeting was held in Phoenix, Arizona, on February 4 and 5, 1968.

> The Committee recognized and reaffirmed unanimously the distinct need for two separate organizations: the American College of Physicians primarily in consideration and evaluation of medical and scientific knowledge and medical education; the American Society of Internal Medicine primarily in consideration and evaluation of the socioeconomic aspects of the practice of medicine and their application to the delivery of health services. The Committee agreed there are also areas of mutual responsibility in the provision of the best possible medical care.

> This Committee acknowledged that each organization must be sensitive to activities and programs of the other. Therefore, it recognized the need for closer cooperation involving areas of common interest. Subsequent meetings will seek to identify those areas and to develop methods for effective action.

Following the adoption of this statement there was obvious satisfaction over the progress made toward better working relations between these two organizations. The Liaison Committee was to meet at least twice annually. The ACP Medical Services Committee was charged with working out methods of communicating with ASIM committees with similar activities. Everyone agreed there would be considerable overlapping of activities, but an atmosphere of increased cooperation prevailed.

The ACP-APA Task Force was made a standing committee of the College at the November Board of Regents Meeting. The pilot projects to promote education of residents in psychiatric techniques and services in the hospital setting continued. In Houston, a full-time psychiatrist with offices in the Methodist Hospital was available for consultation and teaching on all services. A liaison between the Faulkner Hospital and the former Adams Nervine Institute was established in Boston which provided psychiatric consultation to all services. The Nashville approach of providing seminars for small groups of internists continued to be successful. No word was received from the NIMH on the resubmitted grant proposal.

Late in November, 1966, a milestone was reached by the Commission on Professional and Hospital Activities [CPHA] as the 1,000th hospital enrolled in the Professional Activities Study (PAS] program. By November, 1967, 113 more hospitals had been added and 8.6 million patients discharged annually were included. The Medical Audit Program [MAP] had an enrollment of 663 hospitals with discharges totalling 5.7 million patients yearly.

Another milestone was reached by the CPHA in July as the Commission held a ground-breaking ceremony for a new $2.3 million headquarters building in Ann Arbor. I was then President of the CPHA Board, and had the honor of turning the first shovel on construction. The 84,000 square feet structure was scheduled for completion in June of 1968.

The editors of the *Annals Of Internal Medicine* were starting their eighth year of editing the journal. During the previous seven years, improvements had been made in its physical appearance, in the number, quality, and diversity of articles submitted and published, in the breadth and depth of the critical review of manuscripts, and in the circulation to paid subscribers.

Several new features were incorporated into the pages of the *Annals* while other older features continued to be successful. The "NIH Clinical Conferences" alternating with the "UCLA Interdepartmental Conferences", and the "Diagnosis and Treatment" series were continued on a monthly basis. "Editorial Notes", established late in 1966, was broadened, and the number of subjects treated was increased from two or three to five or six. The "Letters and Comments" section became more active and it was hoped that the volume of correspondence would likewise increase. Under the aegis of Dr. Huth, the section on books continued publishing a wide range of reviews and notices that the editors believed was one of the most useful features of the *Annals.*

A new feature, "Abstracts of Articles", was begun in July of 1967. A summary and the complete identifying reference of each article in the same issue of the *Annals* was printed in 3" x 5" boxes on one side of a page at the end of the editorial section. No single innovation, reported the editors, had produced such an avalanche of letters expressing approval and appreciation.

A *Supplement,* the first in three years, was published in September and presented the *Proceedings* of the *Colloquium, "The Changing Mores of Biomedical Research"* held at the 48th Annual Session of the College in San Francisco. This Colloquium received favorable comment and about 500 of the extra 2,000 copies printed were distributed free of charge during a six week period following publication.

Interlingua abstracts were discontinued in July. Not a single written comment or inquiry was received, indicating that foreign subscribers had no trouble reading the journal in English. (At this time the largest number of foreign subscribers were Japanese.)

The *Annals* again led the three other monthly journals in internal medicine in the number of papers cited in the abstract serials, the *Year Book* series and *Abstracts of World Medicine. The American Journal of Medical Sciences* had a new editor, Dr. Arnold Weissler (FACP) of Ohio State, and the publication was being completely overhauled. *The Archives of Internal Medicine* also acquired a new editor, Dr. Morton Bogdonoff (FACP) of Duke University and a major change in format was planned. Dr. Franz Ingelfinger (FACP) had just assumed the editorship of *The New England Journal of Medicine,* and all were striving vigorously to compete with the *Annals* for papers and readership.

The *Annals* editors did not wish to rest complacently on the past but believed that the journal would continue to improve. Several aspects were of immediate concern including both the physical characteristics of the publication and the scientific and intellectual content. As the public importance of the College grew, so too was it important to have the *Annals of Internal Medicine* present the very best in medical journalism. The editors, therefore, proposed to hire the best possible professional consultant on publishing layout to review the present format and to advise changes for its improvement. They also wished to review as carefully as possible the primary objectives of the *Annals* and the best means to attain them.

The editors viewed the essential purpose of the *Annals* as helping physicians to become better physicians. To this end the journal brought to its readers new medical knowledge directly from the investigator and interpreted and reviewed other new knowledge that had been reported previously. To achieve these objectives the journal attempted to present, in its original articles, reviews, and editorials, a wide variety of both experimental and clinical subject matter. Because the editors believed that the best physician was also a citizen well-informed on the problems-of-the-day of his profession and of the society which he served, the *Annals* attempted to provide a reasonable discussion of issues in medicine that lay outside the boundaries of scientific literature.

In support of this essential purpose, the editors reiterated that the first responsibility of the *Annals* was to its readers and not to authors who submit papers for possible publication.

Scientific validity was only one of the criteria for choice. Others included: novelty, usefulness, timeliness and relation to material already published both in the *Annals* and elsewhere. To the authors whose papers were chosen, the editors accepted the responsibility of insuring that the published version was mutually agreed upon and accurately reproduced.

The circulation of the *Annals* continued to grow at a steady pace from a total of 28,079 in 1964 to 38,205 in 1967. Unfortunately, the Headquarter's fire hindered plans for a solicitation campaign and growth during 1967 was below the anticipated rate.

The basic subscription rate of the journal had been $10 since 1949. During this period, the cost per subscription to print and mail had risen from approximately $6 to $12.72. Postage rates were scheduled to increase in 1968 along with other costs. The Board of Regents therefore, approved a base rate increase to $15 effective in April, 1968. Coupled with this, and in order to offset the rising costs of publishing and other operations of the College, an increase in the advertising rates, effective January, 1969, was to raise the per page rate per thousand of circulation from $11 to $14.

For a couple of years, the *Annals'* Editorial Board met at the site of the Annual Session. Attendance was disappointing. To improve the frequency and value of the Board's advice on editorial policies and plans, smaller and more frequent meetings were then scheduled at College Headquarters. Every two months, three members of the Editorial Board met with the editors. In the course of the year, all 18 members would have met with the editors at Headquarters.

Several new features were incorporated into the pages of the *Annals*. Three questions and answers taken from the *MKSAP,* with references, were featured each month, one each in separate subspecialty areas, beginning in January. These were quite popular. An additional feature was the regular announcement each month of the feature articles coming in the next issue.

The quality of papers submitted to the *Annals* continued to be excellent, due mainly to the rigorous and critical review process. The number of manuscripts also increased with 799 received in the calendar year 1966; 910 in 1967; and close to 1100 in 1968, providing a greater choice of papers. The journal also recorded its largest six-month circulation increment ever during the first half of 1968.

In December, 1967, the Internal Revenue Service issued new regulations which classified income from medical journal advertising as unrelated to the tax exempt purpose of a 501[C]3 association. Starting with 1968, the College would be liable for a substantial federal income tax, unless Congress reversed the action of the Treasury Department. Attempts to cancel or postpone the new Internal Revenue regulations were unsuccessful, making the College taxable on its net advertising revenues. The tax liability for 1968 was about $170,000. It was necessary for the Finance Committee to find a way to replace this lost income. Although advertising rates were increased the next year, it was not possible to recoup this amount through higher advertising rates.

The *Annals* had been printed by Lancaster Press since 1934. During these 35 years of steady growth, the printer had done a very satisfactory job. With a circulation of 45,000 in 1968, and increasing about 10 percent a year, the printing of the *Annals* had become a very large job. In recent years, the printer had experienced increasing problems in meeting publication deadlines. In addition, increased use of four-color work in both the advertising and the editorial sections created more problems in printing quality. It had been necessary to issue credits to advertisers. The complaints were so numerous that the editors feared the loss of considerable advertising revenue. Budgeted gross advertising income in 1969 was $1,247,000, making this by far the largest source of operating revenue for the College. The editors indicated that the quality of the color illustrations in the editorial sections hardly justified the extra cost involved. After an evaluation of the facts, the editors concluded that Lancaster Press had not grown sufficiently to keep pace with *Annals* requirements, and recommended that the College change printers. Cost data indicated that there would be no appreciable increase in printing costs (unless a better grade of paper was used) and, indeed, there might even be a cost saving. No firm decision was made but I was authorized to change printers if it was in the best interest of the College and the journal.

## Millis Commission Report on Graduate Medical Education

In November, 1967, the Committee on Medical Services reported their recommendations about the Millis Commission Report on Graduate Medical Education in a fully analyzed report and a point-by-point response. (The Board of Regents, in November, 1966, had already endorsed the general goals of the report.):

Because educational programs properly differed from one institution to another, the Millis Commission had recommended that each medical school faculty and each teaching hospital staff, acting as a corporate body, should explicitly formulate and periodically revise their own educational goals and curriculum. To do so would be a healthy exercise for medical educators and a fundamental step toward the solution of many educational problems. The Committee on Medical Services recommended that the Board of Regents endorse this item, which it did.

A second item for approval related to statements in the chapter on comprehensive health care. Addressing the question of why there are not more primary physicians, the Commission had suggested that there were three major reasons:

1. general practice, once the mainstay of medicine, had gradually lost prestige as the specialties grew in honor and accomplishment. While deciding upon a career, the young physician might never see excellent examples of comprehensive, continuing care, or highly qualified and prestigious primary physicians. It was certain, however, that the young physician would see and observe a variety of specialists and discover that they usually enjoyed higher prestige, greater hospital privileges and more favorable working conditions than did general practitioners;
2. educational opportunities that would serve to interest students in family practice and provide interns and residents with appropriate training were fewer in number and often poorer in quality than the programs leading to the specialties;
3. the conditions of practice for a general practitioner or physician interested in family practice were thought to be less attractive than the conditions and privileges enjoyed by specialists.

The Committee made no recommendation on this statement, and the Board of Regents concluded there were differences of opinion on this philosophical position. The Committee called to the Board's attention, however, that two previous resolutions were adopted by the Board dated November 13, 1965, and April 17, 1966.

The Committee reviewed a third item in the Commission report which concluded that 1) The classical rotating internship among several services, even though extending over a longer period of time, would not be sufficient for primary care training; and 2) Knowledge and skill in several areas were essential, but the teaching should stress continuing comprehensive patient responsibility rather than the episodic handling of acute conditions in several areas. The Board of Regents endorsed this position.

A fourth recommendation endorsed by the Medical Services Committee stated that there should be some experience in handling emergency cases, and that competence in specialized pre-surgical care should be required in the primary care program. This recommendation was also approved by the Board. Having reviewed the fifth item, ''There should be taught a new body of knowledge in addition to the medical specialties that constitute the bulk of the program,'' the Board of Regents withheld endorsement. It found itself more nearly in agreement with the sixth item, ''. . . it is difficult to find this body of knowledge for it is not yet adequately developed.'' The Board would agree that when such a new body of knowledge was defined it should be developed and identified for inclusion and integration in internal medicine training programs.

The seventh item stated, ''The level of training should be on a par with that of other specialties, a two-year graduate program was insufficient. It follows that there should be a specialty Board certification examination and diplomate status for physicians highly qualified in comprehensive care.'' The Board of Regents could not endorse that recommendation because it implied that a new specialty had to be established.

The Board of Regents approved another recommendation with slight changes.

We recommend that each teaching hospital that is *not affiliated with a medical school,* organize its staff, through an educational council, a committee on graduate education, or some similar means, so as to make its programs of graduate medical education a corporate responsibility rather than the individual responsibilities of particular medical or surgical services or heads of services. *This function in medical school affiliated hospitals is the responsibility of the faculty of schools of medicine and medical school affiliated hospitals.*

Another recommendation was approved which stated that internship as a separate and distinct portion of medical education, be abandoned and that internship and resident years be combined into a single period of graduate education called a ''residency.'' The following statement was also endorsed:

We, therefore, recommend that graduation from medical school be recognized as the end of general medical education and that specialized training would begin with the start of graduate medical education.

In response, the Board of Regents added the following:

Since many medical school curricula now begin or offer specialized training before the completion of four years of medical school and since some specialized training programs make an effort to include general medical experience during postdoctoral years, the Board of Regents approves this recommendation strongly emphasizing, however, that a flexible interpretation of the recommendation should be paramount.

Another Millis Commission recommendation was that the specialty board, in amending its regulations, would not increase the required length of residency training. The Board of Regents believed that this statement was unrealistic and that at the present time, four years of training after the MD degree was essential in internal medicine. The Board felt that individual specialty board requirements might vary and that these requirements should be determined primarily by the individual board concerned.

Several other recommendations by the Commission were indicative that teaching programs should be conducted only in approved hospitals, considering the current requirements of residency training programs. The Board of Regents approved, in principle, the creation of a Commission on Graduate Medical Education but urged more study to determine proper membership for such a commission: appropriate selection procedures, terms of office, etc.

The Regents, in summary, found the Commission's deliberations and recommendations parallel with interests of the ACP. The Millis Commission had concerned itself with the supply of broadly educated practicing physicians and the regulation of formal graduate training for all physicians including generalists and specialists. The Regents found themselves in agreement with the goal of an increased supply of broadly educated practicing physicians, and encouraged continued experimentation in efforts to increase the number and quality of all types of physicians with special emphasis on practicing general physicians.

They remained unconvinced that there was a "new body of knowledge calling for a new type of physician training, requiring new and separate departments for graduate medical training." Such new departments, the Regents felt, would only further fragment graduate training and lead to a deterioration in the quality of physicians. The proposed new type of physician should be a general internist rather than a new "specialist" and the need for prestige for this "new physician" by the formation of an American Board of Family Practice was not demonstrated.

A Graduate Medical Education Commission with responsibility for overseeing all of graduate medical education was recommended by the Millis Commission. The Regents agreed in principle but decided that details of the formation of this body needed clarification, especially whether or not it was responsible only to itself or to some other agency.

The Millis Commission recommendation that each teaching hospital be reorganized so that its programs of graduate medical education would be a corporate responsibility, rather than the individual responsibility of a particular head of a service, generally approved as long as the Committee on Graduate Education involved in this action would be advisory and coordinated with the executive branch of the institution involved.

The Board of Regents complimented the members of the Commission for their fine work, writing,

> Many hours were devoted to this pressing problem concerning the provision of medical care for the people of this country and the Commission thoughtfully considered the various complexities while providing suggestions and stimulation to all who are concerned. Selected from a group of outstanding educators and others with diverse talents and interests, they served well and deserve the thanks of all.

Several recommendations from the Committee on Military Affairs and Disaster Medical Care were approved by the Regents in 1968. A motion was passed recommending that the Far East Annual Regional Meetings be resumed as soon as feasible, utilizing the program format and ACP representation as previously established with the understanding that the College would send one or two of its officials to participate in the meeting. In addition, the ACP was to be officially represented at the European Annual Meeting of the Military Forces. Credit for attendance at the ACP Military Meetings was given to ACP Members and participation (i.e., presentation of papers) noted. The Committee recommended that College members be urged to be prepared to render individual and community emergency care, practice preventive emergency measures through instruction to patients and utilize measures such as immunization. Members should also be encouraged to participate on emergency care committees at medical centers. The Regents recommended the full use of the skills of physicians, nurses and paramedical personnel in civilian emergency care immediately upon their return to civilian life.

## Annual Session 1968

At the Annual Session in 1968, the Board also adopted the following resolution: "The Governors of the American College of Physicians are urged to encourage their members of the College to take an active role in the planning and development of emergency medical service."

The Board concluded a critical review of the status of ACP Teaching and Research Scholarships in 1968, with a view toward adopting definite criteria for the awards that would be helpful to the committee as well as to the applicant. The need for revision of the prospectus was stressed and the following criteria were adopted:

1. Scholars should be citizens of the US and Canada only.
2. Graduation from medical school should be not less than five years nor more than nine years prior to the scholarship appointment date.
3. Academic rank at time of appointment should not be higher than Assistant Professor.
4. Evidence of scholarly accomplishment, particularly teaching ability, must be documented.

It was noted that the procedure for endorsement of scholarship applications by College Governors was not being followed with any degree of uniformity. The Board approved the recommendation that the Chairman of the Department submitting the application should notify the Governor of that jurisdictional area about the proposal.

Ten ACP Teaching and Research Scholars were being supported by the College in 1968. Reports about each of these were received by the Committee, which was gratified by the high quality of teaching and research being done by these brilliant young physicians. The Committee, encouraged by the response to the program, agreed that stipends should be increased at all levels beginning with the 1969 appointments. The Board of Regents concurred and approved increases from $7,500 to $8,500, $9,500 to $10,000 and $11,000 to $12,000 respectively.

The Credentials Committee reviewed policies relating to membership elections from Mexico, a country which administered no certifying board examinations. In the past, there had been relatively few candidates from Mexico. These candidates were screened and their publications (usually in Spanish) reviewed by their Governor. With his endorsement, the Credentials Committee waived the Board requirement and elected the candidates from Mexico immediately to Fellowship. In contrast to this procedure, candidates from areas other than the United States (e.g., Canada, Puerto Rico, Panama) were elected either to Associate Membership or Fellowship, depending upon the qualifications of the candidate. The Credentials Committee wished to be consistent and obtained approval from the Board of Regents to modify the current handling of Mexican candidates, and to elect candidates to the category of membership most appropriate to the individual's qualifications.

In somewhat related action, the Board of Regents permitted Honorary Fellows the use of the initials FACP (Hon) after their names and, likewise, Corresponding Fellows; FACP (Cor).

The report of the Cancer Committee included the following:

1. The National Office of Regional Programs on Heart Disease, Cancer and Stroke had made a contract grant to the American College of Surgeons. The purpose of the grant was to establish a multidisciplinary committee of surgeons, radiologists, pathologists, internists, and pediatricians to aid in determining the competence and qualifications of cancer centers. Physicians would play an important role in the Regional Centers' programs on cancer. The Committee on Cancer considered it important that the College take an active part in this national effort. It recommended to the Board of Regents that a letter be sent to Dr. John North (ACS) offering the cooperation of the College. In conjunction with that recommendation, the Committee proposed an outline of standards for medicine in the Regional Cancer Programs, which was approved.

2. The Committee on Cancer discussed the question of instituting a subspecialty Board for medical oncology. This idea had been under active consideration for some time.

Though the Committee believed that a great need existed for physicians qualified in oncology, it was not convinced that a subspecialty board was required to assure this competence. The Committee recommended that, at this time, such training be included in regular internal medicine programs. The Executive Committee of the Board of Regents referred the Committee's observation to the Residency Review Committee of Internal Medicine without recommendation.

At the Boston Session in 1968, additional resolutions of significance were passed by the Regents. After several years of debate by the Cancer Committee, the Board endorsed the Surgeon General's warning on the dangers of the use of tobacco, stating:

The Board of Regents not only strongly supports the warning issued by the Surgeon General of the Public Health Service on the danger of the use of tobacco but, in addition, urges all members of the American College of Physicians and all physicians to participate in educational efforts that will ban the use of tobacco and, further, that the American College of Physicians recommend to the tobacco industry and to the Congress that cigarette advertising be banned on television.

The Board not only endorsed the suggestion that ACP Members urge their patients to stop smoking, but also agreed to encourage a ban on smoking at Regional Meetings, postgraduate courses and at Annual Sessions. This was done for the first time at the Chicago Annual Session in 1969. Dr. Kampmeier was on the Advisory Committee to the Surgeon General which emphasized concern about the effects of tobacco in patients with emphysema, cardiovascular disease and cancer.

In a report of the Committee on International Medical Activities, Dr. George C. Griffith, Chairman, noted that another postgraduate course had been scheduled for Santiago, Chile, in June, 1968, and in Cali, Colombia, December 4-8, 1967. He reviewed the South American postgraduate courses program for the benefit of the new members of the Committee, stating that courses had been held in Rio de Janeiro, Argentina, and Bogota, Colombia, in 1966. For the near future the College intended to concentrate on Colombia, with courses to be given in Medallin, Bogota, and Cali.

## Royal College Participates in Annual Session

In preparation for the Boston Annual Session in 1968, Dr. Daniel Ellis was appointed General Chairman. Dr. Peter Emerson, Assistant Registrar of the RCP(L), acted as liaison officer for program participants from Great Britain.

This was to be an historic occasion, celebrating the 450th Anniversary of the RCP(L). Dr. Kampmeier was asked to submit an historical article about the ACP for the *Journal of the Royal College of Physicians of London.* It was titled, "The Past, Present and Future of the ACP".

In terms of physician registration, interest, and enthusiasm, the 49th Annual Session of the College, convened in Boston and planned in conjunction with the Royal College of Physicians of London, was an unqualified success. The College recorded its largest Annual Session attendance to that date, including 3,159 members and 2,073 guest physicians, for a combined total physician registration of 5,232. Nonphysicians numbered 2,952 making a grand total of 8,184 registrants.

The Convocation, one of the most colorful ever, was presided over by the Presidents of the ACP and the RCP(L). Also attending were either the President or a representative from the Royal College of Physicians of Edinburgh; the Royal College of Physicians and Surgeons of Glasgow; the Royal Australasian College of Physicians; the Royal College of Physicians of Ireland; the Royal College of Physicians and Surgeons of Canada, and the South African College of Physicians, Surgeons, and Gynecologists.

Dr. R.H. Kampmeier, ACP President, presented to the RCP(L) three chairs to be used by the President and other Officers in the dining hall of their new Headquarters in Regent's Park, London. The President of the Royal College, Sir Max Rosenheim, MD, reciprocated by presenting the ACP with an antique silver tea caddy—commenting on the appropriateness of the gift inasmuch as the meeting was taking place in Boston, site of the famous "Tea Party".

At a special reception and dinner prior to the opening of the Annual Session, representatives of the various Royal Colleges were presented with framed etchings of the ACP Headquarters building in Philadelphia.

Complementing the colorfulness of the 49th Annual Session, the scientific program was excellent. The new plan of scheduling basic science and clinical science papers together according to anatomical disciplines resulted in a better distribution of physicians at the presentations. The TV programs attracted overflow crowds. The "Meet the Professor" sessions, a new feature on the program in 1968, proved valuable and popular. Tickets were available at the meeting free of charge and there were 3,900 requests from 1,900 people for only 150 available seats. As a result, "Meet the Professor" sessions and facilities would be expanded for the 50th Annual Session in Chicago.

A questionnaire was sent to randomly selected registrants following the 1968 Annual Session. The overwhelming majority preferred hospital clinics on television rather than live at the hospital. The scheduling of the basic science and clinical papers together was well received. Respondents indicated that they visited the exhibits regularly and would appreciate having them open on Sunday afternoon (which was done in Chicago in 1969). Physicians responding indicated that most stayed the full five days of the Session, but the majority did not attend the Convocation.

In the past the ACP had given awards for distinguished research or service. There were some clinicians whose contributions as teachers had equaled or exceeded others' accomplishments in research and medical service; and had exerted a profound influence on American medicine through their intellectual offspring who became professors. The Board of Regents therefore, at the 1968 Annual Session, established the American College of Physicians Distinguished Teacher Award,

> to be bestowed from time to time upon a physician who demonstrated the ennobling qualities of a great teacher as judged by the acclaim and accomplishments of his former students who have been inspired and have achieved positions of leadership in the field of medical education primarily as teachers of succeeding generations of students.

At the Spring Meeting of the Board of Regents, Dr. H. Marvin Pollard, President-Elect, proposed that a Governors conference be organized. This precedent-setting recommendation resulted from his discussions with many Governors at Regional Meetings, who expressed a strong desire for a special session of the Board of Governors involving a one or two-day meeting. The program could include discussion of teaching and visual aids, and other subjects of potential use in future Regional Meetings. In addition, it would permit an interchange of ideas about how the work and responsibility of the Governors could be expedited. The first Governors Conference in the history of the College was approved and scheduled for two days in the Fall of 1968.

The National Society for Medical Research [NSMR], according to the 1968 liaison report, appeared in good financial condition. Its activities increased during the year in a number of areas, and new educational material was prepared, distributed, and used extensively. It seemed likely that there would be no congressional action on pending legislation concerning the regulation of use of experimental animals during 1968. However, a motion was passed by the organization requesting that the Board of Directors of NSMR take an "aggressively constructive" position by preparing acceptable amendments to presently proposed federal legislation and at the same time draft legislation of its own for introduction in Congress.

The American Association for the Accreditation of Laboratory and Animal Care [AAALAC] continued to receive applications for accreditation, and its activities were publicized to the scientific community through a brief article published in *Science*. The AAALAC's finances were adequate for present needs. The ultimate fate of the Association depended largely upon what kind of federal legislation would be passed with respect to use of experimental animals.

A trade strike in Michigan halted progress for several months on the CPHA's new 84,000 square-foot headquarters building in Ann Arbor. Vigorous efforts were being made to gain occupancy before the end of 1968.

On other fronts, the CPHA established a Regional Medical Program Liaison Office to handle the increasing amount of work being done for and with Regional Medical Programs [RMP]. A study of the management of acute coronary occlusion in North Carolina was done in conjunction with the North Carolina RMP and the North Carolina Society of Internal Medicine.

The Commission also began offering a computerized Cancer Registry Information System in 1968 which would automate record handling procedures for hospital registries and could also consolidate data obtained from local registries to meet the needs of regional registries.

The status of the ACP/APA grant from the National Institutes of Mental Health was reviewed by Dr. Thomas Durant, ACP representative to the Task Force. The projects at the Faulkner Hospital, in Boston and St. Thomas's Hospital, in Nashville were deemed satisfactory and were to be continued. The Methodist Hospital program in Houston, however, for a variety of reasons, had been difficult to initiate, and therefore the project was transferred to Temple University Hospital, in Philadelphia. Two programs on psychiatry were planned for the Chicago Annual Session. One was to be a demonstration of interviewing techniques particularly related to adolescent medicine. The other was a panel concerned with the use of computers in psychiatric care. A program on psychiatry was also scheduled for the next annual meeting of the APA.

An Ad Hoc Committee on RMP was appointed after some meetings between College Officers and Dr. Stanley Olson, Director of the Division of Regional Medical Programs [DRMP]. Dr. Olson had stressed that the relationship between the College and the DRMP was important, but that communications were even more important at regional levels. The charge to the Ad Hoc Committee was basically exploratory in nature, and at the April, 1969 Annual Session, the Board would determine whether it should be continued.

The American Board of Internal Medicine [ABIM] was active on several fronts in 1968. Regarding subspecialty Board eligibility, the ABIM approved accepting Fellows of the Royal College of Physicians and Surgeons of Canada for subspecialty board examinations without going through the full mechanism of ABIM certification.

The ABIM announced that it favored a commission on graduate medical education provided it was organized properly, stating: "that this might well be organized under the National Academy of Sciences." Such a commission " . . . should have representation from the public and not be just an isolated professional organization".

Concerning the Board's examinations, the ABIM continued to work closely with the National Board of Medical Examiners [NBME]. It was attempting to incorporate some of the NBME's more refined techniques for assessing medical competence in patient management, hoping to improve screening for the oral exam. The Board continued to foster the small regional site arrangements for oral examinations and noted it was keeping up with the work load effectively.

Interest in combined certification in medicine and pediatrics, put into effect in 1967, was far greater than anticipated. The ABIM received numerous inquiries from medical schools which were setting up programs for combined certification. Despite this early enthusiasm from the medical schools, very few residents actually went through this program.

When the California College of Osteopathy was changed to a medical school, the ABIM agreed to accept their candidates for the Board, if they met all other qualifications. The AMA and other organizations were pressuring the Board to open the doors to osteopaths, providing they had proper internship and residency training. The ABIM remained opposed, because the quality of osteopathic training programs did not portend a reasonable level of success in the examinations. The Board thought that the necessary quality was lacking in osteopathic schools in general.

In closing, the ABIM reported to the ACP Board of Regents a statistical analysis of its past record: "In 1967, somewhat over 2,000 written examinations were given, the largest number since 1962." Fifty percent of these passed; 64 percent of US and Canadian graduates and trainees passed. Fifty-seven percent of all people taking the examination for the first time passed. The analysis of five years of experience from 1962 to 1967 showed that of university-trained US and Canadian graduates, 73 percent passed the written examination on this first attempt. These were people who had their postgraduate training in university hospitals. Those taking their training in VA Deans Committee Hospitals had a 61 percent success rate. Those training in community hospitals, not closely connected with universities, had only a 51 percent success rate. The figures for foreign medical graduates in all kinds of institutions varied from 20 to 30 percent. In 1967, 1,463 oral examinations were given. Of those having their training in university hospitals, 71 percent passed; in VA Deans Committee Hospitals, 65 percent; foreign physicians, 68 percent. This reflected the fact that the poorer ones were screened out by the written procedure. In other words, a foreign medical graduate who passed the written did just as well on the oral examination as one of our own residents.

The National Coordinating Council on Drug Abuse Education and Information was formed in 1968 to offer an opportunity for the private sector to work on various aspects of drug abuse. Fifty-five organizations accepted permanent or provisional membership in the first year. Physicians, especially those trained in internal medicine, played a major role in this field. Although there were no requirements for a financial commitment, the Board of Regents approved joining the Council and a contribution of $250 was made.

A career of 34 years of service to the ACP drew to a close at the Annual Session in 1968 with the retirement of Dr. Wallace Yater, the Secretary General.

One of the greatest things in my life has been my association with this College,'' [he said.] Serving as Governor for 15 years, seven as Regent and 12 as Secretary General, I've seen many changes. I've come to know many fine men and their lovely wives. Ed Loveland, the only layman to have been made a Fellow of the College and known as "Mr. American College of Physicians" was a predominant figure for many years. I knew Mr. Loveland probably as well as any man did. Dr. Rosenow, I've known for years before he came with us and I've come to appreciate his sterling qualities and great devotion to the College. This is not to discount the wisdom and judgment of the many Officers, Regents and Governors who have contributed significantly to the progress of the College over the years. My love of the College will never wane. I am by nature a modest man, but there is one thing you cannot deny, I have been the best Secretary General the College has had in the past twelve years. This is not good-bye - I'll be seeing you all.

# Part Five (1968-1969)

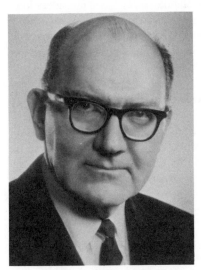

*H. Marvin Pollard, MACP*

Born in 1906 in LaMar, Colorado, Dr. H. Marvin Pollard married Florence Bell and they had one son, William Lee. He died July 15, 1982.

He obtained his MD degree in 1931 and his Master of Science in Medicine in 1938 at the University of Michigan Medical School. He was an intern and resident from 1931 to 1933 at the University Hospital in Ann Arbor. He rose from Instructor in Internal Medicine in 1933 to full Professor of Medicine in 1951, and became Head of the Section of Gastroenterology in 1957 at the University of Michigan Medical School.

He was consultant for the Veterans' Administration Hospital and was also a member of the consulting staff of St. Joseph's Mercy Hospital in Ann Arbor.

A diplomate of the American Board of Internal Medicine, Dr. Pollard was also a member of the following societies: American Medical Association; Central Society for Clinical Research; American Federation for Clinical Research; American Gastroenterology Society; American Gastroenterological Association (President, 1959-60); World Organization of Gastroenterology (Treasurer, 1962); American Cancer Society (President, 1970); American Association for Cancer Research.

He had been a Fellow of the American College of Physicians since 1939. He was Governor for Michigan from 1953 to 1959, a Regent from 1959 to 1967, when he became President-Elect, then President, 1968-69. He was made a Master in 1972.

During his tenure at the University of Michigan he served as Course Director for eight ACP postgraduate courses. He furthered the work of the International Activities Committee as its Chairman, especially its primary function of administering the Latin American Fellowship program supported by the W. K. Kellogg Foundation.

Dr. Pollard always thought that the one-year term of office for the President was not adequate to acquire enough information to conduct the office effectively. He cited the Royal College of Physicians of London as an example of a society which had a longer presidential term. However, he recognized that the Royal College was based in London; where centrality permitted a President to spend a fair amount of time at Headquarters; a logistical convenience not granted to us in the United States, whose Presidents frequently come from distant areas of a larger country.

He also wanted to explore the possibility of appointing a Chairman of the Board in addition to the President, which is the practice in the American College of Surgeons and the American Medical Association. After much consideration, he decided that the College should not change its system.

He thought that liaison with the American Society of Internal Medicine was fairly good, but insisted that the College Governors run their own show at the local level.

## "The Territorial Imperative of Medicine"

Dr. Pollard's Presidential Address was entitled, "The Territorial Imperative of Medicine". He quoted Robert Ardrey concerning the collapse of agriculture in Soviet Russia and concluded that it was due to a lack of dedication among the farmers. There was no way this could happen except from within the system. Pollard then gave examples in medicine where tremendous strides had been made because of individual dedication in spite of governmental encroachment upon the "territory" of medicine.

In some detail, he described how the historic Flexner Report* on medical education evolved. Dr. Pritchard, then President of the Carnegie Foundation, was riding in a train with Dr. Henry Welch, then President of the American Medical Association. He told Dr. Welch he had offered the legal profession funds to study legal education and was turned down. He then offered funds to schools of theology and they also declined. When he asked Dr. Welch if the AMA would accept funds to study medical education, the AMA, already having begun the inspection of medical schools, accepted. Dr. Flexner, headmaster of a small boys' school in Kentucky, directed this study. The study had a lasting impact on medical education; one result among other things, the number of approved medical schools dropped from 162 in 1906 to 76 in 1930.

Another report on medical education resulted from a study by the Millis Commission on Graduate Medical Education in 1962. Dr. Millis, President of Case Western Reserve University, headed this Commission. Dr. Pollard noted that both studies resulted from the medical profession's concern about conditions existing within its own discipline. He cited further the example of the voluntary formation of the American Board of Internal Medicine by joint action of ACP and AMA; formation of the Joint Commission on Accreditation of Hospitals by the AMA, ACS, AHA, and ACP; and the institution of the Residency Review Committee on Internal Medicine by the ACP, AMA and the ABIM.

He identified other areas of governmental intrusion into the province of medicine. Funding of research through the National Institutes of Health had stimulated enormous amounts of research. For a time, federally funded Regional Medical Programs attempted to direct more attention to continuing medical education. This worked out quite well in some places, but Dr. Pollard, accurately, predicted its failure if it could not relate more to patient care, stressing that more

---

*Flexner, Abraham, Medical Education in the United States and Canada. New York, 1910.

dollars should be committed to clinical investigation research funding to make it more directly useful to patients. While the territory of medicine had been invaded in major ways, he still felt the profession could establish its own goals and programs to resist the invasion.

# 1968-1969

First Governors Conference. *Annals* revenue tax. Members and Candidate Members. *MKSAP*-Japanese translation. Essentials for Residency Training Programs in Family Practice. Commission on Medical Education. Specialty representation in AMA House of Delegates.

At the November, 1968 meeting of the Board of Regents, Dr. H. Marvin Pollard, President, reported that he, Dr. Kampmeier, and I were the official representatives of the College at the celebration of the 450th Anniversary of the Royal College of Physicians of London [RCP(L)] in London, October 14-18, 1968.

Continuing his report, Dr. Pollard commented on the general state of world unrest over the past two years, which had resulted in increased concentration on medical services, medical education, and medical research. Stemming from this stimulus, several branches of medicine had initiated efforts to implement the Millis Commission Report on Graduate Medical Education.

Two groups had been attempting to arouse response to the problems relative to this report, one being the Council of Medical Specialty Societies [CMSS]. Dr. Pollard believed that the CMSS, then composed of members from only five specialty societies, was not sufficiently representative to operate optimally. Later in the year the CMSS took steps to expand its membership to 21 specialty societies, each selected because it had the largest number of members in its specialty. A staff soon was developed and the CMSS became important among medical organizations. It was certain to accrue responsibilities in connection with any commission on graduate medical education.

The other group was the AMA Interspecialty Committee, on which the College was represented by Dr. James Haviland. In both bodies the ACP was responsible for representing the specialty of internal medicine.

Dr. Pollard expressed general satisfaction with the work of the ACP/American Society of Internal Medicine [ASIM] Liaison Committee. Not only in his report, but several other times during the reports of various committees, he mentioned that if the membership requirements of the College and the Society could ever be completely brought into alignment one of the major differences between the two organizations would be resolved.

Dr. Pollard gave a detailed report describing the success of the initial Governors Conference held in Colorado Springs, October 25-26, 1968:

On Friday, presentations by a variety of people on medical education elicited interest in the Millis Report. It appeared that "frontiers in medical education" would involve not only postgraduate medical education, but graduate and continuing medical education. A reception and dinner was held on Friday evening, and on Saturday morning the Session was devoted to a panel discussion, "The Role of the Governors". This was a highly successful meeting and plans for its continuation were suggested.

Finally, Dr. Pollard proposed that a Personnel Committee be established which would consist of the President, President-Elect, Treasurer, and Executive Director. He also recommended the formation of a Governor's Committee on College Affairs.

### Annals Revenue Tax

The report of the Treasurer, Dr. William A. Sodeman, described the generally favorable financial status of the College, after which it detailed the most significant financial event in 1968: The Internal Revenue Service [IRS] had imposed federal income taxes on the net revenues of the *Annals of Internal Medicine*. These taxes would amount to approximately $170,000 for 1968 and the budget for 1969 provided for $285,000 in federal income taxes. Although there was hope in some quarters that the new regulations might be reversed in the future, on advice of counsel, the College decided the proper attitude was to assume that the tax was established and would remain in effect. For this reason, the taxes were paid. But as counsel had advised, the College had filed for a rebate. This began a long period of litigation in connection with which I, as Executive Director, and Mr. Fred Dauterich appeared before the House Ways and Means Committee, reviewing completely the implications of this action by the IRS. It was obvious to both of us that the Ways and Means Committee was not particularly worried about the financial problems of the College.

Dr. Pollard and I also testified before the "Nelson" Committee of the Senate (Monopoly Subcommittee of the Senate Small Business Committee). In the interesting one and one-half hour Session, we thought we had demonstrated that the College was not under the influence of the pharmaceutical industry; that we offered many ways for our members to keep informed about drugs, and that we were not opposed to requiring generic prescribing providing that physicians would retain the right to prescribe drugs by trade name as their judgment dictated. Subsequently, the editors of the *Annals* initiated steps to offer the Food and Drug Administration [FDA] a reliable and steady outlet for presenting pharmaceutical information to ACP members.

In my report to the Board, I reviewed additional information about specialty society representation. The AMA's new Interspecialty Committee was a start in the right direction, but in my opinion, the specialties would not really be effective in the AMA until they could elect their own representatives to the House of Delegates.

At a meeting of the Association of American Medical Colleges [AAMC], the Coggeshall Report recommended that a council representing specialty societies should be formed along with parallel committees representing deans, academic societies and teaching hospitals. I recommended that the College do everything possible to urge the AAMC to establish such a council.

At this meeting, one of the College Members, Dr. John Knowles, President of the Rockefeller Foundation, criticized the American College of Physicians and the American College of Surgeons [ACS], asserting that these two organizations were responsible for blocking the development of new doctors for family practice. I noted there was a lack of enthusiasm for its development among many specialty societies, but stated the hope that the Regents would adopt, with good will, the outline of requirements regarding family practice which would be presented later in the meeting. I believed that the College should not be in opposition to any efforts to increase the number of primary care physicians, but should be in the vanguard of those promoting innovative methods of coping with primary care problems.

In conclusion, I reported that I had been president of the Alumni Association of Carleton College and had just been elected a member of that college's board of trustees. I had spoken at a meeting of nursing home administrators and also discussed the *Medical Knowledge Self-Assessment Program [MKSAP]* at the Annual Meeting of the AAMC. I had been invited to discuss the same subject at an ACS conference in January, and to take part in the postgraduate program in British Columbia.

The membership of the College was surveyed in 1968 as to specialties and total numbers. The total membership at the end of 1968 was 14,783 with 4,217 Associate Members; 10,322 Fellows; 43 Masters; 33 Honorary Fellows; 34 Corresponding Fellows; and 134 Affiliate Members. A breakdown in membership categories was also provided:

| | Primary Private Practice | Academic & Research | VA Hosp. Staff, Administration & Public Health | Total |
|---|---|---|---|---|
| Internal Medicine | 8,278 | 1,293 | 948 | 10,519 |
| Cardiology | 533 | 125 | 78 | 736 |
| Allergy | 133 | 8 | 4 | 145 |
| Pulmonary | 75 | 17 | 33 | 125 |
| Gastroenterology | 209 | 39 | 21 | 269 |
| Psychiatry | 201 | 41 | 59 | 301 |
| Administration | | 7 | 372 | 379 |
| Pathology | 70 | 26 | 105 | 201 |
| Physical Medicine | 48 | 19 | 28 | 95 |
| Radiology | 56 | 1 | 12 | 69 |
| Dermatology | 143 | 24 | 11 | 178 |
| Neurology | 72 | 29 | 10 | 111 |
| Pediatrics | 63 | 14 | 12 | 89 |
| Other Allied Specialties | 255 | 98 | 105 | 458 |
| | 10,136 | 1,741 | 1,798 | 13,675 |
| | | Total Military Personnel | | 323 |
| | | | | 13,998* |

*Members not analyzed by specialty: Total 785.

The strength of the ACP was measured by the quality of its membership. However, unless the College did all it could to attract every qualified and eligible medical specialist to its ranks, its influence would diminish accordingly. Some additional information about participation in College educational programs was of notable interest:

| | Total Participation | | | |
| --- | --- | --- | --- | --- |
| | ACP Members | | Non-Members | |
| Boston Annual Session - 1968 | 3,159 | 60% | 2,073 | 40% |
| Regional Meetings - 1967-68 | 3,275 | 58% | 2,334 | 42% |
| Medical Knowledge Self Assessment | 6,375 | 58% | 4,869 | 42% |
| Postgraduate Courses - 1967-68 | 1,202 | 48% | 1,344 | 52% |
| Annals Subscriptions January, 1969 | 14,101 | 31% | 31,856 | 69% |
| Total aggregate participation, all activities | 28,112 | 40% | 42,476 | 60% |

Among those participating nonmembers, it would seem there were many who would be worthy College members. It was disheartening to recognize that many eligible men were not asked to join the College.

The Regents concluded from the results of the 1968 Annual Session survey that the Annual Session had become a very big enterprise and better coordination among persons concerned with parts of the scientific program was needed. After detailed consideration, the Regents agreed that all aspects of the scientific program should be the responsibility of the Committee on Scientific Program. For instance, whereas the Chairman and Committee on Local Arrangements would assume responsibility for setting up television programs, panels, etc., the approval of subjects, format and speakers and decisions on final courses of action in the event of difficulties would be handled by the Chairman and Committee on Scientific Program.

Regional Meetings varied considerably in their educational value, but furnished an important means of communication between officers and members. There was no question that the President, President-Elect and Executive Vice President should act as primary resources in this communication process. The fact that there were now more than 40 such meetings made it unlikely that these three officers could attend all meetings. Some Governors thought they would like to have the representative take part in the Scientific Program, and this was not always possible unless they could select Regents. In any case, there was strong feeling that better indoctrination of official College representatives would be desirable in order to assure a consistent and comprehensive presentation of College activity. A suggestion was made that someone from Headquarters Staff might go to a city a day or two before a Regional Meeting to help with the physical arrangements, but there were reasons that made this impractical. It was decided that more specific help in the form of instructions and checklists would be offered.

In a report of the Committee on Military Affairs and Disaster Medical Care, Dr. George C. Griffiths, Chairman, affirmed that attendance at the annual Far

Eastern and European Regional Meetings being held in association with the Armed Forces should carry the same credit for membership requirements as stateside Regional Meetings. The Committee also recommended that the College give official status to meetings of the Armed Forces Medical Officers, since officials of the College participated in the meetings.

The Committee further recommended, and it was approved, that ACP Governors for the Armed Forces and the Veterans' Administration [VA] should be regular members of this Committee. The Committee would also explore the role of the Governor of the Veterans' Administration, since according to actual practice, the members of the College in the Veterans' Administration's service participate regularly in the Regions in which the VA facility is located. The Committee discussed the role of the Surgeon General of the US Public Health Service [PHS] in relation to the College. This is a quasi-military organization and its personnel included members of the College and research fellows. Action was deferred because of pending Congressional legislation which might change the organization of the PHS entirely. The Committee urged the College to recommend officially that its members take a very active role in emergency medical care in their local communities.

The Subcommittee on Family Practice reported to the Medical Services Committee [MSC] a brief history of the family practice movement and development of ACP policy to 1968. After considerable discussion, the MSC recommended, and the Board of Regents approved, that the following statement supplement its previous pronouncements on this subject:

A. The American College of Physicians strongly supports the efforts of those groups involved in developing adequate, effective training programs for, and making available more generally to, the public the highest quality of personal health care.

B. The American College of Physicians approves generally the draft essentials, "Special Requirements for Residency Training in Family Practice", as a significant step forward. The practical aspects of implementation of these essentials require further study and experience in order to assure that training programs are attractive and effective.

C. The American College of Physicians urges its members to support actively the development of true training programs of this type by ensuring the success of those portions of the program involving training in internal medicine.

Part of the family practice controversy was resolved by the approval of the *Essentials for Residency Training Programs in Family Practice* by the AMA House of Delegates in December, 1968, and by the American Board of Family Practice [ABFP], the Liaison Committee on Medical Specialty Boards of the AMA and the Advisory Board of Medical Specialties in February, 1969.

The MSC discussed future areas of activity for the Committee. They endorsed the suggestion of the Executive Committee of the Board of Regents that continuing consideration be given to the objectives and future plans of the ACP, especially in the areas of delivery of health care and the ACP's role in continuing education development. Although four or five other ACP bodies were concerned with aspects of the rapidly developing health care delivery field, the Committee felt the subject was appropriate to its work, especially at the level of the community hospital. Therefore, it recommended the establishment of a subcommittee on community hospitals to inaugurate efforts in this area.

Finally, they discussed activity in the socioeconomic field. The ACP's primary interest was in education, but the sociology of medicine, and the economic aspects also seemed inextricably linked to educational aspects. Furthermore, this was the most sensitive area of concern recurringly in ACP/ASIM relationships. The Committee recommended to the Board of Regents that the ACP/ASIM Liaison Committee should be urged to aid, as quickly as possible, the development of functional and effective liaison through improved communication between the two organizations. They thought this might be accomplished by establishing some joint committees in which appointments of official representatives from each organization might desensitize some of the overlapping spheres of activity.

The Executive Committee recommended that the Board of Regents authorize the cost of scheduling an annual interim meeting of the Board of Governors similar to the meeting which had been held in Colorado Springs. After hearing the report of the Governors Committee for College Affairs, the Board approved a motion that the committee be called the Governors Committee on College Affairs.

The Educational Activities Committee suggested that consideration be given to changing the time of the Convocation to Monday morning, so that a luncheon could be sponsored following the event. That had never been possible in the past, and it had potential for creating good feeling among the newly inducted Fellows. The Board of Regents approved, and the Convocation was changed to Monday morning.

Dr. Hugh Butt, Chairman, reported *MKSAP* progress: Over 10,500 programs had been distributed and the College had ordered another 1,000 printed. The Board considered making it available to other countries, but no final action was taken at this time. The Board had already approved the general idea of repeating the program within the next three years; committees had been appointed and editorial progress was good.

## CMSS Purposes Outlined

Dr. Haviland reported to the Board of Regents for CMSS describing an organizational meeting at which the purposes of the Council were outlined:

1. To provide and promote communications among specialty organizations.
2. To further advances in medical education and to develop opportunities necessary to attract able persons into specialty fields.
3. To seek joint solutions to common problems of administration and programming.
4. To improve standards for medical care and to encourage responsibility for participation in the operation and management of medical facilities.
5. To assist in the maintenance of medicine as an independent profession.

6. To promote the individual and personal responsibility of specialists to their colleagues and to the public.
7. To provide a means by which specialty groups could have an effective voice outside as well as inside the medical profession.
8. To sharpen the focus on many socioeconomic problems, such as methods of delivery of health services, remuneration and the use of auxiliary personnel.
9. To aid in the prevention of professional obsolescence by the development of effective continuing educational opportunities.

Regarding its composition, the Council determined that any specialty represented by an approved primary board should be a participant in the Council. These should each be represented by that specialty society which most broadly represents the practicing specialists in the field. One representative would be allotted for each 5,000 voting members or a fraction thereof. It was further recommended that the Council be authorized to take action on the basis of a two-thirds vote of those present at a given meeting or when deemed necessary, by a three-fourths vote of its Executive Committee. The Board of Regents approved enlarging the CMSS according to the above plan by inviting other specialty societies to participate.

During a Board of Governors meeting in April, 1969, it was suggested that a standing Committee of the Governors on Regional Meetings be appointed whose purpose would be to collect information about the different Regional Meetings and make recommendations to the Board of Governors. The Board thought that such review of Regional Meetings would offer an excellent opportunity for even better programs and more effective exchange of information. This Committee would consist of six Governors with staggered terms. At this meeting, the Governors voted to recommend that a speakers' bureau be established. This item was referred to the Medical Services Committee. It was also suggested that the Committee on Public Information be informed of this, but no immediate action was taken to form such a bureau.

In November, 1968, the Board of Regents approved in principle the *Special Requirements for Residency Training in Internal Medicine.* It included the following main points:

1. The Chief of Service must be highly qualified and motivated and should serve long enough to provide continuity. The Section Heads should similarly be highly qualified. The requirement that Chiefs should work only in a full time capacity was not mandatory but this was a growing trend which was desirable.
2. There must be an adequate number of medical admissions. The residency must be primarily an educational experience; service responsibility should be limited to patients for whom the resident bears major diagnostic and therapeutic responsibility.
3. Residents, under supervision, must assume responsibility in patient management. Training must include 24 months of primary patient responsibility, which exists during clinical training when the supervised resident

directs the total care of most of the patients under his/her responsibility. The degree of responsibility must be increased progressively.

4. Scheduled bedside rounds should focus on the clinical problem the patient presents. These rounds must be conducted by attending physicians assigned this responsibility. Ordinary rounds made by private physicians on their own patients are not considered as adequate teaching rounds.

5. Well-structured seminars and clinical conferences and reviews of the literature are essential.

6. Residents should be aware of pathological findings on their patients.

7. Social, preventive and rehabilitative aspects of medicine should be stressed. Meaningful patient experience must be available in allergy, cardiology, endocrinology, gastroenterology, microbiology, hematology, infectious diseases, nephrology, nuclear medicine, oncology, pulmonary diseases and rheumatology. Dermatology, neurology and psychiatry are also desirable disciplines for medical residents.

8. Laboratory facilities of special kinds must be available in the community.

9. Internal medicine residencies must have strong supporting services, e.g., surgery, pathology and radiology. There should be an adequate number of residents in a program to provide intellectual exchange and sharing of medical education experiences.

### Annual Session 1969

At the Annual Session meeting of the Board of Regents in April, Dr. Pollard reported that the Executive Committee had recently considered the present and future role of Governors in College activities. The Committee reviewed the current method of electing Governors, the scheduling of their meetings, the relationship of Governors and the Committee on College Affairs with the State (component) Societies of Internal Medicine. No definite changes were proposed, but the Governors were to be encouraged to cooperate with the State (component) Societies of Internal Medicine.

The duties of the Governor continued to be concentrated on the problems of membership, postgraduate programs and Regional Meetings. It had become obvious that future educational activities at the community hospital level, emergency care, comprehensive health care planning in the community, and the development of close relationships with the State (component) Societies of Internal Medicine would be assumed by the Governor and the Governor's Committee for College Affairs in each Region. It was also recognized that from time to time more Governors should be appointed to ad hoc College committees.

Dr. Pollard suggested that since the Committee on Scientific Programs was responsible for all parts of the Scientific Program of the Annual Session, future programming would be improved if the General Chairman and his local committee reported to the Chairman of the Committee on Scientific Programs. By this means, the subject format and speakers could be more closely correlated. This action would add greatly to the duties of the Chairman of the Scientific Program

Committee but would make for a more carefully unified and integrated program. I commented that at this time the size and operation of the Annual Session had become a large undertaking and most of the mechanical, noneducational and nonsocial parts of the program should be handled by the convention staff.

In my Executive Director's report, I noted that the current membership of the College was 14,738 of which 43 were Masters, 10,281 Fellows, 4,213 Associate Members, 33 Honorary Fellows, 34 Corresponding Fellows and 134 Affiliate Members.

## Members and Candidate Members

A significant step was taken at the Annual Business Meeting in Chicago, site of the 50th Annual Session of the ACP, when membership in the College was made available to young physicians who had completed at least two years of postdoctural training in internal medicine, a closely related specialty, or as Medical Officers in either the Armed Services or US Public Health Service.

In a move to "close the generation gap", "Candidate Membership" was granted upon application and recommendation by a Fellow or the chief of a training program; these new members were given all the privileges of regular membership in the ACP except the right to vote or hold office. There was no automatic advancement to regular membership in the College and "Candidate Membership" was terminated one year after the date on which the individual became eligible for regular membership. The Regents went one step further by changing the title of "Associate Member" to "Member" of the ACP.

There were advantages to both the physician in training and to the College in this new category of membership. By the very nature of the resident's work, it had always been difficult to establish lines of communication with practicing specialists outside the hospital. Candidate Membership was an opportunity to associate with and to know members of the College. Additional advantages to the young physician were that, with the payment of modest dues, not only was the *Annals* and the *ACP Bulletin* received by the candidate, but also reduced registration fees for Candidate Members to the Annual Session, Regional Meetings, Postgraduate Courses as well as eligibility for the group insurance programs of the College.

The advantages to the College, on the other hand, were expressed in a tangible way: exposure to the College for the young physician early in his training. College members were given the opportunity to seek out and know young specialists, which was helpful not only to identify possible future members, but to offer opportunities for practice, teaching, research or any advice helpful to those beginning a career in medicine. Dr. William Cooper, Governor for Western Pennsylvania, an especially strong proponent on behalf of young physicians, had for years given over 100 *Annals* subscriptions to residents in his area. Dr. Dale Groom, Chairman of The Board of Governors, also supported this position.

The 50th Annual Session of the College in Chicago was deemed successful in terms of quality of scientific programs, registration figures, and in the acceptance of several new features. A special demonstration and a part of the program was devoted to computer science. A television program demonstrated the "hardware" and acquainted the audience with the jargon. "Input and output," "software," and "programming," were translated into meaningful language from the standpoint of the physician in clinical practice.

A symposium on "The Clinical Use of Computers" furnished additional practical information on the ways computers were being utilized clinically. In addition, a demonstration of "Computers in Medicine" allowed the physician actually to work with a computer at the Massachusetts General Hospital that had been connected with the facilities in Chicago. Automated medical history taking, recording and retrieving information, a computer-aided plan for treating patients, a method for making diagnoses based on sequential decision-making, and many other features, permitted the physician to become "involved". It was interesting to note that the type of questions increased in sophistication as physicians came to the demonstration who had already seen the television program and taken part in the symposium.

The "Meet the Professor" Sessions, so successful in 1968 with their initial offering, were increased to more than 60 sessions of which all were oversubscribed. In place of the traditional hospital visits, 24 "Talks with Teachers" were arranged at various Chicago area hospitals. Also, small groups of registrants were transported to the laboratory of a distinguished investigator to visit informally.

At this meeting Dr. Richard Allyn, Governor for Southern Illinois, organized a demonstration of cardiopulmonary resuscitation and several thousand doctors and others at the Session took part in this program.

At the November, 1968 Regents meeting, approval was granted to change the company which printed the *Annals* if the business office and the editors decided it was in the best interests of the College. After lengthy discussions with several printers, a letter of intent for the printing of the *Annals* was sent to R. R. Donnelley & Sons Company, headquartered in Chicago. The initial contract was for a three-year period, with annual renewals thereafter, to start with the January, 1970 issue.

The prestige of the *Annals* as a preferred advertising medium was noticeable in comparison with the number of paid advertising pages in two competitive journals. The *Annals* rates were based upon a formula of $14 per page, per thousand of circulation. The paid circulation in January, 1969, was 46,000 and it was conservatively estimated that it would exceed 48,000 by the beginning of 1970. The $14 rate was the lowest of all monthly journals published by medical associations. It was proposed to raise the base rate to $16, and with a circulation of 48,000, a new black and white, (noncolor) twelve-issue rate of $765 would be charged representing a 27 percent increase (11 percent for circulation growth and 16 percent actual rate increase). The increase was almost the same as the increase in page size (26 percent) when the *Annals* would be changed from 7" x 10" to 8 1/2" x 11" in 1970.

In 1968, there was a deficit of $34,000 from the publication of the *ACP Bulletin*. This was not deductible against the income of the *Annals* when computing the income tax on the journal's income. In the past, the surplus from the *Annals* had been used to cover the deficit from the *ACP Bulletin*. However, since the advent of the federal income taxes on the *Annals* it was necessary to sell $68,000 of advertising (less 50 percent for federal taxes) in order to obtain enough revenue to cover the $34,000 deficit from the *ACP Bulletin*. The Regents decided, therefore, to sell a limited amount of pharmaceutical and related advertising in the *ACP Bulletin;* only enough to cover the deficit. If advertisers switched $34,000 of advertising from the *Annals* to the *ACP Bulletin,* total income remained the same but $17,000 in federal income tax was saved.

As a result of the announced increase in the annual dues rate for 1969, many members purchased Life Memberships. Towards the end of 1968 and early in 1969 over 1,100 applications were received. The cost of the Life Memberships plus the original initiation fees amounted to approximately $560,000 being added to the Endowment Fund. Although there was an annual dues loss of $58,000, the long-term interests of the College were served beneficially because there would be an immediate and permanent increase of $20,000 in annual income derived from the Endowment Fund.

The College Staff numbered 56, and increasing demands for service to the membership indicated the need for more staff and more space. A feasibility study on the use of computers for the operations of the ACP (dues billing, circulation of the *Annals,* membership records) was conducted and the Regents authorized the Headquarters Staff to proceed with plans to install an Electronic Data Processing [EDP] Department.

The Staff had numbered 29 in 1959. Most of the increase in employees had been in the area of business administration. The expanding Staff necessitated additional space, and preliminary drawings for a new wing were presented to the Board of Regents.

The "insurance building" was to be demolished and replaced by a five-story wing connected to the most recent addition. Dr. Pollard hoped one floor might be used by the ASIM. Architecturally, it would match the present building and would complete the plan of a "U" shaped set of buildings with a garden in the center. Further studies were to be made and presented to the Board of Regents for final authorization.

Before the demolition of the "insurance" building, which had been a farmhouse during the Civil War, the College was informed that it had been designated an historically important building by the Historical Commission of the City of Philadelphia. We had to appear before the Historical Commission, and upon promising that our new building would match the Headquarters building architecturally, the Commission granted permission to demolish the old farmhouse.

The Building Fund, started in 1962, comprised over $1 million in liquid assets available to finance the much needed expansion in Headquarters facilities. The wisdom of the Board in setting up, seven years previously, a funding program for future building expansion was attested to by the fact that in addition to the funds transferred into the Building Fund, there was approximately $150,000 earned on the invested money and over $30,000 of capital gains realized, both of which contributed substantially to the funding program and made it possible for the College to be in a position to proceed without delay with construction plans.

The ACP/APA Task Force, with funds for pilot projects from the National Institute of Mental Health [NIMH], had arranged to move the Houston project to Temple University in Philadelphia. That project was then advertised as a postgraduate course to ACP Members in the Philadelphia area; three non-members signed up for the once-a-week course.

While the Boston and Nashville programs were working quite well, the project in general was not the success we had initially anticipated. The College was authorized to spend $47,000 a year, but in the first year only $15,000 was spent, and in 1969, even less. Three decisions were made concerning the fate of the grant. First, the federal government would be informed of the problems and that money not utilized would be returned. Second, the report pointed out that the College was superbly designed for some activities, but not for others. The Task Force concluded that NIMH grants should be applied for directly by community hospitals. Thirdly, the Task Force would continue its efforts to increase the interest of internists in psychiatry, but would concentrate on the programs at the Annual Session.

A second meeting of the ACP/ASIM Liaison Committee took place in June, 1968 (henceforth, two were to be held each year). One item of concern was the time alloted to the ASIM during the Regional Meeting of the ACP. The Governor for the College must of necessity be in charge of the arrangements for the College, but hopefully he would cooperate fully with the ASIM.

The membership requirements of the two organizations still presented some complications and differences. The dissemination of information between the two organizations remained a problem and methods to improve the process were suggested. The College and the ASIM were moving on closely parallel paths, but better coordination of activities needed to be developed. The problem of communication by comparable levels in the two organizations proved quite difficult at times. Several important items were discussed early in 1969, including the possible development of uniform application forms, the establishment of uniform membership requirements, and the possibility of having better communications between corresponding committees and councils of the two societies. No definite conclusions were reached.

With regard to eventual amalgamation or merger, although it was suggested early in 1969 that each organization canvass its members to determine how the actual membership felt, it was not done. Late in the year, the officers of the respective societies indicated that they were separate organizations and would continue to be separate. While the officers of the two groups agreed, the Governors and Members continued to talk about a merger and the question came up often at Regional Meetings.

The ASIM broadened its activities by increasing the number of its meetings and holding them in association with ACP Regional Meetings and those of other scientific groups. In some localities, it began putting on programs in conjunction with Sections of Internal Medicine of local Medical Societies. In general, the ASIM expressed a desire to participate in more scientific programs.

Another matter, somewhat more difficult to address, was the desire of the ASIM Liaison Committee representatives to have some portion of the ACP Annual Session turned over to the Society for scheduling papers on socioeconomics. The ACP Committee on Medical Services did not wish to relinquish its part in the program and this request was declined.

Specific recommendations and suggestions beneficial to bringing about better coordination and cooperation of the activities of the two organizations, particularly at the state and local levels, were to be explored and presented to the Board of Regents in April, 1970.

When the structure of the Medical Services Committee [MSC] was discussed, it was emphasized that the Committee's main function was the dissemination of educational and scientific information to College members. The close liaison between the ACP Committee and the ASIM Council on Medical Service and Medical Practice was to be maintained.

An example of new liaison approaches was the plan for the second trial forum on socioeconomic matters that was to be presented at the Chicago Annual Session which had been designed by the MSC with advice from the ASIM. The 90-minute program, titled "Medicine and Government - Co-Guardians of Medicine?" was to examine public expectations, government's role, and government's and organized medicine's proposed solutions to this problem.

## CMSS and Intersocietal Representation

There was some urgency expressed by the ASIM that they be represented in the CMSS and the AMA Interspecialty Committee. For the time being, it was agreed the ACP would continue as representative for the field of internal medicine in CMSS.

As specialization became more and more the rule, considerable fragmentation of interest resulted from medical specialty societies having little representation in those organizations influencing the development of effective educational programs and directing the delivery of health services. The CMSS and the AMA Interspecialty Council, in particular, were attempting to implement proposals relative to the Millis Report, recommending a commission for graduate medical education.

The CMSS, now representing 21 societies, met several times in 1968 and agreed that it should represent the major organizations of practicing specialists, offer a forum for the exchange of information and ideas of mutual interest, and that it should speak with a unified voice for the specialty organizations.

The CMSS believed that specialty groups should be officially represented in the AMA House of Delegates. At that time, delegates were elected by the members of the state society. Thus, a physician's geographic area was represented rather than a specialty, although many delegates belonged to one specialty or another. The Council felt that it was desirable to have some proportion of the

House of Delegates officially nominated or elected by various specialty societies. The exact number was not as important as the fact that some members of the House would be responsible to their specialty society and not to the state medical society.

To strengthen the voice of the specialty organizations, the CMSS adopted plans to invite additional societies to join the Council, in particular those with a specialty board. It was anticipated that in the near future, all specialists would be represented.

The AMA Interspecialty Committee, on the other hand, was strictly advisory to the AMA Board of Trustees. Committee members were elected by the Trustees upon the nomination of designated specialty societies with each specialty represented by one society. The College and the ASIM were designated to represent internal medicine.

An ad hoc committee to study the modus operandi of the AMA Scientific Sessions was at work in 1968 to change the method of operating the AMA's scientific sessions and to determine how more direct representation of specialty societies in the House of Delegates might be accomplished. However, no resolution was taken in 1968.

A proposal to set up a commission on medical education jointly staffed by the AMA and the AAMC was agreed upon as the most practical means to get this commission off the ground. The Association of Medical Specialty Boards preferred a freestanding commission but agreed with the general opinion that it would not be feasible to do it in that way.

The financing of the commission received the most active discussion. Dr. William Ruhe, AMA spokesman, wanted the AMA and AAMC to bear the full costs. He argued that otherwise the education program of the AMA would deteriorate and that the AMA might lose interest in the field. Spokesmen for the other associations represented thought that each should bear its share of the expense in proportion to its representation. A small committee consisting of Dr. Ruhe, Dr. Cheves Smyth (AAMC) with Dr. William R. Willard (AMA) as referee, was assigned the task of redrafting the proposals for the organization of a commission on medical education which would include, to a degree, paramedical personnel.

During that year, I was the Secretary of the Medical Intersociety Council, which included about 20 societies, academic and other, of which the ACP was one. The Bylaws Committee presented a proposed Constitution and Bylaws for the continuation of this Council. Dr. James Warren, President, had no strong feelings about continuing the existence of the Council. The Council voted neither to disband or adopt the proposed bylaws, curiously, but adopted a third option—namely to continue as a standby organization. Future meetings would be scheduled at the discretion of the President and Secretary. This is the status of this Council to the current time, but no further meetings have been held.

The results of a survey made by the Postgraduate Committee were reviewed late in 1968 and the information obtained indicated the type of courses desired by physicians. The Committee agreed, and the Board of Regents concurred, that in each year, until there were other indications, the College should offer three courses in general internal medicine, two each in cardiovascular disease, endocrinology and metabolism, pulmonary disease, and renal and electrolyte disorders; the remaining 12 or more would be designed to meet needs indicated in the survey. The final report of the survey was sent to each course director as a guideline in stressing certain aspects of content (where to place appropriate emphasis and especially what was desired in the way of course duration, handout material, etc.). Coupled with this, as new types of courses were added to the ACP program, a member of the Committee or a member of the College selected by the Committee would take the course and provide a special report of evaluation.

Undergoing a trial period with several of the 1968-69 series of courses was a newly designed evaluation form which was distributed to registrants after each course soliciting opinions regarding various facets of the course. These data would also help in planning future courses.

Early in 1969, the Joint Commission on Accreditation of Hospitals [JCAH] was requested by the Board of Regents of the ACP to make provisions for continuing medical education programs in community hospitals. The following statement was drafted and the JCAH approved it in principle and incorporated it into the Revised Standards for Hospital Accreditation:

The medical staff should provide a continuing education program or give evidence of participation in such programs:

A. The program shall be geared toward the improvement of medical care by keeping the medical staff abreast of significant developments in medicine.
B. Medical staff education should include hospital-based activities as well as participation in educational opportunities outside of the hospital.
C. Hospital-based programs should be planned and scheduled in advance and be on a continuing basis.
D. Documentation of these activities should be kept in order to evaluate: 1) scope; 2) effectiveness; 3) attendance; and 4) the time spent at such efforts.
E. The medical audit and utilization review should be incorporated as an important part of the continuing medical education of the staff.

The JCAH was in a period of change in several ways. Demand required over 2,000 hospital survey visits a year, even while hospital accreditation standards were being completely rewritten. While the standards were broadened to cover all elements of the modern hospital and intensified to reflect advancements in the state of the art, they were at the same time being limited to cover just the operation of the hospital itself. The marginal references to the clinical practice of medicine which had crept into standard interpretation (such as laboratory work done before surgery, and specific conditions requiring consultation) were completely eliminated. Hospital standards were contained in what was called Book I; a loose-leaf, flexible enough to incorporate changes.

Other measures for JCAH improvement were being undertaken. The survey procedure itself was thoroughly overhauled, the questionnaires standardized for computer collation, the time of the survey visit extended, the lone surveyor augmented with a professional assistant, the concentration on consultation and on the medical staff interests stressed. In a word, the JCAH was facing the challenge of government inspection and extraprofessional policing by attempting to perfect its program as the intraprofessional voluntary approach to maintaining quality services.

Beyond hospitals, the JCAH continued to offer accreditation services to long-term care facilities in the face of a tepid reception. Through the device of "affiliated accreditation councils," a coordinated approach to voluntary accreditation of health-related services was to be offered by JCAH. A council for facilities for the mentally retarded was planned and one for psychiatric facilities expected soon. Considerable interest was expressed by other categorical groups in the clinical specialties of medicine and in health-related services.

A joint ACP/American Board of Internal Medicine [ABIM] Committee, addressing the question of osteopathy, drafted the following resolution which was approved by both the ABIM and the College: "Resolved that the American College of Physicians would consider individuals who are graduates of schools of osteopathy who have successfully passed the appropriate certifying examination, eligible for proposal for membership in the American College of Physicians."

The ABIM, recognizing the trend of the times toward specialization, revised its examination procedures in 1969. Henceforth, all physicians going into a medical specialty were expected to serve at least two postdoctoral years in a training program which emphasized broad field internal medicine training. In the Fall of the third year of postdoctoral training, a Part I examination based on broad field training would be given. Upon passing this examination and completion of a third year of training, a certificate would attest the adequacy of the physician's internal medicine training. At this point, the decision to enter into practice as a primary physician or take further training in a specialty would be made. After four years of postdoctoral training, a second examination would be taken and if passed, a certificate would be awarded by the ABIM attesting that the physician was qualified to practice the appropriate specialty. Only those who had taken four full years in internal medicine would be eligible to be certified in internal medicine.

In establishing these new requirements and examinations, the ABIM hoped to accomplish two things:

1. that many physicians would feel the three years of training with an examination which attested to qualification in internal medicine would be sufficient training for going into practice. Certainly such men would qualify as primary physicians or general internists;
2. that physicians going into specialties such as cardiology, hematology, etc., would be adequately qualified in general internal medicine in order to fulfill all requirements for certification in the specialty.

In view of the ABIM's actions, the Board of Regents adopted the following resolution: "That a physician who has passed the qualifying examination and has received the certificate offered by the ABIM will have established eligibility in this regard as one of the requirements for membership in the American College of Physicians.''

The financial allotment to ACP Governors for Regional Meetings was revised by the Board of Regents effective January 1, 1969, to allow up to $500 to cover the actual costs of the meeting, excluding social events, but including coffee breaks, regardless of the attendance at the meeting. Social events, such as lunches, banquets and cocktail parties were to be self-supporting. If costs exceeded $500, a registration fee was to be charged to cover the balance of the costs.

Under the new formula, Governors were permitted to charge a registration fee with proceeds to be retained for local use. The balance in the fund and the purposes for which it was held were to be reported to the College Headquarters' office annually. Different registration fees could be charged for members and non-members, but students and trainees were not to be charged. If a registration fee was charged at a Regional Meeting involving more than one Region, it was to be used for the cost of the meeting, and any surplus funds were to be made available to the Governor in charge of the subsequent Regional Meeting. Any expenditure covered by this formula had to be approved in advance by the Executive Director. A financial report, filed by the Governor on a form provided by the Headquarters for each Regional Meeting, was required regardless of the amount of financial aid requested.

The formula for determining the allowance for each Governor's administrative expenses was amended as follows:

Each Governor shall be allowed up to $3 per Member, Fellow and Master, per year, for the necessary costs of carrying on the office of Governor. Reimbursement to be made upon receipt of a detailed statement. Where it is not possible to separate the costs of the Regional Meeting from the administrative costs, reimbursements shall be limited to the combined maximum allowance for both types of expenses.

Other revisions were made in the travel allowances for individuals on College business to bring the stipends more in line with rising costs.

Certain changes occurred in the Professional Liability Insurance Plan of the College Group Insurance Program. Effective October 1, 1969, Liberty Mutual Insurance Company, underwriters of the program, increased the rates. This was a national trend by the underwriters of malpractice insurance and some companies had increased their rates more than a year before the College policy was affected. The other change concerned classifications. In the past, Liberty Mutual had recognized two classifications for insurance purposes: physicians and surgeons. With the advent of cardiac catheterization and other procedures performed by internists, the risks of malpractice increased. A new system of classification was adopted by the carrier and ACP members were asked to complete a questionnaire for rating purposes.

A number of applications for professional liability insurance were received by Liberty Mutual and nonmembers who were associated with College members. Most of these were from surgeons or other specialists whose liability risks were greater than those of internists. The limits for liability for nonmembers insured under the College Plan were therefore established at a ratio of no more than $100,000/$300,000 or as deemed appropriate for the risk.

Chapter Three

# Intersocietal Ferment
# in Health Care Delivery

## 1969-1974

# III. Intersocietal Ferment in Health Care Delivery

## Part One (1969-1970)

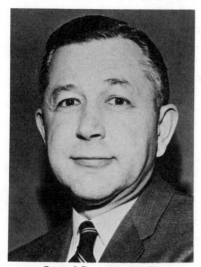

*Samuel P. Asper, MACP*

Dr. Samuel P. Asper was born in 1916 in Oak Park, Illinois. He married Ann Carver in 1942 and they have two daughters, Ann and Lucy.

Receiving his BA degree from Baylor University, Waco, Texas, in 1936, and his MD in 1940 from Johns Hopkins University School of Medicine, Baltimore, he served his internship and residency at Johns Hopkins Hospital from 1940-41. The following year he was a Research Fellow in Medicine at the Thorndike Memorial Laboratory, Boston City Hospital, but interrupted his research to serve with the US Army Medical Corps at the Fifth General Hospital, Harvard Unit, as 1st Lieutenant, then Major, from 1942-1946. Returning to Harvard Medical School as an Assistant in Medicine, 1946-47, he then was appointed as an Instructor in Medicine in 1947 at Johns Hopkins, remaining at his *alma mater* thereafter, as Assistant Professor, 1950, Associate Professor, 1953 and Professor of Medicine in 1960. He served as Associate Dean from 1957 to 1968 and Vice President for Medical Affairs from 1970-1973.

From 1973-1978, on leave of absence, he was Professor of Medicine and Dean of the Faculty of Medical Sciences at American University in Beirut, Lebanon, and Chief of Staff of the American University Hospital. On his return from Lebanon, where he and his wife, Ann, served the community and the university with profound devotion during the Lebanese civil conflict, Johns Hopkins University bestowed on him, in May 1979, the Distinguished Alumnus Award for "superb professional achievement." Few in the US medical community knew the extent of his dedication to the American University in Beirut until much later, but in 1976, he received a Tribute of Appreciation from the US Secretary of State, Dr. Henry Kissinger: "With profound gratitude for his warm friendship, unfailing assistance, and wise and comforting counsel so generously given to personnel of the US Embassy and the American Community in Beirut during the Lebanese Civil Conflict, 1975-76."

In 1979, Dr. Asper became Deputy Executive Vice President of the American College of Physicians. His active membership in many medical societies as well as his former ACP leadership roles were an asset to the College in this new capacity. He was a member of the American Medical Association, Association of American Physicians, American Society for Clinical Investigation, Endocrine Society, New York Academy of Sciences, American Association for the Advancement of Science, American Clinical and Climatological Association, Inter-Urban Clinical and Parapetetic Club, Phi Beta Kappa, Alpha Omega Alpha and Alpha Epsilon, the honorary premedical society.

A diplomate of the American Board of Internal Medicine, he was a member of the Board for several years, serving as Vice Chairman in 1965-66.

He was a specialist in endocrinology, publishing many articles in that field, and served on the Editorial Boards of the *Journal of Clinical Endocrinology and Metabolism* (1957) and *Metabolism* (1963-1969).

Elected to ACP Fellowship in 1957, Dr. Asper was elected Governor for Maryland, serving from 1960-1966; he was First Vice President in 1967, President-Elect in 1968 and President, 1969-70, and Regent, 1970-1972. In 1970, he was made a Master and was awarded the Alfred Stengel Memorial Medal in 1982.

He was a visiting professor and international lecturer on many occasions, received many accolades, including Honorary Fellowship of the Sociedad Venezolana de Medicina Interna in 1970, the Lebanese Order of the Cedars, Officer Class, 1971, and was a member of the historic ACP Teaching Delegation to China in 1979, when he was made an honorary member of the Faculties of Wuhan Medical College and Chunking Medical College.

When he retired as Deputy Executive Vice President in 1981, the Board of Regents approved a commendation, which was presented and read at the Annual Session Dinner in April 1982:

> It is rare that this Board of Regents has the opportunity to express admiration and approbation for an esteemed colleague outside the formal awards ceremony . . . Sam Asper has served . . . with devotion and skill, which will endure in the hearts and memories of those of us fortunate enough to have served along side him. With kindness, understanding, patience and good humor, he moved this College to greater service to its members and extended its influence across geographic, ethnic and language barriers.
>
> Dr. Asper has personified the College in his scholarly, compassionate, steadfast, and loyal dedication to our profession and the people we serve . . .

Dr. Asper does not know the word "retirement", and soon thereafter, he accepted the Presidency of the Educational Commission for Foreign Medical Graduates. Because of his valuable experience, the ACP International Medical Activities Committee asked for his continued assistance as a consultant. I recall, also, on many occasions at meetings of the AAMC and the AMA, Dr. Asper would invariably guide me to any meetings or receptions for international visitors. His sympathy and concern for the international medical community becomes deeper with each new challenge.

A statesman of the first order, Dr. Asper's graciousness extended even to those who served the College in the most mundane tasks. I recall chatting with one of our cleaning women outside the Board Room, where we were looking at the gallery of Presidential portraits. She identified Dr. Asper's portrait by exclaiming,

"Oh! Dr. Asper is the finest gentleman! He always says, 'Hello, Ellen,' and compliments me on how clean and orderly everything is.''

His thoughtfulness was expressed in gracious notes or poems whenever an occasion called for a few words of recognition for someone. At one banquet, he was musing humorously on our many travels together and remarked to the audience that I must be descended from a camel, since I never seemed to require a rest stop. His gentle manner in presenting such remarks invariably elevated the mood of the moment.

> Continuing education is our life-line, [said Dr. Asper, in his parting words as President at the 1970 Convocation] and whatever may come in the reorganization of our way of doing business in coming years, we must not overlook this factor.
>
> What is the best method of continuing education? Some feel it resides in scientific meetings . . . others say . . . rounds, conferences and seminars . . . We must not overlook, however, two fundamental aspects of continuing education. The first of these is to accept our patients, especially those with illnesses we do not understand, as a direct challenge to increase our knowledge for their sake . . . The second is to make use of quality medical journals and texts in steady reading . . .
>
> In our society today, there exists an attitude of anti-intellectualism . . . Surely in medicine we cannot afford an air of anti-intellectualism, for this nation's most urgent problems for the most part, fall in the medical domain . . . The by-word these days is 'cult of relevance' . . . Our scientific community is urged to determine not only what new knowledge is applicable to social welfare, but also to provide methods for its delivery. Yet, important as these new demands for relevance may be, we must not turn away from basic research, for its rewards are great, nor should we insist on 'feckless attempts to apply the inapplicable,' as Dr. Philip Handler, President of the National Academy of Sciences, has aptly said . . . but the bloom of medical science takes on more beauty when the results of medical research are applied to patient care . . . The entry of medicine into a supertechnical age of itself might be alarming, but fortunately it is effectively counterbalanced by a renewed emphasis on patient care and on the social needs of the community . . .*

## 1969-1970

*Annals* Editor, J. Russell Elkinton retires. Non-US citizens admitted as Fellows. Local nomination of Governors. In-house printing and data processing. Quality Care Appraisal [NCHSRD contract]; Manpower; Health Care Costs. ACP joins AEMB and AAMI. JCAH reorganizes.

At the fall meeting of the Board of Regents, President Samuel Asper addressed his major comments to the College's role in health care delivery. He stated that the major issue of the year, worldwide, was the uniform delivery of high-quality care to all citizens, and that the College's large responsibility in this task would become larger. Several committees were seeking in-depth solutions to the problem and when implemented, their decisions could contribute significantly toward achieving the goals delineated by President Lyndon Johnson.

*Annals of Internal Medicine, 73:2, 1970, 325-8.

Dr. Asper had a very strong interest in biomedical engineering, and introduced the subject into Annual Session scientific presentations. He was anxious to demonstrate the use of communication satellites and broadcast television at the Annual Session, selecting some suitable scientific presentations to be broadcast from the Karolinska Institute in Stockholm, Sweden and transmitted via satellite to Convention Hall in Philadelphia.

Though funding for this dream did not materialize, Convention Hall was the scene of a great event in television. The splash-down of Apollo II, the first manned flight to the moon, was shown on large screen television to several thousand people. Several panels on the program were delayed and one panel chairman was mildly annoyed and wanted to proceed with the panel. I agreed that certainly he was free to do so, but that he probably wouldn't have much of an audience. So he, too, watched the splash-down with as much excitement as everyone else.

Numerous biomedical engineering research activities were providing new therapeutic techniques and diagnostic modalities. Considering this a very important development for the internist, Dr. Asper appointed an Ad Hoc Committee on Biomedical Engineering, with Dr. Richard J. Johns, Head of that Department at Johns Hopkins, as its Chairman.

The Board debated the longstanding question of changing the time of the Convocation. Dr. Asper pointed out to the Board that at the Philadelphia meeting in 1970, a Monday morning Convocation would obviate the necessity of transferring people from the Convention Center to a hotel for any reception or social function thereafter, which an evening Convocation would entail. This change was approved. He received strong support for continuation of Annual Governors' Conferences. He also favored an action to extend voting privileges to Members. He submitted that Members were mature people whose eligibility for membership was reviewed with the same care as for Fellowship. Another reason bearing on the matter was that in some of the interdisciplinary societies to which the College belonged, voting strength was determined by the number of voting members in each organization. Since Members did not vote, the College had less representation in such councils.

The Secretary-General, Dr. R. Carmichael Tilghman, reported that the membership of the College stood at 15,467; of which 57 were Masters; 10,700 Fellows; 4,390 Associate Members; 103 Candidate Members; 136 Affiliate Members; 36 Honorary Fellows; and 45 Corresponding Fellows.

In the Treasurer's report, Dr. William F. Kellow indicated that two imminent projects would require substantial financing. A building addition with groundbreaking soon to take place would cost up to $1.5 million dollars, most of which was already available in the Building Fund, a result of the Board's decision eight years previously to fund the building program systematically. The second project, the conversion of some operations to electronic data processing, would cost approximately $90,000.

In the Executive Director's report, I suggested that Candidate Members be solicited by writing directly to residents who were entering training programs. The length of a temporary membership could be tailored to coincide with the time a candidate became eligible for regular membership. I was enthusiastic about the 2nd Annual Governors' Conference and indicated that a fair number of Governors attending believed that relationships with the American Society of Internal Medicine [ASIM] would be improved if there was a possibility of merging the two societies.

I reported lively discussion about how College members could be encouraged to become more active in the affairs of the College. Establishing local chapters would increase the incentive. One of the most important functions of such a chapter would be to nominate and perhaps eventually elect the Governors in the locality.

At their last meeting, the Association of American Medical Colleges [AAMC] voted to invite major specialty societies to become members of its Council of Academic Societies [CAS]. I urged the Board to participate in this new forum for specialty societies. I also noted that the American Medical Association [AMA] was exerting considerable effort to gain the attention of specialty societies and might eventually bow to direct representation in the House of Delegates of the AMA. I predicted that if the specialty societies really became cemented into the fabric of the AMA and the AAMC, it might not be necessary to support other interspecialty councils, but until such representation was available, the Council of Medical Specialty Societies [CMSS] should be supported.

In April, 1969, the category of Associate Member was changed to Member and a new class, Candidate Member, was added to include physicians in training.

In November, the Executive Committee of the Board of Regents stated that it had given long consideration to the category of (Associate) Membership. The first consideration was the new American Board of Internal Medicine [ABIM] examination procedures. The ABIM had decided that there would be only two years of postdoctoral training in the broad field of internal medicine, after which physicians who wished to go into practice could take a qualifying examination at the end of the third year of training. At the end of four years of postdoctoral training, they would take another examination. This was somewhat confusing, but it certainly necessitated revised requirements for College (Associate) Membership to make them congruent with those prerequisites. For this reason, the Committee recommended that passing the qualifying examination would automatically establish a physician's eligibility to become an (Associate) Member of the ACP, and the Board approved. These changes had direct impact on the voting representation of the ACP in various specialty councils. The rules for representation on the CMSS and the AMA Interspecialty Committee, for example, were based on a numerical representation of voting members. These changes by the Board of Regents allowed this new class to become voting members.

The College became a charter member of a new organization, the Alliance for Engineering in Medicine and Biology, contributing $1500, as requested.

The College also joined the Association for the Advancement of Medical Instrumentation with an annual dues contribution of $250. The organization was concerned primarily with medical devices and represented many individuals and medical institutions.

The ACP/ASIM Liaison Committee had met in July, 1969. The Executive Committee suggested that certain committees be made joint committees with representatives from both bodies. Action was deferred for further study.

In reporting for the ACP/American Psychiatric Association [APA] Task Force, I reviewed some of the difficulties experienced in operating the pilot program funded by the National Institutes of Mental Health [NIMH] Grant. It was becoming apparent that the College was not an ideal organization for sponsoring the program in individual hospitals, although some valuable experience had been garnered from the two programs. The Task Force agreed with my contention that individual hospitals should seek grants for such activity directly from NIMH, rather than through the ACP.

The Board approved the request of the Committee on Medical Services to establish an Ad Hoc Committee on Hospitals. This Committee was charged to gather and disseminate information to improve hospital patient care, staff organization, and professional relations, particularly relating to internal medicine and the medical specialties. Areas for suggested development included:

1. Core library resources
2. Guidelines for establishing standards of practice in internal medicine
3. Definition of the place of internists in staff organization and the governing body of the institution
4. Continuing education
5. Coordination of hospital facilities within the community
6. Emergency Room facilities and functions
7. More effective utilization of hospitals and their resources
8. Training and utilization of allied health professionals
9. Ambulatory care problems

The Public Information Committee reported a potential press interview problem that might arise at the next Annual Session. Mr. Donahue, the Public Information counsel, called the Committee's attention to an editorial in the September 18th issue of *The New England Journal of Medicine [NEJM]* which defined acceptable journal contributions. The editor pointed out that the *NEJM* accepted only original contributions and did not reprint articles published elsewhere. Exceptions were made for abstracts of papers published in connection with medical meetings and for press reports resulting from formal and public oral presentations. But it also stated, "Suppose the speaker was interviewed before the talk and provided additional information; here a decision might be difficult." In the *NEJM's* opinion, the material had been contributed elsewhere, if the speaker made illustrations available to the interviewer.

The Public Information Committee discussed the matter at length. It concluded that if the College were to change its policy and refuse to make manuscripts available to reporters in the press room or cease to arrange for press conferences, then accuracy of reporting and even the interest of reporters in our meeting would probably be diminished. The Committee advised Mr. Donahue that for the time being the policy of making manuscripts available to science writers at the Annual Sessions would not be changed.

The recently appointed Ad Hoc Committee on Regional Meetings recommended to the Board of Governors that this Committee should coordinate the Regional Meetings. This suggestion was adopted on April 20, 1969.

Evaluating the results of this arrangement, the Committee submitted the following policy guidelines for approval to the Board of Governors in October.

1. Each Governor should have a relatively free hand in arranging the regional program.
2. Governors could receive up to $500 from the College for each Regional meeting for nonsocial expenses. A registration fee could be charged to members or nonmembers to suit local situations.
3. The Governor, at his discretion, might arrange with other groups to be associated with his Regional meeting.
4. Each Governor should arrange for a yearly meeting in his own jurisdiction.
5. At least every other year, the meeting should be held in a city in conjunction with a medical school rather than convened routinely at a hotel or resort.
6. The word "Regional" should be dropped substituting the word "state" or "area".
7. The Committee would regularly review and offer suggestions for revision of the policy booklet and the ACP Manual section on Regional Meetings.
8. The Committee would develop a checklist which would be helpful to the Governor in arranging meetings.
9. The Committee would welcome suggestions for improving the meetings.

Dr. Hugh R. Butt, Chairman of the Educational Activities Committee reported that the first *Medical Knowledge Self-Assessment Program [MKSAP]* had been taken by nearly 12,000 physicians of which roughly 7,000 were members and 5,000 nonmembers. The anticipated budget for the second program was $115,000 excluding Committee expenses. The Editorial Board for *MKSAP II* recommended the following, which was approved:

a. Each of the nine divisions of the program would have one programmed question in each division.
b. Audio-visual tapes and other audio-visual materials would not be used in the the second program.
c. The translation of the first program into the German language was recommended.
d. If proper sponsors were found, approval be granted for translation of the first program into the Japanese language.
e. In the second program, the membership should have the option to receive data which could help them evaluate their performance in comparison to others. This option would be exercized voluntarily and the Committee believed it was feasible with a guarantee of complete confidentiality.
f. A bibliography would be given similar to the one given in the first pro-

gram, but abstracts would not be made of the bibliography, nor would explanations or answers to questions be given.

Later, Dr. Hinohara, representing the Japanese Society of Internal Medicine, visited me in Philadelphia and expressed interest in translating *MKSAP I* into Japanese. Permission was granted. Because of difficulty in releasing the original photographic material, the Japanese copied from the published *MKSAP*. The quality of these reproductions was excellent. The Japanese have continued to translate and distribute later editions of *MKSAP*.

Dr. Walter B. Frommeyer, Jr., Chairman of the Committee on Scientific Program, reported the results of the random survey of 1,565 attendees among the total of 4,773 physicians attending the Annual Session in Chicago. Of this group 34.6 percent responded to the questionnaire; 59 percent attended the Annual Session every year or every other year; 33.1 percent were in attendance for all five days. Preference for presentations were in the following order: 1) panels; 2) television; 3) Meet-the-Professors; 4) lectures; 5) plenary sessions; 6) talks with the teacher; and 7) colloquia. Finally, 27 percent attended the Convocation and of those 49 percent attended because they were being inducted as Fellows.

Dr. Theodore J. Abernathy, Chairman, of the Committee on Fellowships and Scholarships, reported that this was the last year in which any of the Fellows would be in their fifth year of scholarship. Beginning in 1970 there would be ten worthy young physicians, and from 1971 onward, nine persons in the program. How to identify the type of individual who should apply for these scholarships was a matter of considerable discussion. Of the present list of candidates, more than half had been graduated eight or more years previously from medical school, half were at assistant professor rank in medical departments, and many were being paid at salaries in the range of $20,000 to $30,000. The Board approved amending the brochure to change minimum and maximum periods of training to "no less than four years nor more than eight years of professional training exclusive of required government service." The amended regulations also specified that the Governor should be informed by the proposer of any applications. The supporting letter from the Governor would not be required, and a previous requirement for a personal interview with a candidate was rescinded and made optional.

In my report to the Board in April, 1970, I included suggestions from members who responded to a survey asking for methods of increasing membership activity. The following highlighted these recommendations:

1. Governors might be elected or at least nominated by the members in their local area. The Governors Executive Committee had suggested that the Governors Committee for College affairs might act as a local nominating committee; the official nomination to be made by the College's Nominating Committee.

2. Membership proposals might be acted on by a local credentials committee subject to review by the College's central Credentials Committee. All proposals for election to Fellowship would be the prerogative of the College's Credentials Committee.

3. Establishing Chapters seemed to be necessary to effect implementation of policies which, for example, are developed from recommendations of committees such as those on hospitals and community services. Chapters could also provide an excellent vehicle to work more closely with State (component) Societies of Internal Medicine. Certainly, in some states, it would be entirely feasible to form societies which included all College and ASIM members.

The Regents were somewhat disappointed with the modest response to the Candidate Membership program. It was potentially an extremely good program, and in order to give it further impetus, the name "Candidate" was changed to "Associate". The *Annals* was to be distributed to these members at a reduced rate. Implementing this, I was authorized to send informative circulars by mail to all residents in internal medicine in the United States, pointing out the advantages of Associateship.

Increasing membership activity at the local level was studied early in 1970, and charts of the large specialty organizations and how they elected their Governors were displayed. Although there was agreement that more local activity would be desirable, there was no concensus on how this could be accomplished. However, in the matter of electing Governors of the ACP, the following motion was approved by the Board of Regents:

The present postcard poll should be continued. The Governors' Committee on College Affairs could constitute itself as a nominating committee in each Governor's district, or the Governor could appoint a separate nominating committee.

The Governor would not sit with this committee, but he would name its chairman. Recommendations would be submitted by the local nominating committee to the national nominating committee. The national nominating committee would thus receive more input from the local area for selection of candidates to be presented at the Annual Business Meeting.

### Recertification Approved

The Board of Regents approved in principle the following points concerning recertification presented by the College contingent of the ACP-ABIM Ad Hoc Committee on Recertification:

a. There should be recertification, to be done by the ABIM.
b. Recertification should be accomplished by examination and not by attendance at postgraduate meetings, etc.
c. The frequency of recertification was not decided but less than every 5 or 6 years did not seem realistic.
d. Recertification should be a form of receiving an accolade and not be in any way punitive.
e. It should be voluntary.
f. It was suggested that for the most part the examination should be the one currently being used by the ABIM.
g. Recertification should be available at all levels, including the qualifying examination.

h. There was agreement that there would be no change in the individual's original certification because of results of recertification.

i. Identification of the individuals who are recertified would be done by reissuing a different certificate and list them appropriately in the Directory of Medical Specialists.

The Board of Regents considered the undue financial burden inflicted on the President of the American College of Physicians, who was required to spend a considerable amount of time away from his office on ACP business. It, therefore, decided that the ACP President should receive adequate remuneration, a sum of $5,000 during the presidential year. In addition, when traveling on College business, the expenses of the President and his spouse were to be covered at a rate of $100.00 per diem. In addition the Wedgewood Room at College Headquarters was designated as the "President's Office." Except for regular meetings of committees or the Board of Regents, however, Presidents did not use the room frequently. Thereafter, it was used as a Committee room and eventually converted to additional office space.

## Annual Session 1970

The Philadelphia Annual Session was the third largest in history with only the 1968 Boston and 1966 New York City meetings drawing larger registrations. A total of 7,560 registered; 4,892 of these were physicians.

For the first time, the annual Convocation was held as the opening program on Monday morning of the meeting. The convenience of gowning in the same building and then being able to go directly to scientific programs met with enthusiastic approval.

The demand for the "Meet the Professor" [MTP] sessions seemed almost insatiable. The 87 scheduled sessions were filled to capacity. As in each year since their introduction, the MTP's were to be expanded for the 1971 session in Denver and a fee of $1.00 per ticket was charged. Proceeds from the sale were used to supply coffee during the sessions.

A proposal presented by the Executive Committee to the Board of Regents, "The Appraisal of Quality in Hospital Care Provided by Internists: A Feasibility Study" described a request for proposal to enter a contract with the National Center for Health Services Research and Development, [NCHSRD].

Historically, this has been expressed by organized physicians in various ways, e.g., (1) monitoring of entry into the profession; (2) promoting and assuring quality in the basic and continuing education of physicians; and (3) supporting various accrediting procedures for medical care facilities. Recently, interest has been renewed in the direct assessment of patient care by peer review. The College, with its support of the Commission on Professional and Hospital Activities, [CPHA] has contributed greatly to this development. Over a decade ago, the College pioneered in proposing a manner in which a review of quality of care could be conducted. More recently, it initiated a self-test of knowledge to assist internists in identifying their educational needs. The College, in its position of distinguished leadership, could greatly influence the emerging nature of voluntary quality review by the profession.

The document continued with a review of the 1967 National Advisory Commission on Health Manpower recommendations and in summary, stated,

> The American College of Physicians has the opportunity to provide expanded professional leadership in improving and extending systematic peer appraisal of quality. Because of limitations in our current experience in quality appraisal, a well-designed feasibility study, incorporating refinements in method, would be most meaningful.

In general, such an effort could evaluate community-wide hospital care provided by internists based on criteria for care. The Board of Regents expressed a deep interest in this feasibility study and in the Summer of 1970, a two-year contract with the NCHSRD (HEW) was signed.

According to the contract, three hospitals were to be selected: one general hospital primarily serving a rural community, another in a metropolitan area which did not have strong medical school affiliations, and third, an urban hospital with very strong emphasis on referral type of practice. Each would have at least 20 internists and, in order to have a common source of record information, it was recommended that all be subscribers to the PAS-MAP of the CPHA.

## Health Services and Manpower Statements

"Community Planning for Comprehensive Health Services" was the focus of a Board of Regents policy statement issued at the Annual Session. Prompted by the unprecedented need for expanded medical care facilities and increased personnel training in the health professions, rising costs of medical care, the potential availability of sophisticated equipment and the explosion of medical knowledge, and prefaced by statements on each of these items, the ACP resolved:

> That prompt measures be taken by both private and public hospitals of the nation to combine their facilities to avoid duplication and to coordinate the availability and utilization of health services and personnel to the end that total community health needs may be effectively attacked.

> That the Armed Services, the Veterans' Administration, and the Public Health Services at all levels, coordinate and combine their health services to the maximum extent possible; and that mutual sharing of facilities with the communities be implemented.

The Board approved the statement prepared by the Committee on Governmental Activities entitled, "The Urgent Need for Federal Support of Programs to Provide More Physicians," which advocated the following:

> a. increased, sustained, and better planned support of teaching programs.

> b. that research support be expanded to increase the quantity and quality of teaching as well as to produce new knowledge which can be applied to the better care of more patients.

> The American College of Physicians strongly recommends that programs in teaching, research and medical services be supported in a balanced way so that the

urgent manpower crisis can be alleviated as quickly as possible to improve the availability and quality of medical services to all Americans.

The third statement, "Suggested Organization and Functions of a Department of Medicine in Community Hospitals," was presented by the Ad Hoc Committee on Hospitals:

> The primary purpose of the medical department of the community hospital is medical care and service to the community. Nevertheless, medical care and medical education are interdependent, a concept which is a basic feature of the organization of the medical staff and of the function of the medical service.

The body of the statement comprehensively reviewed recommendations regarding 1) departmental organization, including the role of the chairman of the Medical Service and composition of the membership of the medical service; 2) facilities; 3) functions of the medical service, including provision of patient care, evaluation of the medical service. Control of the quality of medical care, privileges and discipline of staff members and guidelines for residency programs.

> [The statement suggested that] . . . the Department of Internal Medicine should be organized to provide the best possible care for the patient. It should also supply, by proper organization tailored to fit the community hospital involved, a real contribution to regional health care, including education of medical personnel and the public.

With the increased emphasis on peer review and auditing of medical services provided in hospitals, the Ad Hoc Committee on Hospitals recommended to the Board of Regents that the ACP give strong approval to the general principles of peer review and medical audit and urge establishment of both in all hospitals. It was further recommended, and the Board concurred with both recommendations, that the Joint Commission on Accreditation of Hospitals [JCAH] include in its standards for accreditation, a requirement that a hospital staff show evidence of an ongoing program of effective medical audit.

Dr. Richard Allyn, Chairman, reported that the Ad Hoc Committee on Hospitals, was approached by the Postgraduate Institute in Massachusetts for help in validating a core library which had been developed. The Board of Regents authorized the cooperation of the College with the project, and the names of approximately 50 specialists in each of the various categories in internal medicine and allied fields were made available for a questionnaire mailing. Each specialist was requested to indicate textbooks and journals in his or her particular field which were of importance to the practicing internist. The data were to be analyzed to determine the validity of the "Core Library for Internal Medicine". The regulations of the Joint Commission on Accreditation of Hospitals [JCAH] required a library, and it was obvious that some "core" material should be immediately available in every hospital. Work on this project progressed through 1970.

The Ad Hoc Committee on Hospitals had been set up in 1969. In view of the amount of work it was currently doing and that projected for the future, the Board of Regents made it a standing committee at the November, 1970 meeting.

The educational participation requirement for continued ACP Membership was evaluated. The questionnaire sent out to the Associate members in 1966 had revealed that there was sufficient evidence of educational participation by Associate members to make the requirement unnecessary. The Board of Governors, however, continued its review by appointing an ad hoc committee to prepare recommendations for the Board of Regents. At the April, 1970 meeting, the Board of Regents tabled action pending the outcome of discussions about recertification.

The Committee on Educational Activities also studied the question and reported that it would be fairly easy to track participation in College educational activities, but it virtually meant monitoring participation in continuing education produced by other organizations besides ACP. Meaningful continuing education activity, if required, could not be restricted to College educational activities only. At one time, the ABIM tried to do this, found it difficult and turned to the examination. The Committee doubted that many Governors, if it became their duty, would actually recommend termination of College Membership if the educational requirements were not met. Governors would vary in degrees of leniency in considering requests for waivers, and the College would find it difficult to actually dismiss a member. There was also little chance that a dismissed member would ever again attend any College educational activities.

The Board of Regents approved a motion stating that compulsory participation in educational activities as a requirement was not necessary or desirable for maintenance of membership in the College.

In April, 1970, the Committee on Governmental Activities in Medicine recommended to the Board of Regents a set of principles that the ACP or its surrogates could support when the advice of the College was sought by governmental agencies concerned with health care. The recommendation stated,

> The medical profession and the general public holds the American College of Physicians accountable as the leader in clinical practice involving all phases of internal medicine. What are we doing at this time - we would be asked - to make certain that sound policies for the delivery of quality health care are built into the practices of government agencies responsible for such care?

> Within Health Education and Welfare [HEW], there is a movement to "the least cost mechanism" within a given geographic area - rather than the original concept of reimbursement for cost, no matter how much those costs differed within the same geographic area. In addition, new HEW regulations will require participating hospitals to have Prospective Review, inquiring for example, into how often the physician actually saw the patient, what laboratory tests were performed and which were ordered, and so forth. Retrospective review appeared to have real value only when the same individuals reviewed both utilization and quality, and this was seldom done.

With this background, the Committee recommended, and the Board of Regents approved, the following as principles to clarify College policy in these matters:

1. That quality control and continuing or in-service education must be included in the "least cost" mechanism for the determination of charges for the delivery of health care.
2. That the physician is the key to the cost of health care, not just in the fee

that he charges for his services, but because he is responsible for the total health care picture. It is the physician who decides which patients to admit to the hospital, what laboratory and radiologic examinations to perform, what consultants to seek, and when to discharge the patient. Since the government simply hasn't the capacity for effective audit of physicians, the key to making the programs of Medicare and Medicaid work is the physician and his medical society. There could be a strong movement toward economy by orienting physicians to the cost of all the procedures, diagnostic and therapeutic, which they perform. This is an additional reason for placing physicians on Boards of Trustees of hospitals. Physicians will not and cannot control costs for which they are not held accountable.

3. That, since by training and by temperament, the internist is particularly well qualified to work with others in the health care field, the members of the ACP should be encouraged to participate as broadly as possible in:

a. Utilization review committees
b. Peer review committees
c. Boards of Trustees of Blue Shield and Blue Cross Plans
d. Hospital Boards of Trustees
e. and in other similar activities.

The Committee continued to develop methodologies for the maintenance of standards of quality care in internal medicine and reported to the Regents in November, 1970. In agreement with Article III of the ACP Constitution (Section 1, Paragraph (c), which states that one of the purposes of the College is "maintaining both the dignity of internal medicine and the efficiency of its function in relation to public welfare," the ACP's Board of Regents endorsed the principle that its Officers, Fellows, and Members have a responsibility as citizens to become as well acquainted as possible with their elected representatives (local, state, and federal). This responsibility carried with it the duty to be knowledgeable of the facts of any given issue, whether it be primarily medical or nonmedical and to be willing to transmit these facts to their representatives in the interests of the public.

It was with regret that the Board of Regents accepted the resignation of Dr. J. Russell Elkinton, Editor of the *Annals*, effective July, 1971. Dr. Elkinton became Editor in 1960 and under his leadership, "one of the outstanding medical journals of the world", as he referred to the *Annals* in his first editorial, not only remained in that group but grew to even greater eminence in medical journalism. This was due in large part to Dr. Elkinton's decision to continue to seek the critical advice of many skilled and knowledgeable men in all parts of the United States in selecting manuscripts for publication. The growth in circulation during the 11 years of his tenure was remarkable, from 24,000 in 1960 to over 53,000 at the time of his retirement in June, 1971. The number of manuscripts submitted for publication had risen from 500 annually in 1960 to over 1,000 in 1970.

Dr. Marshall N. Fulton, FACP, Chairman of the ACP Committee on Publications paid tribute to Dr. Elkinton in an editorial that appeared in the *Annals* in July, 1971.

The American College of Physicians owes a great debt of gratitude to this distinguished Fellow, now a Master of the College. As Editor of its official journal for nearly 11 years, Dr. Elkinton has left his indelible mark, not only in his contribution to American medical journalism, but specifically in adding to the prestige of the American College of Physicians in furthering one of its main purposes, namely, that of maintaining and advancing the highest possible standards in medical education.

A questionnaire was sent to every tenth subscriber to the *Annals* early in 1970 and 55 percent responded. It was of interest that the mixture of articles of clinical nature and of basic science were thought by respondents to be in correct proportion. An increase in information concerning new drugs was requested by 44 percent of the respondents. The new format of the *Annals* was gratifying to most, although a sizeable minority had objected to the increase in trim size as being both harder to hold and to place on library shelves. The majority, however, approved as the journal was better looking and easier to read.

Some difficulties were encountered in making the press schedule work with the new printer, R. R. Donnelley & Company. Delays were attributable both to the printer and the College, but familiarity and experience soon rectified many of the initial problems.

There was a substantial drop in the number of pages of advertising in the *Annals* in 1970. A general decline had been recorded in medical advertising throughout the industry, and some advertisers were transferring more volume to the journals that dispersed advertisements throughout the editorial content.

The format of the *Annals* divided the advertising approximately between two-thirds in the front of the book and one-third in the back. Many of the large pharmaceutical companies complained about the College's policy of "stacking" advertisements, maintaining that with 50 to 100 consecutive pages of advertisements, readers tended to skip to the editorial content in the center of the *Annals*. This problem was discussed in 1970 and the Publications and Finance Committees were instructed to arrive at a policy and report to the Board of Regents in 1971.

Some journals were carrying classified advertising material, including openings for internships, residencies and graduate physicians. The Board approved this measure in principle to expand College services to members and subscribers and to provide a source of additional income. The Director of Administration and Finance was instructed to pursue the matter and report to the Board of Regents.

The *ACP Bulletin* was to receive a new format with the January, 1971 issue. A new page size, 8 1/4"x 11" conformed with that used in most similar magazines.

At the Board of Regents meeting in April, 1970, the Ad Hoc Committee to Study The Objectives of the College presented changes for incorporation in the Mission Statement of the Constitution and Bylaws. The report was referred to the Constitution and Bylaws Committee for appropriate wording. In preface to the objectives, the Committee stated:

Whereas education continues to be the primary and unremitting concern of the College, if the College is to maintain a position of positive leadership for internists and is to be the effective spokesman for internal medicine and its subspecialties, then the objectives of the College as set forth in Article 3, Section 1, must be interpreted and developed more broadly.

The following objectives set forth some but not all of the expanded program areas for the College in the future:

a. Advancing the standards of education and training for preliminary education of physicians, graduate training in internal medicine, and continuing education of internists.
b. Establishing and improving standards of practice in internal medicine.
c. Defining and developing the role of internists in the delivery of health care.
d. Serving as a forum for medical specialties.
e. Aiding the promotion of an adequate provision for research.
f. Helping to define and develop social policy as it affects health.
g. Serving as the spokesman for internal medicine by virtue of effective and constructive collaboration with other organizations of similar purpose.

The structure of all ACP committees was also reviewed, and the Board of Regents approved the following changes in committee structure: Committees on Membership, Meeting Sites, Pensions, the Consulting Committee on Scientific Program, and the Ad Hoc Committee on Regional Medical Programs were discharged, and their functions absorbed by other committees. Committee names were changed to reflect the nature of their functions: Medical Services to Committee on Community Service; Finance and Budgets to Committee on Finance. The terms of all Committee members were changed to two years with a maximum of three terms and the Chairman was no longer required to be a Regent.

The new Committee on Community Service was to be concerned with the implications of scientific and sociologic advances for medicine, devoting special attention to the effect of these advances on medical teaching, research and the delivery of health services. Where appropriate, the Committee was to study and develop recommendations for College positions and programs which dealt with a variety of communities making special demands for health services including the disadvantaged, ghetto and rural groups. ACP activities were to be expanded, when indicated, in the following areas: medico-legal considerations as they affect the internist; matters of information and public relations as they pertain to internal medicine, and the development and maintenance of standards in internal medicine as innovations appear in health care delivery.

Membership for noncitizens was discussed by the Credentials Committee in 1970. The Bylaws stated, under Article VI Section 1, "Qualifications" subsection, "Noncitizens may be elected to Full Fellowship in the College, when such a candidate meets all other requirements except residence and citizenship." Heretofore, candidates in the noncitizen class were those who had received their training in the United States or Canada, and indicated their intention of returning to their country of origin. This clearly did not allow election of noncitizens to Membership and thus eliminated the possibility of a noncitizen Member returning to his native country where, in the absence of a Governor, further supervision, proposal and endorsement for advancement to Fellowship would be impossible. On the other hand, certain fully qualified noncitizens who entered the country were barred from Fellowship because of citizenship. The Board of Regents authorized the Credentials Committee to interpret that section of the Bylaws on qualifications broadly and make it a policy to elect to Fellowship selected noncitizens on a permanent visa status in the United States, provided these noncitizens were fully qualified in all other respects.

The Residency Revolving Loan Fund of the College was considered a very valuable College service to young physicians. However, a good deal of trouble was encountered in the repayment of loans. The Board approved the following requests from the Fund Committee and administrative changes were adopted to effect more efficient operation of the Fund. The Committee announced that,

> Strenuous, but considerate efforts will be made to obtain payment of loans upon maturity and to insure interest payments when due. A letter, appropriately worded and signed by the Chairman, will be sent to each grantee prior to and, in the event of nonpayment, six months after maturity of the loan. A study is being made of the "Graduate and Professional Student's Financial Statement" of the College Scholarship Service, Princeton, N.J. From this, we will consider revision of our present questionnaire on whether it would be preferable to obtain the evaluation of financial need from the service. This is the practice in many colleges and graduate schools. If the evaluation were done by the service, it would involve no cost to us, but a three dollar fee to be paid by each applicant.

> In the future, monthly reports prepared by the Committee Secretary with the cooperation of the ACP accounting office will be sent to each member of the Committee and any questions or reservations as to the evaluation of applicants' needs will be sent to the Chairman prior to committing the loan.

> Up to the present there has been no information about the careers of our grantees other than for those who had become Fellows or Associate Members of the College. It was voted that a questionnaire be composed and sent to each grantee who had received a loan ten or more years previously; and that this be a continuing process. It is probable that the Fund can support itself for the remainder of 1970 with its estimated working capital of $33,361. However, this will not be possible if the $25,000 appropriated in 1967 is withdrawn or if the receivables do not materialize as estimated. It was therefore voted that the Board of Regents be requested to authorize the Committee on Finance to honor its previous commitment of $25,000; and that additional emergency funds, not to exceed $5,000, be made available to the Residency Revolving Loan Fund upon demonstration of need to continue the program for 1970.

As a result of the feasibility study on the use of computers in the operations of the College, the Board approved a contract with the Sperry Rand Corporation, Univac Division, to lease a Univac 9200 Model II Computer with appropriate peripheral devices, judging its bid to be the best in performance and economy.

A comparative analysis was made of in-house versus outside printing costs. Relative costs of both options were comparable, but internal control and in-house capacity to respond to immediate needs for many items were considered sufficiently justifiable to introduce an in-house printing operation.

At the November, 1969 Board of Regents meeting, the reduced dues rate of $20 for Mexican and Latin American Members was eliminated and these Members were put on the same dues schedule as residents of the United States and Canada. As of April 1, 1970, 37 of 74 Mexican Members had not paid their 1970 dues and the headquarters office was informed by the Governors that the new dues rates were a financial hardship for many of these Members. It was therefore approved that dues for Mexican Members be 50 percent of the basic rate with a minimum of $20 and the Initiation Fee be $50 instead of $80 - retroactive to January 1, 1970.

## JCAH Reorganizes

The JCAH completed development of its administrative organizational structure and personnel strength to meet the expanded role given it by decisions of its Board of Commissioners. Under the Office of the Director, three major divisions were created: the Division of Programs administered the Accreditation Programs, including hospitals, long-term care facilities, rehabilitation facilities, facilities for the mentally retarded and psychiatric facilities. The Division of Research and Education contained a Department of Research which was developing new hospital standards and survey instruments, and a Department of Education, only partially activated, which provided professional orientation, personnel training and public information. The Division of Central Services served the organization's administrative necessities.

The Accreditation Council for Psychiatric Facilities was created in February, 1970, and had its first organizing meeting that same month. It was sponsored, under JCAH auspices, by the American Academy of Child Psychiatry, the American Association on Mental Deficiency, the American Psychiatric Association, the National Association of Private Psychiatric Hospitals and the National Association of State Mental Health Program Directors. Funding came from Council member contributions and a two-year Federal grant during the developmental phase. The program anticipated the establishment of standards for all forms of psychiatric facilities and services and hoped to offer an accreditation service to them by 1971.

The rapidly expanding activities of the Joint Commission aroused, in the minds of its Corporate Members, a question of future financial support. Each Commissioner's seat had cost sponsors slightly more than $14,000 per annum. The Board of Commissioners had taken careful steps to assure that each new accreditation council formed had in hand sufficient funds to support completely its first two years of operation. By that time, the field survey program of the council would be expected to generate sufficient survey income to support operations, while council member organizations would support general council activities. Furthermore, each council's agreement with the Joint Commission would provide a contribution of 10 percent of its gross survey fee income to support the basic budget of the Division of Research and Education. This together with outside contributions from granting sources would finance the division's services to all programs. It, of course, remained for JCAH member organizations to support Commission expenses and the costs of the Office of the Director and its necessary activities of supervision and direction.

Several innovations were introduced by the Residency Review Committee in Internal Medicine [RRC-IM]. A Long-Range Planning Committee was formed to consider issues relating to graduate medical education. A revision of the Essentials of an Approved Residency in Internal Medicine had been formulated, which was approved by the Board of Regents and by the ABIM. In 1970, approval by the House of Delegates of the AMA was still pending. In addition, some revisions of the procedures used by the RRC-IM in data acquisition and evaluation were introduced, and consideration of the substantial problems related to foreign medical graduates was initiated.

The Committee agreed to take on review of straight medical internships and of rotating ("mixed") internships which consisted largely of training in internal medicine, so that graduate training in internal medicine in a given institution could be evaluated as a whole. Under consideration was the evaluation of subspecialty training in departments of medicine.

Efforts had been made to define with somewhat greater precision the ways in which private patients could contribute more effectively to graduate training in internal medicine. Closer coordination with the examination procedures and results of the examination had evolved, and proved helpful in program evaluation. The Committee was making attempts to improve communications between the Committee and the Council on Medical Education of the AMA. The evolutionary nature of the field was a continuing challenge for the Committee, and these initial steps formed the basis for a process of ongoing productive change.

## Part Two (1970-1971)

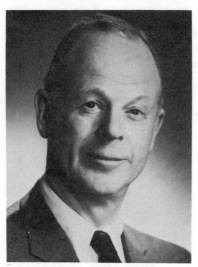

*James Haviland, MACP*

James Haviland was born in 1911 in Glens Falls, New York; he received his BA degree in 1932 from Union College in Schenectady and his MD in 1936 from Johns Hopkins University School of Medicine. He married Marion Cranston Bertram in 1943 and they had four children, James, Elizabeth, Donald and Martha.

Following his internship at Johns Hopkins Hospital, he served his residencies in internal medicine and pediatrics at Johns Hopkins from 1936-1938 and 1939-40, and an additional assistant residency in medicine at the New Haven Hospital in Connecticut in 1938-39. He was appointed to instructorships in medicine at the Yale University School of Medicine in 1938-39 and at Johns Hopkins University School of Medicine in 1939-40. He was Chief of Services for the Crippled Children Program of the Washington State Department of Health from 1940 to 1942. He was a Lieutenant Commander in the Medical Corp, US Naval Reserve, from 1942 to 1946.

Returning to private practice in 1946, he remained associated with academic medicine as a teaching clinician. In addition to his practice, he served as Clinical Assistant Professor in Medicine at the University of Washington School of Medicine from 1947 to 1952; Assistant Dean from 1949 to 1953; Clinical Associate Professor of Medicine from 1952 to 1956; Acting Dean from 1953-54, Assistant Dean from 1954 to 1959 and Clinical Professor of Medicine from 1956 to the present. He is on the staff of Swedish Hospital and the King County Hospital (now Harborview Medical Center), as well as the University of Washington. He is also on the consulting staff of several other hospitals. He was Consultant in Internal Medicine to the U.S. Public Health Service Hospitals, and the VA Hospital in Seattle from 1950 to 1959.

He has been a trustee of the Seattle Artificial Kidney Center and the Seattle Symphony Orchestra. He is a Fellow of the American Geographic Society in New York and the American Heart Association, and was President of the King County Medical Society, Washington, in 1961. He was a member of the AMA's Council on Medical Education from 1966 to 1976, serving as its Chairman from 1974 to 1976. He was also a member of the Residency Review Committee for Internal Medicine and served as its Chairman for several years. He is a member of the Pacific Inter-Urban Clinical Club; American Federation for Medical Research; American Clinical and Climatological Association (President in 1980); American Association for the History of Medicine and is a member of the Institute of Medicine of the National Academy of Sciences. He belongs to Phi Beta Kappa, Sigma Xi, and Alpha Omega Alpha.

He has been an active member of the American College of Physicians as a Fellow since 1950, was Governor for Washington and Alaska from 1956 to 1965, and served as Assistant Marshal and Marshal of the College from 1959 to 1964. He was a Regent from 1965 to 1969; President-Elect in 1969-70, President in 1970-71, and became a Master of the College in 1973.

## "We Are One"

In his Presidential Address entitled, "We Are One", Dr. Haviland asserted his belief that although medicine was troubled by divisive forces, both internal and external, "apparently irreconcilable differences can be adjudicated, when those of goodwill, earnest intentions and integrity try". He perceived the College as an adjudicator, with the potential to aid the profession in achieving the highest quality in education, research, service, tradition and ethics.

He had witnessed the College at work "through a series of trying situations . . . hot on the heels of one another", problems ranging from family practice to comprehensive health care planning to the "era of disagreement with the ASIM", and had seen their outcomes. "I came to realize," he said, "that apparently irreconcilable differences tend to disappear, and suitable solutions seem to present themselves, when [we] gather round the table, intent on making progress." From his undergraduate (Union) college's motto, he quoted, "Under the laws of science, knowledge and wisdom, we all become brothers". All seek the same goal, service of the highest quality".

> This is an age of social turmoil in which our citizenry has become preoccupied with integration, segregation, discrimination, consumer representation, and many more appellations . . . Medicine, too, has been preoccupied with troublesome problems: . . . delivery systems, physician distribution, financing, undue public expectations, inadequate communications and even problems unearthed by our own *ACP Medical Knowledge Self-Assessment* tests! . . . Our greatest assets work to our detriment . . . our desire to be fairminded and attuned to the problems of our age . . . make us vulnerable to the efforts of those with different concepts and goals.

> We in medicine *are* one. The concept of oneness brings a challenge of struggle, a debate over different points of view, of transcending petty personal differences for the common good.

He emphasized that the internists of the ACP are "particularly suited for a unifying role, [having a] good reputation based on a sound program, attracting the thoughtful, the objective, the forward-looking and the humane".

He expressed a sense of urgency, noting the cries that within 10 years the medical profession will become hopelessly split.

> When voices in our government say, 'Medicine is too important to be entrusted to doctors', medicine is in deep trouble. This is no time . . . for petty squabbling. It is a time for our ranks to be closed. [The College, he felt, had a great opportunity to lead, but if it could not lead, it could at least participate.] Let us make it a reality with all its provocative, struggling, vital and dynamic connotations - we are one.

Dr. Haviland served to promote better ACP relations with outside organizations such as the AMA, ASIM, AAMC and the government. As reflected in his numerous organizational activities, he was a leader of considerable stature in intersocietal affairs. His diplomatic style of communicating earned him great respect in the medical community, not only personally, but also as the official representative of the ACP.

Dr. Haviland was always conscious of the College's financial constraints. At one meeting he tried to persuade the Board of Regents to travel tourist class to save money. Dr. Robert Petersdorf opposed this move. Dr. John Layne was amenable, but said he would go first class and pay the difference. The Board decided to make no change in the travel arrangements. I told Mrs. Haviland about this, and she laughed and said, "How do you think Jim got elected to the Mercer Island Water Company Board , if he didn't understand finance?"

Jim and I spent much time together at meetings of the AMA. He was an elected member of the Council on Medical Education and, for several years, its Chairman. During that time, I was Chairman of the Advisory Committee on Continuing Medical Education and had to report periodically to the Council. Developing a conjoint board to certify specialists in nuclear medicine was very much a problem for several years. Surgeons, internists, pathologists and radiologists were involved. That this Board was at last established is due in large measure to Dr. Haviland's patience. What to do about family medicine was another problem finally resolved with much help from Dr. Haviland. It, too, was established as a primary board. We saw a good deal of the Havilands and Marian and Esther became the best of friends.

Dr. Haviland played an important role in persuading the Board of Regents that it should adopt a positive attitude and make an offer to help promote that portion of the family practice program which required training in internal medicine. This helped the program to receive support from all the specialties.

Dr. Haviland took more interest in College operations than most of the Presidents, and was much concerned about the manner in which things got done. He led the Board of Regents to become concerned with all aspects of the organization. Consequently, sometimes difficult relations improved between the Board of Regents and the Board of Govenors and between the administration and both Boards.

He showed great patience and persistence as President. The local Denver committee for the Annual Session wanted to plan an evening at the rodeo, which he and I were not enthusiastic about. He made his objections known, but left the decision up to them. When it finally occurred to everyone that it was not possible to have what was essentially a private party at the rodeo, the local people planned a party at the hotel and provided entertainment by the Koshare Indian Dancers, who had performed at the previous Denver session. This was a most unusual spectacle, performed by a group of teen-aged boys from a neighboring town who had made a study of old Indian ceremonial dancing. They make their own costumes and advance in the troup from year to year. The program also included Max Morath, a famous "Ragtime" pianist. Both performances had an appreciative audience.

# 1970-1971

Executive Director renamed Executive Vice President. Dr. Edward Huth new *Annals* Editor. ACP Chapters. *MKSAP II.* Library for Internists (I). State of the Art Lectures. AAMC supported on "Conquest of Cancer" statement. ACP meets HEW Sec. Egeberg. Visiting Professors to Hospitals; A-V films. ABIM oral exams discontinued.

At the Annual Session of 1970, Dr. James Haviland launched his year as President, outlining his concerns and plans: The operation of the Board of Regents, particularly the lack of time for free discussion of policy matters, was a special concern. He observed that too much time was spent in "nuts and bolts" housekeeping details, which a smaller group, such as the Executive Committee could handle more properly.

He announced some special items of interest: The College had been invited to attend a meeting of colleges of physicians of English speaking countries. Dr. Roger Egeberg, Assistant Secretary for Health, Department of Health, Education and Welfare [HEW], had invited the ACP to send six representatives to Washington to discuss health needs of the country. Finally, Dr. Haviland read a letter of resignation from Dr. Russell Elkinton, Editor of the *Annals,* to take effect July 1, 1971.

I urged the Board of Regents to do what it could to make the ACP the inclusive body for all specialists in internal medicine. Recognizing trends toward specialization, I expressed hope that the Council of Medical Specialty Societies [CMSS] might become, eventually, the advisory committee to the American Medical Association, replacing the AMA's own Interspecialty Council. Since the CMSS was composed of designated representatives of the specialty societies, rather than elective nominees of the AMA, specialties would receive more adequate representation. The CMSS (originally the Tri-College Council) now represented 21 specialties.

Regarding Chapters, I stated that although the Board of Governors had been against their formation, I could find no way for the College to increase the participation of members in College affairs within the limited number of national offices and committees.

## Montreal Meeting for Long Range Planning

The Executive Committee of the Board of Regents held a two-day long-range planning meeting in Montreal in June. A wide spectrum of subjects was discussed, and in several actions, the Committee:

1. Authorized entering into a contract with the National Center for Health Services Research and Development [NCHSRD] of HEW. This action would provide two years of support for a feasibility study on "The Appraisal of Quality in Hospital Care Provided by Internists."
2. Approved the presentation of a scientific exhibit at Annual Sessions of the College.

3. Adopted a motion that all committees submit reports and recommendations for action before October 1, to permit the Executive Committee to consider them for action on October 19. This would give the Board of Regents time to consider actions of the Executive Committee in a more deliberate manner. The remaining committees would meet on November 6, before the Regents November meeting.

The Executive Committee also devoted time to studying current programs and new program proposals.

1. The current status of educational activities was reviewed in detail.

   a. The *Medical Knowledge Self-Assessment Program II [MKSAP]* would be ready in January, 1971.
   b. Postgraduate Courses were deemed successful and popular, but the College needed better methods to evaluate their effectiveness.
   c. The success of Regional Meetings varied considerably in quality and effectiveness.
   d. The Committee recommended continued exploration of films and tapes, hoping that soon the College could offer physicians single topic programs teaching techniques and procedures and patient counseling aides.

2. The Committee also recommended that the College develop socioeconomic policy positions. Considering problems and implications in health care and cooperation with government and with professional groups, the Committee noted that the recent College statement, "Organization and Functions of a Department of Internal Medicine in a Community Hospital" had been most effective.

3. The Committee endorsed the American Board of Internal Medicine's position regarding "the desirability of promoting internal medicine as the ideal training for (one) who intends to be a primary or family type of physician". It urged the College to " . . . exert leadership in promoting the idea of voluntary recertification". The Committee felt strongly that the time had arrived when the idea of assuring continued competence of ACP members could be realized.

4. The recommendation to study additional approaches to certifying the competence of internists suggested several possibilities:

   a. participation in clinical competence testing which could be an extension of *MKSAP;*
   b. peer review of a helpful, non-threatening type, and
   c. attendance at meetings, PG courses, etc., on a voluntary basis.

5. The Montreal meeting included discussion of the future relation of the ACP to the specialty of family practice. Physicians with three years of training in family practice who passed a certifying examination and did not engage in obstetrics or surgery would practice similarly to general internists. The educational programs of the College would certainly help such

physicians improve their skills. The Committee considered their being included in College membership, but no action was recommended.

6. Relations with the American Society of Internal Medicine were considered to be satisfactory. Interactions in the Section Council of the AMA offered additional potential for American Society of Internal Medicine [ASIM]-ACP cooperation.

7. The Committee concluded that international programs were limited by available funding, but those the College could support were effective. The postgraduate courses seemed to be particularly useful, notably in Colombia and Chile.

8. The delivery of health care was undergoing important changes and exploring new directions. The Committee reviewed contributing factors suggesting areas needing College involvement:

   a. More specialization could be expected.

   b. Models defining effective triage in health care delivery needed to be developed to distinguish the well from the sick, and to give each its proper emphasis.

   c. The aphorism "Good health is a right, not only a need" was an accepted principle.

   d. Few real advances or changes in the delivery system were observable, in contrast to marked changes in technology.

   e. Future hospital care would be extended to community care.

   f. There would be less private fee-for-service care.

   g. Use of allied health personnel would probably increase. Nurses seemed to be the choice of most internists to serve as physicians' assistants.

   h. It was predicted that there would be universal prepaid health insurance.

   i. The potential benefits of patient interface at non-MD levels of primary health care were emerging, utilizing medex corpsmen, public health nurses, physicians' assistants, Canada's model of "outpost nursing", etc.

   j. The ACP should consider the development of continuing educational programs for non-ACP physicians and allied health professionals.

   k. The College must gather information from the many types of group practice engaged in evaluating health care, including the experiences at Mayo, Kaiser Permanente; Straub, and other clinics.

In conclusion, the Committee reviewed the implications of these issues on staff functions and financial resources. Clearly, the size of the staff and ACP's financial resources would need to increase rapidly as the College became more active in future programs. Some of the related questions for study were assigned to individual committee members; others were referred to an appropriate College committee.

The Committee on Community Services, appointed at the April, 1970 meeting of the Board of Regents, superseded the Committee on Medical Services of 1964, absorbing its members. The new Committee agreed that the following four points adequately represented its responsibilities and areas of interest:

1. To be concerned with the implication of scientific and sociologic advances for medicine, with special attention to their effect on medical education, research, and the delivery of health services.
2. To study and develop recommendations for College positions and programs dealing with a variety of groups making special demands for health services, such as the elderly, the urban disadvantaged, and individuals living in remote rural areas.
3. To expand ACP activities in:

   a. Medico-legal considerations affecting internists.
   b. Information and public relations pertaining to internal medicine.
   c. Development and maintenance of standards in internal medicine, as innovations appear in health care delivery.

4. To make recommendations to the Board of Regents as to what further actions should be the business of this committee.

The Committee suggested that programs at Annual Sessions might be organized to bring information about community medicine to the internist. The Committee met in June, 1970, and discussed several issues affecting primary care and allied health professionals:

1. In view of current emphasis by many groups on primary care, it suggested that the College should study the role of the internist in delivering primary care. A subcommittee was appointed to study ways in which the College could work more closely with the American Academy of General Practice [AAGP] and the American Academy of Pediatrics [AAP].
2. Regarding allied health professionals, specifically physicians' assistants, the ASIM had circulated a questionnaire to its members to determine their feelings about the kind of professionals they could work with effectively. The response indicated a fair consensus that any allied professional with less training than a registered nurse would not be adequate. A document presented to the Committee which comprehensively defined the role of physicians' assistants was approved in principle; it was referred to the Executive Committee of the Board of Regents to be discussed with ASIM, AAGP and the AAP.

The Educational Activities Committee had been investigating the film media for a number of years with the intention to produce audio-visual material for use in the continuing education of physicians and in patient counseling. A subcommittee was appointed in April, 1970, which reported to the Board of Regents in November, recommending:

1. that the College have the copyright to these audio-visual materials;
2. that procedural films (lumbar puncture, etc.) should have first priority because of simplicity of production;
3. that the Executive Director explore further with ROCOM, a division of Hoffmann-LaRoche, means of sponsoring a program of procedural films for which hospitals and departments in medical schools would be the chief consumers;

4. that the Executive Director also explore further work with Media Medica, Inc., with Dr. Bernard V. Dryer as the architect;

5. that, to further promote self-learning programs, as with the *MKSAP,* the College should embark on the program of audio-visual materials and offer these to the physician and any other consumer as a direct marketing effort without premarketing questionnaires to determine demand for such materials;

6. that single-topic and other types of physician education films be given second priority;

7. that patient counseling films be given third priority;

8. that the Executive Director explore with the Staff what functions of the program the College should do in-house, such as taking orders for subscriptions.

In April, 1970, single topic 8mm cartridge films, *Medical Skills Library,* were demonstrated to the new Ad Hoc Committee on Hospitals prior to the Annual Session. Designed for use in hospital emergency rooms, these single subject films, running five to ten minutes, would focus on clear and concise instruction in the performance of selected medical procedures. The Committee prepared a list of 12 commonly mismanaged medical emergencies, relating to treatment or final disposition of the patient; 12 rare medical emergencies, and 12 common technical procedures which were used in the practice of internal medicine. From these, in April, 1971, the Committee presented the following single topic subjects to the Board of Regents:

1. Lumbar spinal puncture
2. Thoracentesis
3. Abdominal paracentesis
4. Bone marrow aspiration
5. Sigmoidoscopic examination
6. Arterial puncture
7. Joint aspiration and injection
8. Tracheotomy
9. Laryngeal intubation (endotracheal)
10. Liver biopsy - percutaneous
11. Bladder catheterization
12. Tonometry - eye

The Committee on Educational Activities announced that *MKSAP II* had proceeded on schedule and the final review of questions had been completed in September, 1970. The Prospectus was scheduled for distribution in January, 1971. The program differed slightly from the previous *MKSAP* in that physicians were invited to volunteer their scores for the development of norms. Candidate Members were offered the program at cost ($7) while other housestaff could were charged the same price as regular ACP members ($20).

In reviewing the April, 1970 nine-point policy on recertification, the Committee reaffirmed its position that recertification should be accomplished by written examination determining knowledge, contending that current educational activities, including the self-assessment programs, would prepare a candidate for re-certification adequately. At this time there were no other practical or effective methods available.

After discussion, the Committee recommended that compulsory attendance at educational programs should not be necessary for continuance of ACP membership. This recommendation was approved by the Board of Regents subsequently.

A survey in 1966 had shown that College members in general surpassed currently accepted levels of continuing education required by other societies. Keeping track of educational activities not sponsored by the College was considered to be too difficult. The Committee was concerned that exceptions to compulsory attendance would be made and the interpretation of those exceptions by individual Governors would vary so much that objective evaluation would become impossible.

The Committee further recommended that the Ad Hoc Committee on Hospitals develop a Program of Visiting Professors to the Community Hospital. Visiting professor and hospital protocols were developed by the Ad Hoc Committee and approved by the Board of Regents in November, 1970. Until it was determined how much interest such a program would generate, a roster of potential professors would not be prepared. The Committee decided, instead, to inform the Governors of the College about the program and ask them to indicate the names of some hospitals in their area which might be interested in the program. Target hospitals were those which did not have a program in continuing education conducted by a Director of Medical Education. Inasmuch as the program was intended to be self-supporting, it would be the hospital's responsibility to determine the amount of the honorarium to the consultant.

A proposed protocol for visiting professors to hospitals was approved by the Executive Committee. The two-part format approved would include one form to be used by the hospital requesting a visiting professor and the other by the visiting professor.

## Library for Internists

The Chairman of the Committee on Hospitals, Dr. Richard Allyn, reported in November, 1970, that work had begun on the Core Library Project. Experts in all specialties were being asked which textbooks and journals in their specialty should be in the basic library of all internists. The Core Library list was also intended to give needed guidance to hospitals, not only to fulfill Joint Commission on Accreditation of Hospitals [JCAH] standards, but also to enable them to make available adequate reference textbooks and journals to their medical staffs.

The Committee was also exploring several other areas, including the role of internists in emergency care and liaison activity with the Association of Hospital Medical Education. The medical audit program in three hospitals had been established by a contract with the NCHSRD. Dr. David Jones was appointed on a part-time basis to be coordinator of this program. The three hospitals chosen were in York and Allentown, Pennsylvania, and Baltimore, Maryland. Dr. Jones would report to the College, but would work geographically out of the York Hospital.

An Executive Session of the Board of Regents, in November, included extended discussion of administrative issues regarding the top level administrative structure of the College; projected ACP developments; the need for job descriptions and salary scales; the use of outside consultation in management analysis; as well as the problem of the search for, and training of, successors to any of the top level administrative posts. The length and depth of the discussion indicated the Board of Regents' expression of its deep sense of responsibility for the total well-being of the College.

Several actions relating to the administrative structure and function of the ACP were taken:

1. The Executive Director's title was changed to Executive Vice President.
2. The Executive Vice President was authorized to seek physician staff assistance at a salary commensurate with responsible physicians of like status and similar experience in other organizations.
3. An ad hoc committee was appointed to study the administration of the College, including functions of the Administrative Staff, the Board of Regents and the Board of Governors.

In November, 1970, the Scientific Program Committee evaluated the entire Annual Session program. Of the 1,765 questionnaires sent to members and guests, 833 (47.2 percent) were returned. Responses were reviewed with considerable interest by the Committee and the Board of Regents: 84 percent thought the panel discussions should be conducted in an informal manner without slides, 81.9 percent had viewed the 30-foot widescreen color television presentations and thought they were instructive.

In the future, special efforts would be devoted to the TV Hospital Clinics in order to ensure continued improvement in this part of the program; the Philadelphia TV programs had not been as effective as the Committee had hoped. The following suggestions and comments were made:

1. Technical difficulties should be worked out. It was noted that the problems in Philadelphia were not only technical but included poor presentation of scientific material.
2. The TV chairman should work closely with the Executive Vice President.
3. Programs should be artistic as well as informative.
4. Tapes could be dubbed into programs.
5. The programs should be better than the advertisements.
6. Visual aids should be used whenever possible.
7. More time should be spent on the audio-visual material and rehearsals.

State of the Art Lectures, a new feature organized by Dr. Robert Petersdorf and Dr. Arno Molutsky, were to be added to the program at the 1971 Annual Session. Well-done lectures could be a "formal didactic boost-in-the-arm" for education. Eight one-hour lectures were scheduled to be given by outstanding people who would be paid a reasonable honorarium. All lecturers would be asked to direct their remarks to individual aspects of a broad central subject. Awardees were encouraged to present lectures.

The Board of Regents voted that the Awards Committee would make awards without considering the speaking ability of the candidate. The Scientific Program Committee could invite any of the awardees to participate in any part of the program.

At the November, 1970 meeting, Dr. Haviland gave a comprehensive status report about the Council of Medical Specialty Societies and the AMA Interspecialty Committee. Much overlapping in personnel and functions limited the potential effectiveness of each group. Two distinctive questions had emerged:

1. Should there be a separate and freestanding organization like the CMSS?
2. How could medical specialties best relate to the AMA? Most agreed the AMA was in need of strong support or at least advice from the specialties. In 1970 there was still no official specialty society representation in the AMA except in the planning of scientific programs.

Several interesting membership matters were discussed. The Board of Regents decided that being a physician accepted for training in internal medicine established eligibility to become an Associate. "Candidate Member" was redesignated "Associate" in April, 1970.

The Board of Regents decided to continue the Governors' Fall Conferences on an annual basis for another three years, after which time they would be evaluated.

## Annual Session 1971

At the 1971 Spring meeting of the Board of Regents, Dr. Haviland reported that at a recent meeting, the ACP/ASIM Liaison Committee had accomplished a workable plan for the two organizations to cooperate in the AMA's Section Council in Internal Medicine. He announced the appointment of Dr. Edward Huth as Editor of the *Annals of Internal Medicine* as of July, 1971, following Dr. Elkinton's retirement. Since Dr. Huth had served as Assistant and Associate Editor since 1961, continuity of editorial excellence was assured.

Dr. William F. Kellow, Treasurer, reported that the Headquarters' new wing construction was near completion. Nearly $300,000 had been received from members through the building fund assessment and from voluntary gifts. The endowment fund's market value was $3,888,000, resulting in earnings of $170,000.

In my Executive Vice President's report, I described the impact of the new American Board of Internal Medicine regulations on membership. Residents would be examined at the end of three years of training, eliminating the qualifying examination which had been given at the end of two years of training. Passing candidates could be fully certified as qualified internists in practice or could continue in Fellowship training in one of the subspecialties. I suggested that these physicians should be eligible for Membership upon being certified. Direct Fellowship could still be attained by more mature physicians who might become interested in the College at a later date. I also announced that since we began approaching residents directly concerning Candidate Membership (hereafter to be called Associate), almost 1500 had become Associates. From this time on there continued to be a rapid increase in the number of young physicians who showed interest in becoming permanent Members.

I continued to urge consideration of formally established Chapters in ACP Regions as a means of increasing membership participation in College activities. I also suggested that the College either appoint a Chairman of Local Arrangements in each city where the Annual Session would be held, or designate the Chairman of the Scientific Program Committee as General Chairman. The operation and preparations of the Annual Session had become so complicated that it was not realistic to expect a busy physician to be concerned with all of the technical details of conducting a large convention.

## Recertification

The Board of Regents reviewed the ACP-American Board of Internal Medicine [ABIM] nine-point document on recertification which it had endorsed in principle in April, 1970. Originally developed by the ACP-ABIM Committee on Recertification, the document had been studied and commented upon by the Board of Governors. The Board of Regents referred the following information back to the ACP-ABIM Ad Hoc Committee for consideration:

1. Both Boards agreed that recertification was a desirable objective, but thought it could not be accomplished effectively or objectively by any method of allocating "credit" for attending meetings, reading, etc.
2. Any such examination should test the internal medicine specialist's clinical ability to care for patients. Various methods of testing were under study. The possibility of an "open book" type of examination was being explored. It could be the type of computer-based examination currently being tested by the National Board of Medical Examiners and the American Board of Internal Medicine. The Carnegie Foundation and the Commonwealth Foundation had given a grant to ABIM and National Board of Medical Examiners [NBME] for a three-year study of this method which showed some potential for being more related to clinical competence than technical knowledge.
3. The possibility of peer review or some form of medical audit was discussed at great length. All studies in this field would be watched closely to determine their potential as an alternative method of recertification.
4. The Board of Regents held that a physician who took a recertification examination and failed should be permitted to take it annually until he or she passed. It also agreed that original certification should be unaffected if the recertification examination was failed.
5. Anyone who passed the recertification examination should not be permitted to take it again for a minimum of six years.
6. The ACP would continue to intensify efforts to help those who failed.

7. "Recertification" was considered a satisfactory term and could not be described any more accurately or more satisfactorily by any other word.
8. The American Board of Internal Medicine was to move ahead strongly, designating a committee which would have the responsibility to develop the method, the timing and all other matters connected with the recertification procedure. It was emphasized that the ABIM would be offering voluntary recertification for specialists.
9. Any official announcements should be made only upon mutual agreement between ABIM and ACP.

The American Hospital Association [AHA] invited the College to participate in a series of workshops similar to one it had cosponsored with the American College of Surgeons [ACS], whose purpose would be to increase understanding among the three major bodies influencing the conduct of hospital affairs; physicians, administrators and trustees. The Committee on Hospitals, with Board of Regents approval, cooperated in scheduling two of these conferences with the American Hospital Association. The conferences were well attended by invited physicians and administrators, but very poorly by trustees. Although those who attended thought the conferences useful, the AHA decided not to continue them because of their failure to attract the trustees. The Committee on Hospitals suggested that the project might have had better success if the trustees had been invited directly by the College rather than through the hospital administrators.

## Cancer Control Program

In April, 1971, several matters brought to its attention by the Cancer Committee resulted in the Board of Regents' endorsement of a statement issued by the Association of American Medical Colleges [AAMC] in response to federal proposals to create a "special and extraordinary program" for cancer control.

The Committee on Educational Activities approved a motion opposing the recommendation of the Committee on Cancer regarding the goals and recommendations contained in the Report of the National Panel of Consultants on the "Conquest of Cancer" authorized by S. Res. 376, and urged the Board of Regents to support the action taken by the AAMC as endorsed by the Executive Committee of the Board of Regents on March 2, 1971. It further recommended, with Board approval, that the College President alert the press that the College took a strong stand in support of the AAMC position. Following the meeting of the Committee on Cancer, Mr. Benno Schmidt, the Executive Secretary of the Panel of Consultants, telephoned Dr. Haviland to ascertain the opinion of the Committee on Cancer, which he conveyed to the Yarborough Congressional Committee. This statement was interpreted as being the College position. The main point at issue was whether a new freestanding Commission on "Conquest of Cancer" should be established outside the National Institutes of Health [NIH]. This idea was opposed by the AAMC. The Regents therefore thought that the College should make an additional statement and also endorse the AAMC policy statement.

The Board of Regents considered further the question of the College making its own policy statement regarding these proposals for a stepped-up program to find the cause and cure for cancer. This resulted in the following:

> The American College of Physicians supports the expansion of research to find the cause and cure for cancer as expressed by President Nixon in his State of the Union Message. The College strongly urges, however, that this expanded effort in cancer research be carried out under the aegis of the NIH organizational structure under the supervision of its Director.

The Board of Regents voted to continue support of the CMSS, which was undergoing rapid expansion and changes in function.

## ACP Chapters

During the Board of Governors meeting in April, 1971, a significant resolution concerning Chapters was adopted. The following was also approved by the Board of Regents:

> The Masters, Fellows and Members within the jurisdictional areas may constitute a Chapter, the presiding officer of which will be the Governor. The Governor may appoint committees deemed necessary to conduct the business of that Chapter within the structure of the Constitution and Bylaws of the College. One committee will be known as the Governor's Committee for College Affairs.

Local option would decide the structure, scope and membership of this committee as well as other committees of each Chapter. In approving the above, the Board of Regents stipulated that the formation of each Chapter must be approved by the Board of Regents.

Upon the recommendation of the Awards Committee, the Board of Regents voted to discontinue the Honorary Fellowship sponsored by the Lilly Company. In recent years it had become associated erroneously with Honorary Fellowships bestowed by the College. The Lilly Company had also, on a few occasions, encountered the same confusion on the part of some of the recipients. The Board of Regents thanked the Lilly Company for its support of these Fellowships for so many years. Honorary Fellowship was to be continued for any of the Presidents of the several Royal Colleges, if they personally attended the ACP Convocation.

A significant action recommended by the Finance Committee was taken: "That the practice of having the Investment Committee make recommendations of portfolio changes to the entire Finance Committee and then wait for response before consummating the transactions be discontinued." It was recommended that sole responsibility should rest with the Investment Committee upon consultation with the investment counsel and that members of the Finance Committee be informed of what had been done.

## Health Care and Continuing Education

On November 9, 1970, a meeting was held at HEW at the invitation of Dr. Roger Egeberg, FACP, Assistant Secretary for Health. The purpose was to bring input to HEW from the ACP. In attendance were Dr. James W. Haviland, Dr. Hugh R. Butt, Dr. Maxwell Berry, Dr. John Gamble, Dr. John A. Layne and Dr. Edward C. Rosenow, Jr. This group developed the following statement, which was approved and issued by the Board:

Tenets:
1. The ready availability and accessibility of quality health care are the basic rights of every citizen.
2. In our opinion, it appears that health care will be delivered most effectively by teams of health professionals working in close cooperation with physicians.
3. Physicians should be aware of the costs of health care. There should be incentive for physicians (as well as all citizens) to control these costs without jeopardizing the quality of care.
4. Continuing education is an indispensible ingredient of good health care.
5. Evaluation of health care must be done in a positive and constructive manner, with dignity, and must be directed toward the improvement of the quality of care.

The American College of Physicians believes these items merit special concern and continued consideration:

1. Resolutions passed by the Board of Regents concerning:

    a. Direct support of medical education and medical research, and fair payment for teachers of medicine for services rendered to patients.
    b. The importance of community planning for comprehensive health services.

2. Delivery of health care:
    The College favors multiple, innovative pilot projects geared to the specific requirements of individual localities. This would include group practice models, the use of Health Maintenance Organizations [HMOs] and the attainment of more equitable distribution of health care and personnel.
3. The College is interested in primary care whether delivered by a family physician, an internist, a pediatrician, or similarly trained physicians.
4. With regard to medical education:
    The financing of health education is of the utmost importance, and the College believes that a better balance or mix in the support for education and research should be obtained. The College also believes that methods such as direct capitation and the assignment of a percentage of gross health expenditures to research and development are two alternative pathways that are feasible in the support of health education. The College is concerned about legislation of the type which was introduced into Congress last year (but was not made a law) and which would have Congress determine how the individual medical schools should be organized and how they would teach. The College believes that this is not a congressional function.

    The College believes that student loan funds should be augmented and draws attention to a new and intriguing vehicle, the Educational Opportunity Bank, as yet untried. The College also feels that continuing education, its scope, development and financing, must be considered in the field of medical education. The College is vitally interested in the field of peer review. It is concerned at the specificity and marked limiting characteristics of some of the proposed legislation, and believes that peer review should be truly peer in its administration and that the educational aspects must be stressed.

This document was made available to the Committee on Governmental Activities in Medicine which met on March 26, 1971. The Committee returned to the Board the following report and recommendations:

1. Physicians have not fully utilized relationships with Congressmen and Senators to advise them on matters of health legislation. Congress no longer pays much attention to floods of telegrams and letters - unless some degree of personal acquaintance exists. The health decisions of 1971 and 1972 will be made in Congress.
2. Many ACP members have doubts as to how interested the College is in the various health measures before Congress.
3. While there is at present much discussion concerning what type of delivery system of health care is best, the basic factor in quality health care is the quality of the physicians.
4. The ACP agrees that desirable peer review, in essence, is the review of the quality of care that the patient receives.
5. Although the College has not been in a position to concern itself with the "hardware" of health delivery systems, such as HMOs, it has helped prepare its members for innovative changes by sponsoring on its programs, panel discussions dealing with Biomedical Engineering, Computers in Medicine, and Multiphasic Screening, among others.
6. The College wishes to be consulted about new health delivery systems and is ready to help advise when asked. We believe that there should be a continuing dialogue among the Congress, federal health agencies, and the College.
7. Through its educational programs and publications, the College hopes to improve the efficiency of the internist and to increase his productivity in helping to care for an increased number of patients.
8. Strong support must be given to all efforts to educate the public about what each individual can do about his own health. There are many people greatly concerned about the pollution of the environment, yet insufficiently concerned about the pollution of themselves.

Therefore, the Committee recommended to the Board of Regents that the policy of the American College of Physicians should be:

1. That the ACP is strongly in favor of the delivery of better and augmented health services for all Americans. This would involve experimentation with different types of techniques.
2. That the main thrust of the College should be in educational efforts directed to improve the quality of care received by the patient through continuing efforts to upgrade the education and training of physicians and allied health personnel.
3. That the prevention of disease depends largely upon eradication of poverty, improvement of nutrition, better education for our children, better housing and better working conditions for our citizens and the correction of many other social and environmental ills. Also involved is the education of the public in how to avail themselves of medical care and how to use effectively the medical care and advice they receive.

The Committee on International Medical Activities suggested that funds should be sought to support at least one Latin American Fellowship. In 1970, the Kellogg Foundation informed the Board of Regents that, by recent action of the US Congress, present federal regulations of the activities of foundations would prevent them, henceforth, from making grants to individuals, which resulted in a decision to discontinue their support of Latin-American Fellowships. In 1971, the Foundation reported to the College a new method of indirect support; although it was possible that the Latin American Fellows could be supported by grants made to the American College of Physicians or to the host medical school in the United States, it was the Foundation's intent to make grants directly to Latin American medical schools, permitting them to make their own arrangements for training in the United States of their candidates for Fellowship.

The previous program had been exceptionally successful and had resulted in advanced educational opportunities for nearly 170 Latin American junior faculty members, almost all but one of whom had returned and assumed permanent faculty appointments in their own countries.

The Committee members thought that they could and should continue to serve in reviewing, advising and assisting in preceptorship arrangements, and in verifying the adequacy of proposed stipends and other allocations.

This Committee also reviewed the ACP relationship with the International Society of Internal Medicine [ISIM]. This organization had been going through a reorganization plan favoring a federation of national societies rather than an individual membership society. The Committee recommended that two ACP members be appointed to the international committee of ISIM and that ACP staff give support to the next Congress in Boston, in September, 1971.

## Major Disaster Care

The Committee on Military Affairs and Disaster Medical Care developed the following recommendations on Major Disaster Care which were approved by the Board of Regents:

1. That the College use all possible means to urge its membership to participate actively in the organization of emergency medical care and disaster planning in their local community and state governments, and to be prepared to participate actively in providing emergency medical care or other types of relief in time of disaster.
2. That the internist formally accept both civic and professional responsibilities by directing attention and interest to the varied ways in which the physician may participate in emergency and disaster care, other than simply standing by to apply the skills of his specialty.
3. That it be established as a matter of policy that a member of the Committee on Military Affairs and Disaster Care serve on the Committee on Community Service, and possibly the Committee on Hospitals (when the functions of this new Committee were better defined), either as a regular member or to attend in liaison capacity. This was important, as the emergency medical care which might be expected in the event of a major disaster would be no better than the or-

ganization and delivery of emergency medical care for day-to-day minor disasters (e.g., highway accidents, which in total, constitute the greatest disaster in the United States).

4. That the College appropriately publicize the peaceful activities of the Military Services' assistance in major natural disasters in the United States and foreign countries.

The Board of Regents approved the report and motion made by the Chairman, Dr. Thomas V. Mattingly, that the Committee on Military Affairs and Disaster Medical Care be abolished. The concerns of this committee would be taken up by other standing committees.

The Publications Committee heard the last report of the retiring Editor of the *Annals,* Dr. J. Russell Elkinton. During the previous 12 months, 1,152 manuscripts had been submitted; approximately 10 percent of these were accepted for publication. Total subscribers numbered 53,000. Gross revenue from advertising was $1,168,000, resulting, after taxes and administrative costs, in net income to the College of $331,000. In closing, he expressed enthusiastic approval of the appointment of Dr. Edward J. Huth as the new Editor. He thanked the Board for the opportunity of serving as Editor for over ten years. At the request of Dr. Huth, Dr. Elkinton was named Consulting Editor on a half-time basis.

### Alcoholism

The Public Information Committee developed the following American College of Physicians Statement on Alcoholism, which was approved by the Board of Regents:

Alcoholism is one of the major problems of our time with both social and health implications. The American College of Physicians strongly supports the efforts being made to curb excessive use of alcohol and urges all members of the College and other physicians to participate actively in educational programs regarding its hazards and in treatment programs for persons with this illness.

Alcoholism is a disease. As such, it merits the attention of all physicians, who should take an interest in noting the early signs of addiction in their patients. Strong efforts should be made to help patients in the early stages of the habit. While proof is not available, it is reasonable to believe that success in treatment will be more frequent at this stage than later when overt evidence of alcoholism is present.

The cause of alcoholism is not known. It is likely that psychologic and social factors are of great importance. Physicians who are interested and consider the possibility of impending alcoholism in their patients can do much to prevent alcoholism.

Many physicians are in a position to extend their influence by learning what there is to know about the disease, and through education and participation in community efforts, to help control it.

The treatment of advanced alcoholism is unsatisfactory, but this fact does not relieve the physician of responsibility. He treats many chronic illnesses for which no completely satisfactory treatment is available. If the alcoholic patient is regarded as a patient in need of help, and if individualized treatment is applied, many can be rendered asymptomatic and others greatly helped.

All physicians and most particularly internists, should become more interested in treatment, education, and research in this important field of medicine.

The Residency Revolving Loan Fund status report indicated that during the life of the fund only $3,940 had been written off or was uncollectable; less than 1 percent of the loan granted. The Board of Regents approved a recommendation that loans be restricted to Associates or Members of the College.

### ABIM Oral Exams Abolished

The Chairman of the ABIM, Dr. Richard Ebert, announced to the Board of Regents in November, 1971, its decision to abolish the oral examination and establish a single two-day written examination. This was to be given after completion of three years of training in internal medicine (including a straight internal medicine internship). Passing candidates would be certified as diplomates of the ABIM. It was hoped that many physicians would enter the practice of internal medicine after certification and become eligible for full membership in the College.

The Board was aware that abolition of the oral examination would be criticized on the ground that the action might lead to de-emphasis on training in basic clinical skills. To avoid this possibility, the Board would demand certification of clinical skills, including ability in history taking and physical examination, prior to admission to the examination. This would be done at the local level.

No changes were made in the plans for the examination in the subspecialties to be offered in 1972. Two years of training in the subspecialty and certification in general internal medicine were required for admission to the examination.

The Board was aware that the recent changes in procedures had aroused a certain amount of criticism. Much of this had been constructive and of assistance in planning the recent actions. One unfair criticism was the charge that the Board was de-emphasizing training for the practice of general internal medicine. On the contrary, it was hoped that the new procedure would increase the number of doctors prepared to assume responsibility as primary care physicians. The establishment of the subspecialty examinations was a recognition of the fact that a certain number of consultants in special fields, such as hematology or endocrinology, were necessary in modern medicine. It was in no way an invitation for a mass movement into the subspecialties.

Dr. Ebert submitted the following position statement to the Board of Regents:

The prerequisites now are three years of training in internal medicine, that is, clinical training - this can be a straight internship, another year of residency followed by another year of residency in internal medicine or a Fellowship. At the end of this training period, the examination can be taken which will be a two-day exam and if successfully completed, will fully certify the individual as a diplomate in internal medicine. This will permit listing in the Directory of Medical Specialists. As part of this examination, a substantiation of his clinical competence will be carried out by those in charge of his training program. The exact method whereby this will be done has not been established and Dr. Petersdorf is heading a committee that will establish this by June, 1971. The intent is that the emphasis on clinical skills will be maintained although the present oral examination will be dropped.

However, the Board does not wish to leave the impression that it is depreciating the importance of bedside clinical skills in certification of an internist. After three years of training, the physician will have a substantiation of clinical skills done at the local level and then will take a two-day examination, and if successful in all of these, will be certified. There will be no advanced degree or examination in general internal medicine in the old way. It will be possible for individuals who had two years of subspecialty training to take subspecialty examination in their specific fields. There were controversies that arose concerning training. It's still technically possible for an individual to take two years' training in general internal medicine and to take further years of training in the subspecialty and to be certified in both general internal medicine and in a subspecialty.

The recommendation of the Board, and this is quite strong, is that the individual take three years of training in general internal medicine before entering into the subspecialty field, which would take two further years. I think this briefly summarizes the recent action of the ABIM. The intent of the Board might be stated as follows:

There is a need for internists who serve as primary physicians and the certification as a diplomate in internal medicine. There is also need for a smaller group of highly trained subspecialists to serve as consultants. The distribution of highly trained subspecialists and general internists will be determined by a number of forces, including the system of delivery of health care in the future. I think we're in a position to meet the demands of the health care system by these certifications.

The Residency Review Committee reported that the adoption of the revised *Essentials of Approved Residencies in Internal Medicine* had been useful to the Committee, which at that time met three times a year and reviewed a total of 300 programs. It was working on improving its methods to assure that collected data had to do mainly with clinical competence.

During the year 1970-71 several items of interest to the Governors were considered by the Board of Regents:

1. An interesting idea came up at the Governor's Conference proposing that a Governor be permitted the privilege of recommending for advancement to Fellowship members who had attained 55 years of age and had shown consistent loyalty to and attendance at College activities, but who did not meet all criteria for advancement. These requirements would be waived. This motion, however, was defeated.

2. A change in nominating procedures for the office of Governor was approved. The incumbent would appoint a local nominating committee. A post card poll would be conducted. Results of the poll would be given to the local nominating committee; which would recommend one or more candidates to the central nominating committee for selection.

3. There was no action and little interest in setting up local Chapters at the time of the Governors Conference. However, at the April meeting the Board approved developing Chapters on a purely voluntary basis.

4. The following items were considered important areas for College concern:

a. Education.

b. The ACP as spokesman in all aspects of internal medicine.

c. Advance standards of training.

d. Standards of the practice of internal medicine.

e. The promotion of standards for continuing education.

f. The College as an umbrella organization for subspecialties.

g. The role of the internist in the delivery of health care.

h. Study of all social policy factors which affect health.

In November, 1970, a document on Allied Health Professionals (Physicians' Assistants) was presented to the Board of Regents and adopted in principle. It was a preliminary draft and the Regents expressed reservations about parts of the report, but the Committee was urged to continue to pursue its work in this area and continue deliberations with the other organizations involved, namely, the ASIM, the American Academy of Family Physicians [AAFP] and AAP.

Ground-breaking on the new five-story Headquarters addition was delayed because of zoning problems. Approval was received and construction, which was to take about 12 months, began early in March, 1970.

The Mead-Johnson Residency Scholarships were discontinued. The final report of 14 scholars was reviewed by the Fellowships and Scholarships Committee. These had been granted since 1954 and were deemed invaluable for recipients. The Board of Regents expressed thanks to Mead-Johnson for its contributions over the years, and regretted their discontinuance.

## Part Three (1971-1972)

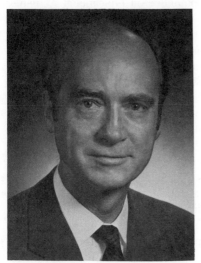

*Hugh R. Butt, MACP*

Dr. Hugh R. Butt was born in Belhaven, North Carolina in 1910. He married Mary Dempwoll in 1939 and they had four children, Selby, Lucy, Charles and Francis.

Dr. Butt's undergraduate studies were completed at the Virginia Polytechnic Institute, and he received his MD degree from the University of Virginia, Charlottesville, in 1933. He interned at St. Luke's Hospital in Bethlehem, Pennsylvania, and was a Fellow in Medicine at the Mayo Foundation from 1934 to 1937. In 1937, he received the Degree of Master of Science in Medicine from the University of Minnesota. He became a Professor of Medicine at the Mayo Foundation in 1952.

A member of the American Board of Internal Medicine from 1952 to 1960, Dr. Butt was its Vice Chairman in 1959-60. He served on the Editorial Board of the *Archives of Internal Medicine* from 1950 to 1960, and on the Residency Review Committee from 1952 to 1960, becoming Chairman in 1959.

He served as President of the American Gastroenterological Association in 1960-61 and as Chairman for the American Association for the Study of Liver Diseases in 1961-62. He served in many organizations, including the National Cancer Institute Board of Scientific Counselors, of which he was a member from 1958, and Chairman in 1961-62; the Mayo Clinic Board of Governors from 1953 to 1959, Vice Chairman from 1955 to 1959; Mayo Foundation Board of Trustees, Vice Chairman from 1962 to 1966; University of Virginia Medical School Board of Trustees from 1963 to 1967; National Cancer Advisory Council from 1965 to 1970, and Consultant since 1970; and the Subspecialty Board of Gastroenterology Chairman from 1966 to 1969.

His societal memberships include the Association of American Physicians; American Society for Clinical Investigation; American Clinical and Climatological Society; Central Society for Clinical Research; American Institute for Nutrition; American Gastroenterological Association; American Association for the Study of Liver Diseases and the American Medical Association. He is a Fellow of the Royal College of Physicians of London. He is also an Honorary Fellow of the Royal Colleges of Physicians of Edinburgh, Glasgow, and Ireland.

Dr. Butt was very active in the development and establishment of the Mayo Medical School in Rochester, Minnesota, and was instrumental in raising funds for the expansion of laboratory and research facilities at Mayo. He continues an active career as consultant and advisor to many similar projects.

Dr. Butt has been a Fellow of the American College of Physicians since 1940, serving as Governor for Minnesota from 1959 to 1965, and as a Regent from 1965 to 1972. He was Chairman of the Committee on Educational Activities from 1965 to 1970. Largely due to his fine work on this Committee, the College developed what has become a very successful educational program, the *Medical Knowledge Self-Assessment Program [MKSAP]*.

As President he was a dynamic, creative and somewhat aggressive person. He understood perfectly the division of administration and policy, never interfering with Staff functions.

When he was elected President, Dr. Wilbur, a mutual friend remarked to me "Every executive should have a president like Hugh once in awhile." I think he meant it might be a difficult year, but it proved to be one of the most pleasant years during my tenure. I recall one committee meeting in which he kept saying that "the College was beginning an interest in continuing medical education." Each time, I told him that continuing medical education had been about the only business of the College since its beginning in 1915. I finally rapped on the table to emphasize the point. After the meeting he said, "Ed, you are right and you should not let me say things like that." I replied, "I'll try if I know what you're going to say ahead of time." He laughed and we left together in a state of good humor.

I remember well an occasion when we first started meeting with the American Society of Internal Medicine officers about a possible merger. Dr. Otto Page, President of ASIM, at one meeting said their governing body was made up of practitioners, while the Board of Regents was made up of academicians. Hugh asked him how he practiced. Otto said, "In a group of five internists". Hugh said that he also practiced in a group of over 600 physicians and depended entirely on patient care practice for his income. This broke the ice and got discussion underway on a good note.

During the time the College was preparing the first *MKSAP,* Dr. Butt, at a banquet in Washington, DC, sat next to John Gardner, then Secretary of Health, Education and Welfare. Mr. Gardner asked Hugh if he knew about a medical society that was preparing a self-assessment test for its members. Hugh said he knew something about it and asked Mr. Gardner what he thought of the idea. He replied that if the public knew that a medical organization was so interested in helping its members stay current, there would be much less criticism of the profession. Mr. Gardner was later a recipient of the Loveland Award and gave the convocation speech in 1969.

About the time we were announcing *MKSAP I,* one of our Fellows, Dr. Don Williams from Edmonton, Canada, sent us a quotation from St. Paul's letter to the Galatians which we found most appropriate and used in some of our promotional material:

> For if anyone thinks he is something, when he is nothing, he deceives himself. But let each one test his own work and then his reason to boast will be in himself alone and not in his neighbor. For each man will have to bear his own load. (Galatians 6: 3-5)

Everyone who had anything to do with *MKSAP* knows how important Hugh's forceful leadership was in getting it started. Dr. Butt described three major premises on which *MKSAP* was based: "Physicians want to learn and increase their excellence. They would like to know their deficiencies providing no one else knows them. All of us have some paranoid tendencies and need careful reassurance. How true!" When presenting the program, his deliberate pause after the third premise invariably drew laughter from the audience. He then promptly told them their laughter indicated they recognized the paranoia. On one occasion, an agitated physician told me that while he trusted me and the College, he could not be convinced that the FBI or some other governmental agency would not be able to ascertain his test score. The wisdom Dr. Butt showed in insisting on complete privacy of results was confirmed by the responses of physicians subscribing to the program. They demonstrated strong trust in the College.

Dr. Butt's wide ranging creative interests included modern art, sculpture and music. He is also a recognized connoisseur of wines. Once, during a telephone conversation with me from his home, he excused himself to open the door for air conditioning installers. When he returned, I asked if he was air conditioning his house. He laughed and said, "No, my wine cellar". On every visit to Philadelphia, he brought Esther and me a bottle or two of wine, which he presented with a short discourse on its characteristics, and we enjoyed an ever increasing appreciation for good wines.

Dr. Butt's presidential year was marked by major contributions to self-assessment as an effective approach to continuing education. His driving concern for this subject is reflected in the perspectives he offered in his Presidential Address at the completion of his term.

"Certainly the public has a right to demand that their physicians maintain their professional excellence at all times," he began. To support such excellence, "We must have within our professional lives, a system of continuing education with potential for solid improvement of our skills". Internists must not only support, but "actively lead and participate in peer review or audit review or any other means that may ensure better practice." Recertification "should not be opposed", but rather internists should "guide it, develop it, and control it", making it a "voluntary and nonpunitive educational tool which preserves the dignity of the profession".

He urged physicians, when speaking to the public, to support medical schools and basic biomedical research. The public should be advised constantly that medical practice will not advance without research, and must know that we strongly support it. He also felt that it was the responsibility of the profession to "open the door" into the health care system "so the patient can be seen". In addition, internists should be ready to participate in programs which would make 24-hour service readily available to all patients. Dr. Butt called for the profession to recognize that it needs help and must "encourage and train paramedical help, such as nurse practitioners, physicians' assistants, and others . . . Allied health professionals are now the largest group in the medical community. We must work together productively".

It is only through education, much of which we can provide, that people will learn to demand and support what is needed for excellent health care. They must understand that medical care from better trained physicians in larger numbers with adequate plans for continuing education is essential to good care.

He spoke hopefully of the increase of specialty group practices, which afford the internist excellent opportunities to serve as a primary care physician and as a family friend and advisor.

"The American internist, 1972", he suggested, should be known by more active participation in community affairs, such as advocacy of community health and involvement in problems of pollution, sewage, drug abuse, and interpersonal relations. The internist can encourage people to take responsibility for their own health. "Medicine can be a midwife for social change; another responsibility we must accept."

# 1971-1972

Headquarters south wing. ACP organization and future directions. Clinical Pharmacology Committee. A-V films. ACP/ASIM "Intent" to merge rejected. San Joaquin Foundation, "Study of Internists' Practice". Physicians' Assistants. Emergency medical care. ACP/AHA Resource Utilization Conference. CCME, LCME, LCGME.

This was an unusually busy year for the College. The Board of Regents met four times. Several special ad hoc committees were appointed to study a number of subjects and make recommendations.

The Board received their reports in November, 1971:

A. Medical Educational Opportunities for Minority Groups, Dr. John R. Graham, Chairman
B. Direction of Medicine, Dr. William F. Kellow, Chairman
C. Tenure of Board of Regents, Dr. William A. Sodeman, Chairman
D. Role of the Past President, Dr. Maxwell G. Berry, Chairman
E. Role of the American College of Physicians in the Future, Dr. Maxwell G. Berry, Chairman
F. Committee on Committee Structure of the Board of Regents, Dr. Wright Adams, Chairman
G. Relationship of the Board of Regents to the Board of Governors, Dr. John A. Layne, Chairman

### A. Medical Educational Opportunities for Minority Groups

This committee concluded early that any proposals addressing minority problems must not only be formulated at a high level with adequate input from the minority groups, but must also avoid an attitude of reverse discrimination. Acquiring data about what was needed was an enormous problem. Recent civil rights laws made it difficult to determine how many minority physicians there were. Less than 100 black physicians were members of the College; only some 15 minority physicians were members of College committees.

1. The committee was charged to study:
   a. medical educational problems of minority groups,
   b. minority group participation in College affairs (officers, boards, committees, courses, regional activity), and
   c. what constituted good medical care for minorities.
2. The Postgraduate Committee was asked to cosponsor courses with Meharry and Howard Medical Schools.
3. The Committees on Hospitals and Community Services were asked to pay special attention to needs of minorities.
4. The Postgraduate Committee planned a course with Meharry. Meharry also agreed to having the ACP arrange for a visiting professor for a week or two. At year's end, funding for this was to be sought.

To enhance continuing education for the ghetto physician and improve continuity of care for the ghetto patient, Dr. Leonidas Berry offered a plan to conduct a project in a selected hospital in Chicago, in which the "ghetto" physician would be allowed to follow his or her patients who were admitted to the hospital staff service. Few patients from the ghetto are admitted to private service and actual care is usually given by the hospital staff. The community physician, under the project plan would be permitted to follow the patient in the course of hospital care, interacting regularly with the staff physicians who were administering care. This presented a number of problems, however, which the College could not solve, so no effort was made to implement it.

### B. Committee on Direction of Medicine

This committee considered a number of questions related to medical practice:

1. How would medicine be structured in the 1980s?
   Solo practice was diminishing, primary care would be done by teams of health workers working in ambulatory health centers.
2. Who would be the primary physician in the 1980s?
   Opinions were varied. Some felt that primary physician training, in order to prepare for group practice, should emphasize internal medicine, pediatrics, psychiatry, emergency medicine, administration, management economics and personnel procedures, with strong support by nonphysician health professionals. Others felt that ambulatory care centers would prevail, utilizing broadly trained specialists in internal medicine, pediatrics, obstetrics and psychiatry.
3. How would specialized medical care be furnished?
   The committee predicted minimal change, with trends continuing toward appropriate specialists working in group ambulatory settings, and through "walk in" clinics in coordination with hospital emergency departments, to solve health care delivery problems.

4. Were medical schools preparing physicians to practice in the 1980s?
   The schools were deemed to be doing well in training specialists, but were not addressing questions of shorter training periods or whether new primary care training programs were needed.
5. Did residencies need to be restructured?
   Those favoring broadly trained specialists for primary care did not see a need for restructuring. All agreed, however, that internal medicine training programs should require experience in pediatrics, psychiatry, office gynecology, rehabilitation, and community medicine, and more training in ambulatory settings.
6. How will costs be met in the 1980s?
   Inevitably, more and more care would be prepaid. Federal financing would probably be focused on coverage of catastrophic illness, co-insuring private policies at various levels of need, and providing incentives for health maintenance and preventive medicine.
7. What measurements of continuing medical education and health care standards were likely to develop before 1980?
   Physicians would be required to attend postgraduate medical programs and they would be urged to accept recertification. Systems of peer review would require better organization and standardization of medical record systems.
8. How would changes in medical care and medical education affect the American College of Physicians?
   The College should redefine the types of physicians it wants in its membership. The committee recommended that the College offer membership to all physicians who accept the role of personal, primary, or family physician and who have strong training in internal medicine.

   Continuing medical education should continue to have high priority, especially for those engaged in primary care. The College should seek opportunities to become an important spokesman for internal medicine and its allied medical specialties. These efforts should be carefully coordinated with other medical organizations.

   The College should be a leader in establishing methods of measuring medical performance.

Additional factors emerged from study of this question:

1. Allied health professionals were pressing for improved professional status, not regarding themselves as merely workers under physician supervision.
2. Public attitudes no longer regarded health care delivery systems as solely a physician leadership role.
3. In some geographic areas, upgrading chiropractors' education to some types of primary health care would receive public acceptance.
4. The general practitioner and the internist with a subspecialty probably would be unable to fill the expanding need for primary physicians.

5. Family practice was being firmly established, but it was impossible to project whether this move would fill the need for primary physicians.
6. The "emergency care physician" specialty movement was growing rapidly at the community hospital level. Residency programs, where available, were being filled. Potentially, well-trained physicians could potentially gain specialty recognition in this field, which currently was filled with physicians who enjoyed working in emergency medicine but might not be particularly well qualified. Unquestionably, emergency care in the United States was highly variable in quality, often disappointing public expectations.
7. The trend toward more specialization would continue. General primary care would have to be made just as attractive to draw more physicians.

The report was referred to the Committee on Community Services, to review and prepare flexible policy statements incorporating these concepts.

### C. Tenure of Board of Regents

The Board accepted the Committee's recommendation to change the tenure of Regents to one term of five years, replacing two terms of three years each.

### D. Role of the Past President

The Committee successfully recommended that:

1. The Immediate Past President should serve one year as an active member of the Board of Regents.
2. The four most recent Immediate Past Presidents, including the one on the Board, the President-Elect and the Executive Vice President, should constitute an Advisory Committee of Consultants to the President to:

    a. act as advisors at the President's request,
    b. respond to agenda prepared by the President,
    c. meet at the Annual Session, and other times at the President's request, with reimbursement.

### E. The Future Role of the American College of Physicians

1. Graduate Medical Education. The Committee submitted that the College needed much closer relationships with the American Board of Internal Medicine [ABIM]. It recommended that the Chairman of ABIM be invited to report to the Board of Governors and Board of Regents at the Annual Session. A recommendation that the College and the ABIM explore means of developing an in-training examination was referred to the Educational Activities Committee.
2. Undergraduate Education. Current representation on the Association of American Medical Colleges [AAMC] Council of Academic Societies

[CAS] and representation by two Regents on the AMA's Council on Medical Education were considered adequate and should be maintained.

3. Continuing Medical Education. All College programs should include significant educational opportunities for subspecialists. The Committee also gave strong support to further expansion of audio-visual programs.
4. International Education. The Committee urged that the College support all practical efforts to insure that foreign physicians training in this country would return to their own country on completion of training. It should be their express policy to encourage exchange of physicians at educational and practice levels, and to work with the State Department and other appropriate agencies to support strong international ties. Some methods of permanent funding for such activity would be necessary.
5. Chapters. The Committee concluded this was the only way larger numbers of our members could be active in College affairs, and considered it an effective means of getting things done at the local level.

The Committee, having concluded its work, was discharged with thanks in April, 1972.

### F. Committee on Committee Structure of the Board of Regents

1. This Committee recommended that both the Personnel Committee and the Ad Hoc Committee on Administrative Relationships, appointed in April, 1971, be discharged with thanks. It further recommended that the functions of the latter committee be assumed by a new permanent Standing Committee on Administration, consisting of the President, President-Elect, Secretary General, Treasurer, Chairman of the Finance Committee, Executive Vice President and a representative from the Board of Governors.
2. Functions of the Board of Regents. Three options of management were presented to improve efficiency in the Board's functions.

   a. The Executive Committee should perform most of the "housekeeping" chores of the Board and act as a steering committee.
   b. The size of the Board should be decreased.
   c. The Board of Regents should meet more frequently.

The first two options were not accepted and the Board voted to meet more frequently in order to handle the increased level of business. To improve their familiarity with information on their agenda, the Board also decided that committees should meet sufficiently in advance to provide reports before the Board's meeting date.

### G. Relationship of the Board of Regents to the Board of Governors

From 1970 to 1972, relationships between the Boards of Governors and Regents were examined extensively. The annual Governor's Conference was introducing important changes in the role of the Governor. Matters of importance to the College were subjects of serious study at these conferences.

The method of electing the Governor had changed so that each Governor was nominated and elected within his jurisdictional area. In addition, following one year served as Governor-Elect, Governors now served one four-year term rather than two three-year terms. In the absence of the Governor, the Governor-Elect, as an ex officio member of the Board of Governors, would act as the substitute.

The officers of the Board of Governors were the Chairman, who would be an ex officio member of the Board of Regents, empowered to vote, and Chairman-Elect.

The Executive Committee, composed of eight Governors including Chairman and Vice Chairman, exercised all powers of the Board subject to approval at its next meeting.

The Committee recommended Bylaws and policy changes regarding the duties of Governors. It was discharged with thanks and the report was referred to the Committee on Constitution and Bylaws to prepare changes in the Bylaws and the ACP Manual of Policies and Procedures. A special committee was then appointed to draft the changes. The changes, in summary, stated the following:

1. Duties of Governors (Bylaws).
   a. The Governor is responsible for endorsing candidates for action by the Credentials Committee. The Governor is also responsible for recruiting candidates who are eligible for membership.
   b. Local or Regional Meetings are the responsibility of the Governor, who transmits and interprets College policies to his constituents and assures implementation. He also promotes professional development of the membership.
   c. To assure regular review of their efforts in implementating College policies, each Governor should report local activities in writing to the Board of Governors.

The Bylaws, approved in April, 1972, defined all Governors as constituting the Board of Governors, each as the official representative from his jurisdiction:

2. The Committee also reviewed the Board of Governors' section of the "ACP Manual of Policies and Procedures" and recommended revision of the entire section. While retaining its comprehensive information for the Governors, regrouping information for better understanding of their duties was essential. The reorganization was to include: 1) Organization, 2) Membership, 3) Regional Meetings, 4) Other local activities, 5) Finance.

The Board of Governors, conferring in Philadelphia in October, 1971, requested that the duties of the Governors' Committee on College Affairs be described in more detail, and submitted the following for inclusion in the Procedure Manual:

It is recommended that the Committee have at least two meetings a year, held at such times that the Committee may assist the Governor in deciding on endorsement for the various categories of membership prior to the meeting of the Credentials

Committee. In some of the larger regions, a Governor's Advisory Committee may also be established. Members of this Committee are appointed by the Governor and should be experienced and knowledgeable in College affairs. Members of this Committee have, in the past, served on the Governor's Committee for College Affairs. This Committee also may be helpful to the Governor in making policy decisions, and may, if the Governor so decides, serve as a local Nominating Committee.

The Board revised the jurisdictional division of the Southern California Region: Region I included the counties of Los Angeles, Kern, Ventura, Santa Barbara, San Luis Obispo; Region II, the counties of Orange, Riverside, and San Bernadino; Region III, San Diego and Imperial Counties.

## Study of Internists' Practice

The Committee on Community Services reported progress on the survey of what internists do in their day-to-day practice, which was conducted to give guidance to the College in its educational programs and to the Residency Review Committee in Internal Medicine [RRC-IM] and the ABIM. The survey sought not only to find out how internists are being trained and how this coincided with what they actually do in practice, but also to determine how much primary care the internist, whether general or subspecialized, actually provides.

The committee also sought approval for a second cooperative project with the San Joaquin Foundation for Medical Care, entitled "Computer Based Evaluation of Medical Care by Foundations", which had the following stated purpose:

The problem of evaluation of medical care rests in the translation of excellence, as designed by those who continually practice excellence, into concise standards for a given disease which can be applied to computerization. The ACP has the prestige and ability to constitute a group of physicians who can define such standards. This has been done on a local piecemeal basis here and there throughout the country. Only an organization such as the ACP can define such standards with the hope of reliability, and general internal medicine will encourage other academic societies to accomplish this in their respective fields.

The project plan was described as follows:

1. Groups consisting of five physicians, four of whom would be outstanding practicing clinicians chosen to represent degrees of experience and geographic distribution, the fifth member being a full-time academic clinician, would define criteria for acceptable medical management of a specific group of diseases as delineated in the College's self-assessment program.
2. Representatives of the San Joaquin Foundation would meet with each of these groups to explain the purpose of developing the criteria and how to define these criteria so that computerization could follow.
3. Criteria would be developed so that under-utilization as well as over-utilization were defined in order that the best possible care of the patient would be ascertainable.
4. A member of the College should be appointed to give overall supervision

to this program. That person should attend each of nine meetings to provide coordination and continuity.

5. The San Joaquin Foundation would pay for the expenses of its participating personnel.
6. The College should provide the expenses of its participating members. It was very likely that a government contract could be obtained to cover these costs, estimated at $30,000.
7. Since there were certain time requirements, it was proposed that the first meeting of one of these groups be organized immediately, with funds appropriated by the ACP. Approving, the Board stipulated that "subspecialty societies may be consulted for names of suitable committee appointees. They may be informed about any standard set".

The College had sponsored a tour of the British Isles in 1971. The President reported in November that 280 physicians and their spouses participated. In Dublin, David Mitchell, President of the Royal College of Physicians of Ireland presided over an excellent scientific program and hosted a delightful reception and dinner in this historic headquarters building. During the reception, he installed Dr. Butt and Dr. R. Carmichael Tilghman, ACP Secretary General, as Honorary Fellows in the Irish College. A similarly interesting program and reception occurred in Edinburgh, over which Dr. J. Halliday Croom, President of the Royal College of Physicians of Edinburgh, presided. At the Glasgow College of Physicians and Surgeons, President E. M. McGirr conferred an Honorary Fellowship on Dr. Butt during the conviviality of a reception and dinner. Traveling on to London, the group attended the Scientific Program at the Royal College of Physicians of London, arranged by Lord Rosenheim. An elaborate dinner was given for more than 300 Americans and their English hosts. On another evening, a reception was provided at the Royal Society of Medicine. Sir and Lady Hedley Atkins hosted this event.

The outpouring of friendship and hospitality to ACP members by these sister colleges reminded us of our lasting debt to these colleagues.

The Secretary General, Dr. Tilghman, reported a total membership of 19,940, of whom 76 were Masters, 11,553 Fellows, 5,204 Members, 43 Honorary Fellows, 57 Corresponding Fellows, 195 Affiliate Members and 2,812 were Associates.

In November, I reviewed the initiation of two very important new systems at ACP headquarters. Membership lists and subscription lists were converted to computer service. Henceforth, *Annals* subscription addressing would be computer generated. A sophisticated communications center was also introduced. All telephones became dictating stations and most typing was done through use of tape-driven word processing machines.

I agreed with the Board's move toward closer liaison with subspecialty and allied medical groups. While acknowledging its importance, I urged that the College carefully avoid dilution of its own very strong programs. Moves to expand such activity would require constant evaluation of Staff support for new projects. Priorities should be reviewed periodically to prevent inordinate expansion of

Staff without commensurate cost effectiveness.

I submitted that the newly developed Governors' Committee for College Affairs did not go far enough in conception to achieve more active participation by the membership. More formal local organization was essential to achieve this.

### American Board of Family Practice

The Board of Regents acted on significant recommendations from the Board of Governors.

1. Action to recognize the newly formed American Board of Family Practice was deferred.
2. A four-part resolution on education was approved, which read:

   a. The American College of Physicians endorses the philosophy of a liberal medical education;
   b. The College goes on record as favoring preservation of the the internship year;
   c. The College urges that medical students not be encouraged to make premature career commitments;
   d. The College favors preservation of the broadly trained, Board certified internist;
   e. Subspecialty recognition be secondary to demonstration of broad internal medical competence.

3. The Board of Governors unanimously approved a motion from the Ad Hoc Committee on Direction of Medicine at the Toronto meeting that the College should become involved in the economics, organization, and costs of medical care, to fulfill its primary mission of education in quality care. The Board of Regents referred this issue to the Committee on Community Services.

### Physicians' Assistants

At the Fall Meeting of the Board of Regents, 1971, an important document was presented by the Community Services Committee, "Essentials of An Approved Educational Program for The Assistant to The Primary Care Physician". A basic description of the profession and the College's interpretation of the role of the Physicians' Assistant [PA] was published in the *ACP Bulletin* in May 1971. The final detailed document was a collaborative report of the American Academy of Family Physicians [AAFP], American Academy of Pediatrics [AAP]; ACP; American Society of Internal Medicine [ASIM] and AAMC and was approved by the AMA's Council on Medical Education and the House of Delegates.

Objectives

In summary, the objectives of the program emphasized development and maintenance of standards of educational programs and guidelines for self-evaluation of such programs. They also included criteria for program approvals and publication of approved programs.

Description of the Occupation

Delineation of the medical profession and its role in paramedical functions stressed that the PA is a specifically trained, skilled person who would perform services under the responsibility and supervision of a doctor of medicine or osteopathy in a highly flexible context, depending upon the nature of the physician's medical practice setting.

The assistant's education should emphasize diagnostic and therapeutic training for tasks which could be performed under the physician's supervision, thus allowing the physician to extend his services through more effective use of his time, knowledge, skills and abilities. In addition, the assistant would play a valuable role in the collection of data necessary to diagnostic and therapeutic decision-making and patient care planning. Other criteria included development of subjective qualities essential in relating to patients, such as respect for the person and privacy of the patient, and calm and reasoned judgment in critical situations.

Because the functions of the primary care physician are interdisciplinary, training of the physician's assistant would necessarily include varied services applicable to total patient care, such as transmission and execution of the physician's orders, performance of patient care tasks and diagnostic and therapeutic procedures which could be delegated by the physician.

Acknowledging a broad variability in functions affected by the primary practice setting, the document established general criteria for training.

The report established additional criteria for the implementation of educational programs, including essential requirements for accreditation, clinical affiliations, facilities, financial resources, faculty, student selection, academic records, curriculum and program administration.

The plan provided for annual reports from accredited institutions to the collaborating medical organizations and for a standing committee on which approved programs and the collaborating medical organizations would be represented. The Committee would propose changes in standards and criteria and submit them to the collaborating societies for approval.

The Board of Regents was satisfied that, with strict supervision of the educational programs by the sponsoring medical organizations, the physicians' assistant would be well trained, and approved the "Essentials".

At the November meeting, Dr. R. Carmichael Tilghman, Chairman of the Committee on Credentials, indicated that of 622 candidates for Membership, 197 were recommended for election to direct Fellowship, 389 were elected Members and six were recommended for reinstatement. There were 147 candidates for Fellowship, of which 86 were recommended for advancement.

The Committee on Educational Activities, Dr. Walter B. Frommeyer, Jr., Chairman, reported that the following issues were still under study: 1) peer review programs to evaluate medical services; and 2) evaluation of the effectiveness of postgraduate courses.

The ACP-American Psychiatric Association [APA] Task Force suggested that it continue to meet at least twice a year and add liaison representation from the Committee on Postgraduate Courses and Educational Activities Committee. The ABIM and the RRC-IM collectively supported the position that psychiatry is of great importance to internal medicine. The ABIM was giving full Board credit for rotation through periods of training in psychiatry. The American College of Physicians provided two scientific sessions on psychiatry at its annual meeting.

The *Medical Knowledge Self-Assessment Program* was receiving wide acceptance. Fifteen thousand copies of *MKSAP II* were ordered at first printing. Five thousand physicians returned the answer sheets in time for machine grading and 4,000 physicians chose to have their scores pooled for representive data collection. Fifty percent of those returning their answer sheets requested subspecialty scores. Another 5,000 copies were subsequently printed and *MKSAP II* was expected to be sold out completely. The program was self-supporting and contributed significantly to the financial resources of the College.

Audio-visual single-topic procedural films would be completed by late December or mid-January and could be shown at the 1972 Annual Session. Topics included arterial puncture, placement of a central venous line, venous cut-down, intubation, emergency tracheotomy, and lumbar spinal puncture.

The Committee on Fellowships and Scholarships reported that teaching and researching scholars who had concluded their scholarships in June, 1971, had done extremely well, attesting to the usefulness of the program. Current traveling scholars were also doing well and five new traveling scholars had been chosen from 13 applicants for the coming year. Established criteria had excluded nine of the 36 candidates for teaching and research scholarships and three scholars were selected from the remaining 27 candidates.

The Committee on Finance, after considering the regular budget of expenses and income for 1971-72, listed the contributions that the College makes to various medical organizations. The largest sum, contributed to support the Joint Commission on Accreditation of Hospitals [JCAH], was $40,000. The other societies, supported at smaller levels, were the National Society for Medical Research [NSMR]; RRC-IM; American Association for Accreditation of Laboratory Animal Care [AAALAC]; National Committee on Drug Abuse; National Interagency Council on Smoking & Health; Student American Medical Association; Alliance for Engineering in Medicine & Biology [AEMB]; Association for the Advancement of Medical Instrumentation [AAMI] and CAS (AAMC). The Finance Committee, in support of the Board of Regents' April, 1971 Resolution, approved $5,000 and Staff support for the Congress of the International Society of Internal Medicine, to be held in September, 1972.

## Headquarters South Wing Completed

The new five-story wing of the College Headquarters, started on March 19, 1970, was completed and occupied on May 1, 1971. Some additional construction remained to be done in 1972, including an adjacent parking area and a driveway around the building. The architects considered the driveway impractical since it would require demolishing an adjoining house owned by the College. This impediment, however, was itself demolished by fortune. A young architectural graduate of the University of Pennsylvania spent some of his evening hours planning a solution to the problem which saved the College about $20,000, and the driveway was built. The total cost of the building addition, $1,318,494, was financed by a special assessment of the Members which raised $544,370, and by the previously cumulated building fund, accrued annually at $100,000.

### Emergency Medical Care

Emergency Medical Care was an important agenda that year for the Committee on Hospitals. Dr. Richard Allyn, Chairman, recommended the adoption of a policy statement which was published in the *ACP Bulletin* in December, 1971, entitled "The Internist's Role In Emergency Medical Care".

The changing pattern of the delivery of health care has involved an increasingly significant role for the hospital in emergency medical care. Emergencies, once primarily related to trauma and surgery, now encompass a broad spectrum of medical diseases, for which sophisticated techniques of management are now available. The internist has been called upon increasingly as a consultant, primary provider, administrator and educator. It is assumed that any internist responsible for emergency care obligations will address himself to the special body of information available in this area of endeavor . . .

The statement addressed specific areas of involvement, stressing the role of the internist in the emergency unit, intensive care units, in-hospital medical emergencies, and in the community.

The internist should participate in planning and supervision of emergency medical care and should be consulted about the design, location, construction, purchase of equipment and operation of the Emergency Department, intensive care units, in-hospital emergency teams, and community emergency services.

In the emergency unit, it advised the internist to provide direct care for his own patients if staff regulations permitted. Commitment to emergency services should involve the internist on committees concerned with resuscitative or other medical emergency procedures, hospital admission transfers, rotation in staffing, formulating recommendations for equipment, and training health personnel.

The statement stressed the necessity for the internist's intimate involvement in all aspects of the design and operation of intensive care units. In the community, internists should seek opportunities to serve on councils and agencies involved in the formation and coordination of emergency medical services.

### Medical Audit Feasibility Study

Another project under the surveillance of the Committee on Hospitals was the Medical Audit Feasibility Study. Supported by Health, Education and Welfare [HEW] funds, the study was operating in three hospitals near Philadelphia. The Allentown Hospital had already completed some of their initial studies on five or six diseases. The plan engaged local hospital staffs to develop criteria for adequate care for specific diseases. After a period of time records would be audited, comparing treatment before and after these decisions to determine how well the staff responded to these locally established criteria. Progress was, not surprisingly, rather slow. The idea was innovative, and even with professional help for detailed work, an additional two years would be required to complete the project. It had, however, demonstrated its acceptability, showing that physicians were interested in doing adequate audit in their hospitals.

The American College of Physicians and the American Hospital Association [AHA] jointly sponsored an interesting resource utilization conference in New York City, on January 21-22, 1972. Representatives from approximately 25 hospitals in New York, New Jersey and Pennsylvania (Region II of the American Hospital Association) participated. Each hospital was represented by a trustee, an administrator and an internist. The conference was a series of workshops covering four resource utilization topics:

1. Manpower utilization: hospital and other supportive personnel for the internist;
2. Effective utilization of financial resources;
3. Space and facility utilization;
4. Planning for future resources.

In November of 1971, Dr. Truman J. Schnabel, Jr., Chairman of the Committee on Publications, reported steady growth in *Annals* subscriptions. Particularly noteworthy, the *Annals* had the largest number of nonmember subscribers (36,008) of any of the journals devoted to internal medicine. Members' subscriptions were 17,250, with total subscriptions being 53,258. The number of student, intern, and resident subscribers had dropped observably, but this was attributable to the introduction of Associate membership in the College, which transferred their representation to the category of member subscribers.

Advertising revenue was stable, but production costs of printing by computerized methods resulted in smaller net revenues available for other College activities. Federal taxes for advertising income had become another item of expense to the College. Cumulative payments since 1968 totaled $750,000. Following the advice of its attorneys, the College continued to pay the taxes, but filed for a refund on the basis that this income was not correctly classified as "unrelated business" income. The law was, at that time, quite specific. In order for a educational institution to derive income from advertising in a journal, the advertising should be directly related to the "exempt" purposes for which the organization had received the designation of a "charitable or educational institution". With the 1968 changes in government regulations, the attorneys believed the College might recover some of the taxes paid, although a date for adjudication before the Internal Revenue Service was uncertain.

## Clinical Pharmacology Committee

The Board of Regents voted to change the Ad Hoc Committee on Clinical

Pharmacology to a standing committee. Dr. Marcus M. Reidenberg, Chairman, presented the recommended charge to the new Committee:

1. To recommend policies and actions for the American College of Physicians to take in the area of education of the medical profession about the rational use of drugs.
2. To advise the leadership of the American College of Physicians about questions for which they desire counsel from clinical pharmacologists.
3. To initiate positions for the American College of Physicians on matters pertaining to clinical pharmacology, broadly defined.
4. To represent the American College of Physicians at meetings where problems in the field of clinical pharmacology are discussed.

## ACP Members and Associates

In a report from the Ad Hoc Committee on Membership, Dr. Herbert W. Pohle, Chairman, presented the following recommendations, which the Board approved. Items 1-4 were referred to the Committee on Hospitals. Other approved changes were referred for incorporation in the Bylaws and the ACP Policy Manual.

1. The American College of Physicians should continue to be an umbrella organization of internists and qualified, certified members of recognized nonsurgical specialty groups . . .
2. The image of The American College of Physicians shall be maintained by insisting that it be an organization that stresses competence, scholarliness, and quality medical care. Its primary goal shall continue to be the continuing education of its members.
3. Since the American College of Physicians is a national organization and not a federation of state chapters, we should preserve our present concept of a central Credentials Committee empowered to make final decisions on all classes of membership free from local pressures. Associates, however, need not be considered by the Credentials Committee.
4. Our present concept of an internist does not preclude his performance of manipulative procedures, e.g., cardiac catheterization, endoscopy, and insertion of pacemakers. These endeavors constitute a small fraction of the internist's total effort and should be performed by a capable physician.
5. After he has started his first year of residency training in internal medicine and has the endorsement of his Chief of Medicine, a trainee may apply for Associateship in the American College of Physicians.

The Committee included detailed recommendations for eligibility requirements for Members of the College which were referred to the Constitution and Bylaws Committee. Among these recommendations, it advised deleting the existing provisions, that a physician could not be proposed for Membership until six years following medical school graduation or for Fellowship for a minimum of eight years following graduation.

Addressing the question of admission of family practice physicians, the committee concluded that the wide variability in quality of training programs precluded a general position on eligibility and recommended that the Credentials

Committee continue to consider proposals based on individual merits. Information on training programs in family practice was still insufficient to establish criteria for membership based on training.

The Credentials Committee was unable to concur with this recommendation, nor did it find acceptable the following additional guideline offered by the Ad Hoc Committee on Membership:

> It is important to interest qualified physicians in the College as soon as they are eligible either for Associateship or Membership. However, Fellowship by advancement from Membership or by direct election should be an honor and mark of distinction that will be achieved only by those who can demonstrate growth and maturity in the application of their knowledge and skill to their specialty. Those considered for this honor must document advancement and growth in knowledge, competence, scholarship, and acceptance by their peers. In cases where local circumstance precludes demonstration of such professional growth in the usual ways, the Governor's endorsing letter must carefully and specifically document the reasons for his conviction that the candidate has indeed grown professionally and is deserving of Fellowship. The Credentials Committee must continue to screen critically all proposals for this honor. As in the past, the Credentials Committee may waive specific Fellowship requirements including written material if documented evidence of continuous growth during the period of Membership is furnished.

The Commission on Professional and Hospital Activities [CPHA] reported that in August, 1971, 1,469 hospitals were subscribing to the Professional Activity Study [PAS]. PAS was now registering over 12 million hospital discharges annually. The "PAS System" (previously referred to as PAS-MAP,) more accurately described the six parts of the system. These were PAS itself plus five additional options: Medical Audit Program [MAP]; Length of Stay Study; Perinatal Study; Study of Patient Charges [SPC]; and Special Studies. The SPC had been made available in July, 1971, and had been formulated in response to increasing concern over the steady rise in hospital costs. Through this system, a hospital could corollate the patient's medical data with his total bill, furnishing comparisons between services, diagnoses, and operations within a hospital.

In October, the College's Committee on Hospitals met at the CPHA headquarters for thorough briefing in the operation of this organization. Dr. Calvin F. Kay, Deputy Executive Vice President, was elected to succeed me on the Board of Directors of CPHA.

The ACP Commissioners to the JCAH, Drs. Wright Adams, Marshall M. Fulton and John A. Layne, reported a major achievement during the preceding year: the successful introduction of a new program of hospital accreditation. Since July, 1971, new standards adopted in December, 1970, and published in March, 1971, became the basis of hospital surveys. The key feature of the new procedure was a substantially more detailed questionnaire which the hospital would complete and return prior to the survey visit. This allowed a computer analysis of the replies and print-outs of specific diagnostic messages concerning the hospital. The analysis was provided to the survey team to assist in its evaluation and consultative attention to each hospital's particular needs. With this information available, the survey visit became more of an individualized educational conference. The data were also stored in cumulative totals, providing a highly useful source of previously unavailable information for the study of trends in American hospital practice.

The Kellogg Foundation was supporting a series of JCAH workshops for medical and hospital professionals about the new standards and their application. Most of these were cosponsored by state hospital and medical associations. These workshops had been received enthusiastically and were well attended. Many more individual practitioners than ever before were acquiring firsthand experience in the voluntary program to enhance the quality of hospital care for their patients.

Dr. John Beck, Chairman of the ABIM, updated the Board of Regents of an in-training examination for candidates being educated in internal medicine. The examination was employed to validate procedures being used in the ABIM's certifying examinations and to define the logistics involved in offering in-training examinations. Having introduced it as a "trial balloon" to measure constituent response towards evaluation during the training period, the Board was surprised by the deluge of requests from program directors and trainees.

Dr. Beck raised a question about which body should prepare and conduct these in-training examinations. The ACP or the ABIM were two obvious alternatives. A precedent had been established in the United Kingdom to utilize a commercial alternative. During the Annual Session, the Educational Activities Committee met with ABIM Directors to study the question further.

## ACP/ASIM Memorandum of Intent

During 1971-72, matters regarding ACP/ASIM relationships were reaching a decisive stage. Since 1967, when high level liaison interaction was adopted, laying aside temporarily the other two alternatives of complete societal separation or amalgamation, the barometer of relationships rose and fell with seasonal regularity, foreshadowing eventual confrontation over the unanswered questions. In 1971, the Liaison Committee recommended that amalgamation should be attempted. At an informal meeting of the respective societies at the AMA in June, 1971, the Liaison Committee and the Officers of the societies decided to pursue a plan of amalgamation to its logical conclusion. Polling the membership by questionnaire was rejected, since even the exploratory suggestion of a merger might mean that some members would resign their membership in their present society.

The Liaison Committee met several times in the fall to draw up a preliminary plan for presentation to the ACP and ASIM Boards. The Board of Regents met in special session in February, 1972, to decide on two questions: 1) Did the Board think it important that the ACP and ASIM affiliate? 2) Did the Board think affiliation possible? The Board moved unanimously on their importance and approved the general plan, authorizing the Liaison Committee to proceed with the lawyers of the two societies to prepare a Memorandum of Intent. (Appendix G)

Soon thereafter the Liaison Committee met again in Chicago, and at Annual

Session meetings in April, 1972, presented the Memorandum of Intent, testing the feasibility of amalgamation. The Board of Governors considered the memorandum during almost three hours of discussion on April 16. Although they conveyed to the Board of Regents on April 18 that "some aspects . . . should be studied further", they recommended approval of the intent "to find acceptable grounds for amalgamation."

> The Board of Governors recommends to the Board of Regents that the Board of Governors approves the intent to try to find acceptable grounds for amalgamation with the ASIM but to postpone any final action of the Board of Governors on this matter until further study and deliberations of the specific articles of intent are carried out.

The House of Delegates of ASIM rejected any change in the locus of power outside the Councilors as described in the "Intent", and communicated other points of disagreement to the Board of Regents through the Liaison Committee:

Whereas the Memorandum approved by ACP specified in Section I that headquarters would be in Philadelphia, the ASIM House of Delegates rejected it and urged the possibility of Washington, DC, as headquarters locale.

The ASIM rejected the specifications in Section 3(1) of the memorandum which would transfer the locus of power from the Councilors to a Board of Directors.

Opposing the Section 3(0) requirement of a two-thirds vote to rescind actions of the policy making body, the ASIM offered the following amendment to Section 3(0): "The Council shall meet at least annually and conduct business by a simple majority vote of the Council and any action by the Board of Directors may be rescinded by a simple majority vote of the Council."

Following review of these Reports, the Board of Regents approved the following statement on April 18:

> The Board of Regents of the American College of Physicians does not find it feasible to amalgamate with the American Society of Internal Medicine at this time, but the College will have continued liaison with the ASIM.

The ACP-ASIM Liaison Committee met immediately thereafter to draft and approve a letter communicating these actions to the membership of both organizations.

The Board of Regents then called a special meeting at 2:00 p.m. of the same day and approved the letter to the membership.

## Annual Session 1972

The 53rd Annual Session of the College was held in Atlantic City from April 16-21, 1972. Attendance was disappointing and no future meetings were planned for Atlantic City. Dr. Hugh R. Butt, President, reviewed the achievements of the past year. He expressed satisfaction with the decision to decrease the tenure of the Regents from two successive three-year terms to one five-year term and hoped that the Governors would soon follow suit. He also expressed the hope that a Past Presidents' group would be formed. He was pleased with the progress of the Audio-Visual Committee in developing single topic medical skills films and initiating work on patient counseling films.

Several weeks before the Annual Session, I received a telephone call from a young woman who claimed that she was a member of the Students for a Democratic Society. She requested time on our program for her society to protest the award we were giving to Dr. Sol Krugman for his work on hepatitis at the Willowbrook Institution for the Mentally Retarded. Feelings regarding human experimentation were running high at that time and this organization found Dr. Krugman's work unacceptable. I explained to her that it was not possible for us to change the program at this late date. Dr. Butt, President, Dr. Sodeman, President-Elect, and I conferred with Dr. Krugman in New York. Dr. Krugman was very pleased to receive the award but was quite willing to postpone its acceptance to avert disturbance of the meeting, if that was what we wished. We told him that if he were willing to accept it under these circumstances, we certainly wished to bestow it as planned.

On my arrival in Atlantic City, I met with the Chief of Police and told him that I expected some student protestors to which he retorted, "Yes, about 400". Some were coming from New York and there was quite a deputation from Boston. Whether any were coming from Philadelphia, he was not yet certain. I asked him how he knew that and he said, "We get information like that from the FBI". Then he explained that as long as we rented the Convention Hall, we were responsible for everything occurring inside the building. If we wanted interior police guards and protection, he would provide them at our expense. In addition, if they arrested anybody on my instruction, then I would have to agree to appear in court to prefer charges. When I had agreed to these arrangements, he arranged to have police officers ready to secure the stage and hall for the Convocation procession.

When the procession began, there were about 300 students ominously gathered in one corner of the auditorium. I was to call the orders from one side of the stagefront. Dr. Krugman's award was placed at the end of the program. As soon as his name was mentioned, noisy pandemonium broke loose. Several people approached the stage; one, a fast moving young man who was dressed and groomed as conservatively as a stockbroker. He tried to vault onto the stage, grasping the decorative hedge across the stagefront. However, it was not fastened down and he fell backward away from the stage. My assistant, Miss Murphy, called police security. They trooped in, removed the young man, and formed a line in front of the stage. The incident was recorded by our convention photographers.

Just in front of me, another interesting scene was being enacted. A young woman was chasing one of the officers, striking out at him. He merely took hold of her firmly, but her people were taking pictures and shouting, "police brutality".

When the Convocation was finished in the restored silence, the Rabbi's Benediction impressed many of us. He called on the Lord in Heaven to make us all mindful that these children were our children. After the Benediction, we immediately announced that one of the meeting halls would be available after lunch for those attending the Annual Session who wished to congregate and talk with the students. Approximately 400-500 people went to listen to their arguments.

At the end of that afternoon, Dr. Krugman took part in a panel discussion which many of the students attended. The moderator said they had already had a chance to expound their arguments and that it would be appreciated if they would ask respectful questions. They responded with some very intelligent questions which Dr. Krugman graciously answered as well as he could. At the end of the discussion, there was a loud ovation for this fine researcher in medicine.

Before the end of the panel, one disturbance provided a little humor. A student was held up at the entrance to the room because he didn't have an identification card. I asked him where he was from and he replied, "Harvard Medical School". I told him I had also gone there but couldn't remember that we took part in such protests. When I asked him why he was so anxious to get into that particular room, he replied, "I just want to go in and tell my friends the bus leaves in ten minutes for Boston". Naturally, we allowed him to enter.

The protest thrust an additional problem on us involving the exhibitors. They wanted assurance that their booths would be protected. I suggested that if they were worried about their booths they'd have to help us by remaining in them. It was an interesting experience, but it had some frightening aspects.

Annual Sessions of the College held in Philadelphia averaged $43 per physician attending as compared to $78 per physician in Denver. Obviously, the increased cost was attributable to transporting Staff, speakers, and materials to cities distant from Headquarters. The Treasurer was pleased to announce that even with the substantial increase in the cost of printing and mailing the *Annals,* there was still a net income from the *Annals,* after federal taxes of $165,000. The Endowment Fund in this year had reached a market value of $4,361,000, compared with a market value of $3,868,000 the year earlier, yielding a total income of $178,000.

For the Credentials Committee, Dr. Tilghman, Chairman, presented 319 candidates for membership and recommended 99 for immediate Fellowship and 195 for Membership. Of 183 candidates for Fellowship, 73 were recommended for Advancement to Fellowship, 80 were recommended for election contingent upon attendance at the 1972 session.

I reported with satisfaction the progress of the new computer systems and described some cost saving developments, including postgraduate bulletin mailings. Six audio-visual films were ready for production and the Medical Skills Library would be be shown at this Annual Session.

My Executive Vice Presidential report also reviewed a new development in medical malpractice. In the past year, the Secretary of HEW had appointed an investigative commission on medical practice. I had attended a meeting in February at which many solutions to medical malpractice problems were offered, but without substantiating data. The Commission accepted my offer to survey the ACP membership to obtain more objective data. The questionnaire, sent through the cooperation of Mr. Claypoole and the Group Insurance Administrators, yielded some interesting results. Responses were received from 7,647 of our members; most were under 40 years of age. Almost two-thirds of the respondents were in private practice. Although at that time most of them were covered by $100,000-$300,000 limits, almost half of these had increased the limits of their coverage in the previous five years. None of the members expressed any undue difficulty in obtaining coverage. Nine hundred and ninety-one of the respondents reported that claims had been instituted against them, most relating to hospital care. Of the entire number of claims made, only 57 were for care given in the patient's home. Interestingly, of those physicians reporting claims, a high proportion said that patients who had filed claims had been under their care for less than a year and a fair number said they had seen the patient only once or not at all. This suggested strongly that many physicians involved in a malpractice suit have little actual contact with the patient. This was especially true in hospital management of patients.

## Coordinating Council on Medical Education

The Ad Hoc Committee on the Future Role of ACP in Medical Education made its final report at the Annual Session. This Committee met in February, 1972 and made recommendations regarding two matters referred to them from Board of Governors: 1) mandatory shortening of medical school curricula, and 2) mobility in the training in internal medicine. These issues, the Committee stated, were fairly well resolved and could be handled by the new Coordinating Council on Medical Education [CCME]. The newly established Council was represented by the AMA, AAMC, CMSS, American Board of Medical Specialties (ABMS), and the AHA. The Committee was discharged and the recommendations were referred to the Educational Activities Committee for further study.

Dr. Marvin Pollard, Chairman of the Committee on Cancer, presented a comprehensive review of the status of the College's current activity in cancer. The American College of Surgeons [ACS] was much more extensively involved in cancer activities than the ACP. He noted, however, that neoplastic disease had been included in our self-assessment program. He urged that the JCAH support the need for paying more attention to procedures, such as "Pap Tests" as part of workups for female patients being considered for surgical intervention for cancer of the cervix. The Committee believed that everything should be done to help the primary physician caring for cancer patients, whether internist or other. Medical house officers also should be expected to order "Pap Tests" regularly. Dr. Pollard then reported on a program sponsored by the National Cancer Institute and the American Cancer Society, which proposed establishing a series of cancer centers. A lengthy discussion followed concerning the role of the College in educating its own members, resulting in a consensus that cancer educational efforts should be increased, not only in publications but at the Annual Session and in postgraduate courses.

A report from the American Joint Committee on Cancer Staging and End Results Reporting revealed that during 1971, after 13 years of work, stage classifications for nine anatomical cancer sites were completed and distributed: breast, larynx, cervix uteri, corpus uteri, pharynx, urinary bladder, thyroid gland, oral cavity, and stomach. The Committee also had published a paper entitled: "Reporting of Cancer Survival and End Results". The Cancer Committee recommended that an editorial for *Annals* be prepared, based on Dr. Pollard's report, emphasizing that criteria for many cancer sites were available in the manual.

The Board of Regents approved the following policy statement about consultants to the Food and Drug Administration:

> A question has been raised concerning the propriety of consultants to the Food and Drug Administration being selected [from] among those clinical investigators who performed studies sponsored by drug manufacturers. The Food and Drug Administration should have the best medical and scientific information in existence. Therefore, it should be able to consult with the most knowledgeable people available. These few people often participate in therapeutic trials, the costs of which are borne by pharmaceutical manufacturers as well as in research supported by government foundations, industry and other donors. Clinical trials by university affiliated investigators are usually desired by both the pharmaceutical industry and the Food and Drug Administration because they are the best quality clinical trials generally done. The criteria for selecting consultants should be scientific merit and knowledge, and not the source of research support for the consultant.

Dr. Walter B. Frommeyer, Jr., Chairman of the Educational Activities Committee, presented a retrospective 3-year summary of activities:

Regional Meetings showed steadily increasing total attendance; at 39 meetings in the 3-year period, attendance totaled 4,621 in 1969-70; 5,120 in 1970-71; and 5,881 in 1972-73. The proportion of membership attending by Region varied from a low of 5.1 percent in Southern Illinois to a high of 70.6 percent in Vermillion, South Dakota.

A comparative report of Annual Session attendance from 1969 to 1972 showed some interesting characteristics. In Chicago, in 1969, from a total registration of 6,704, 17.7 percent of total registration, (2,614), were College members, and physicians, both member and nonmember, represented 65 percent (4,373) of all registrants. The Philadelphia Session in 1970, showed the highest proportion of members attending in the four year period, 19.1 percent (2,991) of 7,719 total registrants. In Denver, 1971, and in Atlantic City, site of the Annual Session in 1972, member attendance dropped to 13.9 and 13.5 percent respectively, with a concomittant drop in total attendance; 2,443 members among 5,624 total registrants in Denver; and 2,681 members among 5,791 total registrants in Atlantic City.

Nearly 15,000 copies of *MKSAP II* had been sold, and it was noteworthy that 1,900 of these subscriptions were from Associates of the College. The Board of Regents enthusiastically approved the development of *MKSAP III*.

The new *Medical Skills Library* single-topic films were extremely popular at this Annual Session and Dr. Frommeyer predicted continuing and increasing support for this effort. He reported that the College was negotiating a contract with ROCOM, a division of Hoffman-LaRoche, to develop further films, especially for patient counseling.

Dr. Richard Allyn, Chairman, reported a large agenda for the Committee on Hospitals. The Visiting Professors to Hospitals Program had elicited about 40 requests from hospitals, but only one or two of these had actually made contact with one of the suggested professors. The Committee was making progress on the development of policies to delineate hospital privileges.

Further efforts to increase the College's interest in emergency health service had been made: 1) by attendance at the Second National Conference on Health Services; 2) by a policy recommendation that the American College of Physicians maintain its friendly interest in the American College of Emergency Physicians; and 3) by actively encouraging internists to participate in all proper areas of emergency care.

The Conference on Resource Utilization in Hospitals, which was co-sponsored by the AHA and the ACP in New York City in January, was successful. A similar meeting was scheduled for San Francisco in the Fall.

Noting that it was estimated that 70 percent of those who die from initial heart attack, do so before they reach a hospital, the committee urged approval of an important resolution regarding cardiopulmonary resuscitation which the Board of Regents approved for press release:

> Members of the American College of Physicians and other internists should actively participate in training programs for teaching all hospital personnel to perform Cardiopulmonary Resuscitation, in cooperation with the American Heart Association, the American College of Cardiology and other interested organizations. This training should include recognition of this cardiac emergency, as well as its treatment by pounding of the chest, mouth-to-mouth respiration, closed cardiac massage, etc. Each hospital should supply to the community, on request, experts to teach these procedures to all citizens and to groups, including Boy Scouts, Girl Scouts, lifeguards, public utility employees, policemen, firemen, ambulance personnel, and members of the Armed Forces. It is further recommended that classes on the subject be established in high schools, colleges and all lifesaving courses.

The Insurance Committee reported that Liberty Mutual representatives were concerned about the increase in the number of credible malpractice suits currently being instituted against insured members. However, Dr. Harrison J. Schull, Committee Chairman, conveyed that an increase in rates which had been forecast for January 1, 1972, did not materialize, due to the Phase II freeze on prices established by the government. Other parts of the insurance program were considered to be functioning satisfactorily. A new program, announced January 10, 1972, concerned the extension of coverage to employees of members. In addition, an amendment to the Physicians' Insurance Trust agreement was presented to the Board for approval. The Committee stressed that the extent of any plan of insurance, by arrangement between the Trust and any insurance company to professional persons eligible under the revised definition of a "Member", could be issued either under the Employee Group Insurance Plan or the Member Group Insurance Plan.

Dr. Thomas P. Almy, Chairman, reported that plans for a future Latin American Fellowship Program had been discussed extensively by the International

Medical Activities Committee. Due to the fact that $10,000 was an insufficient sum to be used effectively to replace the former Kellogg Program, the Committee decided that the money might best be used for four stipends of $2,500, to provide three month refresher Fellowship programs in the US for Latin American medical leaders.

Associate membership having been made available to foreign physicians who were in graduate training in the United States, the Committee recommended the distribution to all Members of the College a letter from the officers of the Royal Society of Medicine, which offered opportunities to join that society. Several foreign internists were approved for Affiliate membership in the College.

Dr. Truman G. Schnabel, Jr., Chairman of the Publications Committee, reported continued growth in *Annals* subscriptions. As of January, 1972, subscribers numbered 56,913, of which 38,206 were nonmembers. The advertising rates were adjusted in January to take into consideration the substantial increase in circulation volume and production costs. The proportion of pages of editorial content to advertising pages was optimal, approximately 66.7 percent for editorial and news, and 33.3 percent for advertising.

Dr. Richard Vilter, ACP representative to the CAS, reported agreement among representatives from the AMA, AAMC, American Board of Medical Specialties [ABMS], CMSS, and the AHA on a number of issues:

1. As soon as possible, a Liaison Committee on Graduate Medical Education [LCGME] would be established, with representation from each of the five organizations, to serve as the official accrediting body for graduate medical education.
2. Simultaneously, a CCME would be established to consider policy matters in both undergraduate and graduate medical education, for referral to the parent organizations.
3. The existing Liaison Committee on Medical Education [LCME] and the new LCGME would have the authority to make decisions on accreditation in their respective areas within the limits of policies established by the parent organizations. It was understood that the RRC-IM would continue to function as currently defined.
4. All policy decisions would continue to be subject to approval by the parent organizations.
5. Policy recommendations might originate from any of the parent organizations or from the two liaison committees, but would be subject to review by the Coordinating Council prior to final action by the parent organizations.

Dr. Vilter further indicated that the CAS was still considering the amount of funding necessary for the operation of the CAS. He stressed the great value of this newly formed Council, which would bring together not only the clinical departments of medical schools, but also the departments of basic sciences in medical schools and, in addition, representation from specialty societies.

In recent deliberations of the ACP-APA Task Force, reported Dr. John R. Graham, the two societies had completed plans for establishing a mechanism to feed back information to their respective organizations. The type of training in medicine which those entering psychiatric residency programs should receive was carefully considered, especially in view of the deletion of the internship from the psychiatric board requirements. Methods for teaching the psychiatric aspects of medical diseases for those in internships and residency programs in internal medicine received continued study. The conclusion resulting from the discussion was that the Task Force should urge, whenever possible, that such training be provided for medical students and residents on the medical service. A suggested College "position paper" was offered for approval by the Postgraduate Courses Committee and the Educational Activities Committee.

## Part Four (1972-1973)

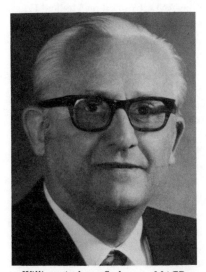

*William Anthony Sodeman, MACP*

William A. Sodeman was born on June 13, 1906, in Charleroi, Pennsylvania. He married Agnes Wagner in 1928 and they have two sons, William and Thomas; both are Fellows of the ACP.

Dr. Sodeman received his degrees at the University of Michigan; his BS in 1928 and his MD in 1931. He also holds honorary degrees from Villanova University, ScD (hon.), 1959; Thomas Jefferson University Medical College, LHD (hon.) 1967, and the Medical College of Ohio, ScD, 1976.

He was an intern at St. Vincent's Hospital, Toledo, Ohio, 1931-32, and a Fellow in Internal Medicine at Tulane University, New Orleans, from 1932 to 1936, when he was appointed to the faculty as an Instructor in Medicine, and served successively as Assistant Professor of Medicine, 1940-41, Professor and Head of the Department of Preventive Medicine, 1941 to 1946, and Professor and Chairman of the Department of Tropical Medicine and Public Health from 1946 to 1953. During his tenure at Tulane, he was also Visiting Professor at Charity Hospital, New Orleans, from 1932 to 1938 and Senior Visiting Professor from 1938 to 1953. The University of Michigan awarded him the Commonwealth Fellowship in Cardiology in 1938-39. On leave from Tulane in 1951, Dr. Sodeman was Visiting Professor in Medical Sciences at the Calcutta School of Tropical Medicine. From 1953 to 1957, he was Professor and Chairman of the Department of Internal Medicine at the University of Missouri School of Medicine. In 1957, he began his long term association with the Thomas Jefferson University Medical College in Philadelphia, first appointed as Magee Professor of Medicine and Head of the Department of Medicine, 1957-58, then Dean and Professor of Medicine, 1958-1967, Vice President for Medical Affairs, 1962-1967 and Dean Emeritus and Professor of Medicine Emeritus, from July 1967 to the present.

Dr. Sodeman's professional activities included Scientific Director of the Life Insurance Medical Research Fund from 1967 to 1970; Executive Director of the Educational Commission on Foreign Medical Graduates from 1970 to 1973. He has also served as Clinical Professor of Medicine and Academic Advisor to the Dean of the Medical College of Ohio from 1974 to the present. He now resides in Toledo, Ohio.

Certified by American Board of Internal Medicine in 1939, he also holds certification in the subspecialty of cardiovascular diseases, 1941, and was certified by American Board of Preventive Medicine in 1950.

Dr. Sodeman was President of the American Society of Tropical Medicine, 1953-54; in an official capacity, he served as President of the American College of Cardiology, 1970-71; he was Chairman of the AMA Council on Medical Education from 1970 to 1974. He was also a member of the American Federation for Clinical Research; American Heart Association; American Public Health Association; American Society for Clinical Investigation; Central Society for Clinical Research; Royal Society of Tropical Medicine and Hygiene and Southern Society for Clinical Research.

The American College of Physicians elected Dr. Sodeman as a Fellow in 1941. He served as Treasurer from 1963 to 1969; Regent from 1969 to 1971; President-Elect, 1971-72, and President in 1972-73.

Because of his long career as a department head and as Dean of Jefferson Medical College, Dr. Sodeman understood the difference between policy and administration; he was a patient presiding officer. I had a chance to observe this quality while attending many meetings of the AMA's Council on Medical Education, of which he was Chairman. The fact that this is an elected office spoke well for Bill's ability to get along well with practicing physicians. He was gregarious, friendly and had a delightful sense of humor. He set a more deliberate pace from that of Dr. Hugh Butt, who preceded him as president and Dr. Wallace Frommeyer, who followed him. He seemingly was never in a hurry and pursued a patient and methodical course in bringing issues to conclusion. I believe he acted on the theory that if one allowed enough time for exhaustive discussion, then any issue would be more acceptable and more easily implemented when finally settled by a vote.

Dr. Sodeman was my sponsor in the J. Aitgen Meigs Society, which has a membership of 36 and has been meeting once a month for dinner and a speaker for more than 100 years. It was my pleasure to serve as its president when the Society celebrated its centennial year in 1980.

During the years of controversy with the ASIM, Dr. Sodeman's impulse to be active in resolving differences was a stabilizing influence in the College and fostered cooperation between the two societies.

It was during his presidential incumbency that I was nearing my 65th birthday.

When he learned of it, he asked me if I'd be willing to remain longer as Executive Vice President. I told him I would not serve an indefinite period, but I would work for another three years, until my 68th birthday, pending their search for a successor, provided the Board reviewed our agreement on an annual basis. I suggested the appointment of a search committee approximately two years before my retirement and that they should plan to announce my successor about one year before I retired. Bill led the Board of Regents in setting up a reasonable method of effecting a smooth transition to a new administration. I also suggested that the Regents should spend some time studying the relationship between the Board of Governors and the Board of Regents and also review the administrative structure.

Bill was very devoted to his wife and his two sons, one of whom became a pathologist and one a gastroenterologist. The years we spent together, especially at the meetings of the AMA, were some of the best of my life.

In an interview during his presidential year, he reflected on his accomplishments and concerns:

He considered his most important accomplishment to be the resolution of a policy for the future relationship of the College with the American Society of Internal Medicine and some of the changes in relationships of the Board of Governors and the Board of Regents. He felt that as chapters became more active, especially in putting on good educational programs, they could improve some of the national meetings by showing what younger members were capable of doing in the educational field.

He thought the Council on Medical Specialty Societies had been an effective organization, particularly helpful to the AMA in demonstrating ways in which the specialty societies could become more directly involved in AMA matters.

Commenting on the perennial question of establishing a new office, Chairman of the Board of Regents, he predicted it could be helpful if its principal purpose was to provide more continuity of leadership.

He urged that only truly professional societies be included in representation on the newly formed Council of Subspecialty Societies in the College. He did not think the American Diabetes Society or the American Heart Association should be represented, being principally fund raising lay organizations.

An interesting incident occurred at the 1973 Annual Business Meeting which caused a potential parliamentary problem. During the election of Governors, Dr. Thomas Hartigan of Nebraska, was named by the Nominating Committee for a second term. Much to the consternation of everyone, a Fellow nominated another candidate from the floor. Dr. Hartigan won, but I asked the nominator of the second person after the meeting if he wasn't from Colorado. He laughed and said yes, but he merely wanted to stir things up a little. Though this was the first occurrence of its kind in the College's history, it supported my argument favoring the election of Governors in their local Regions. Of incidental interest, local election of Governors was first propounded in 1936, when Governor Adolph Sachs, of Nebraska, made the suggestion. It was still not accepted in 1972.

# 1972-1973

ACP/ASIM relationship to AMA and other bodies. Boards functions. Medical Practice Committee. Calvin C. Kay, appointed Deputy Executive Vice President. PSRO. Policy statements: Venereal disease; physicians' assistants; recertification; federal support of medical schools; hospital privileges; cancer detection.

A special Summer meeting of the Board of Regents was held in order to discuss in an informal atmosphere the significance of the failed attempt by the American College of Physicians and the American Society of Internal Medicine [ASIM] to amalgamate.

Dr. William A. Sodeman, President, reported on the official actions of the House of Delegates of ASIM and of the Board of Governors and Board of Regents of the College. He reported that fundamental compromises would have been necessary to effect the amalgamation, which were not acceptable to either the ACP Board of Governors or to the ASIM House of Delegates. Therefore, neither group was wholly responsible for the failure of the effort. The "Memorandum of Intent" was discussed, but inasmuch as it had been devised for the purpose of amalgamation, it was no longer a document which could be implemented and would require no further action. However, the "Memorandum" could still serve as background information for possible future discussions on cooperative efforts.

The Board then discussed the implications of these circumstances for the future relations between the College and ASIM. Neither organization favored very close liaison activity, and a period of reflection and study by both organizations should occur before liaison activity was resumed. When a climate suitable for joint liaison or other related committees had again been established, it was suggested the committee members appointed should be members of both the ACP and ASIM. The general effect of the failure to amalgamate was that the College would adopt the third of three alternatives that has been presented to the College five years previously which were:

1. That the College should attempt to amalgamate with ASIM.
2. That the two societies attempt to work more closely together, through the appointment of a high level liaison committee.
3. That the societies separate completely and pursue independent directions in a state of friendly coexistence.

The first two had been tried with no success, leaving only the third alternative. Without any feeling of competition or hostility, the Board concluded that close cooperation with ASIM on issues of mutual concern would be necessary from time to time, but for the time being each organization should continue to develop its own directions.

## Future Structure of the College

The Board then turned its attention to proposed changes in the structure of the College. There was general agreement that efforts were in order to increase membership participation and interest in College activities. Participation was obviously essential to the College's effectiveness in community service issues, activities at the hospital level, and improvements in educational functions at the local level. Discussion on this matter revolved around several major aspects:

Board of Governors

The Board of Governors was a logical structure to focus on increased local activities and participation by members. The following mechanisms for change were discussed:

1. At the national level the Board of Governors should continue to serve in an advisory and consultative role but final decisions on policies should be established by the Board of Regents.
2. At the local level, the Governor should be formally nominated for office by a local committee or by some other mechanism which would generate nominations at the local level, or the Governor could be elected by popular vote at the local level.
3. Possibly a number of Governors should be placed on the Board of Regents.
4. Individual Governors could serve as liaison officers between the Board of Regents and the Regions. To make this effective, local Chapters would have to be formally constituted with appropriately elected officers.
5. Governors should have a shorter term of office.
6. A number of Regents felt that the Board of Governors' role should remain relatively unchanged, but that Governors' Committees should be required to be more active and also to report regularly to the Board of Regents.

Board of Regents

1. The Board considered possible changes in the method of election of Regents, such as election by the Board of Governors, (as has been the practice in the early years of the College) and was the current practice in the American College of Surgeons [ACS].
2. There was strong feeling that the composition of the Board of Regents should be broadly representative of academic, geographic and a variety of medical practice interests.

Development of Chapters

A brief resume was presented concerning the methods of operation of other organizations, which revealed that almost all had an officially organized local chapter arrangement. However, in none of these organizations were chapters organized uniformly in all parts of the country. If ACP chapters were to be developed, the College would need to consider the following:

1. Local members should elect their own officers and operating Board.
2. They should nominate and elect Governors directly.
3. They should elect Members locally according to nationally adopted regulations.
4. They should nominate candidates to the Central Credentials Committee and to the Board of Regents for election of Fellows.

5. They should be empowered to set local dues which would be collected by the National Office.
6. They should act for the College locally and provide continuous information to the Board of Regents on the implementation of College policies.
7. They should be responsible for appointing appropriate committees for local programs.
8. Toward the development of stronger educational opportunities, Governors or their committees or local organizations should be urged to work closely with Professors of Medicine in their local areas.

In addition to this far ranging discussion, an ad hoc committee of Regents, Governors, Fellows, Members and Associates was constituted to study further the stated purposes of the College and make preliminary reports in November and a final report in April, 1973. The chairman of this committee would be a Regent.

The Board also considered how the College could work more actively with subspecialty societies. An invitational meeting was projected, to be attended by the President of the American College of Physicians and the presidents of internal medicine related subspecialty societies.

The issue of family practice was discussed again at some length, resulting in a general consensus that it was too early to determine which types of training programs and examinations would qualify these new family physicians for College membership. Recently, the American Board of Family Practice [ABFP] had given its first examination and, although it was not as stringent as the one given by the American Board of Internal Medicine [ABIM], the Board of Regents agreed to withhold decisions until more information had been obtained. If these certified family physicians proved ineligible to become members of the College under present rules, then changes in the Bylaws might be required. Ineligibility for the College membership was generally considered to be open to all non-surgical specialties.

An interesting request had come to the College from the American Association of Medical Legal Consultants, which included physicians who were also trained in law. They asked the College to appoint a panel of experts whom they might call on to review malpractice cases. After considerable discussion, the Board declined, concluding that the College would have no real control over the results of such involvement and would not be serving College members specifically. Also, a panel of this type might promote the tendency to base all malpractice decisions on one national standard.

At the November meeting, Dr. Sodeman, discussed the impact of the newly formed Coordinating Council on Medical Education [CCME] on the College. It functioned as the coordinating body for the other committees formed to address different aspects of medical education. A Liaison Committee on Graduate Medical Education [LCGME] and a Liaison Committee on Continuing Medical Education [LCCME] had been established. The Council was also considering a third committee on allied health education. Already existing was a Liaison Committee on Medical Education [LCME], jointly operated by the AMA and the Association of American Medical Colleges [AAMC]. There were no plans at that time to place this committee under the aegis of the Coordinating Council. Dr. Sodeman was involved in the CCME as a member of the AMA Council on Medical Education, but there was no direct representation by the American College of Physicians on these bodies. The LCGME, however, included Dr. Edward Rosenow, as a representative from CMSS, Dr. Jack Myers, as a representative of the American Board of Medical Specialties [ABMS] and Dr. James Haviland, as an AMA representative. While the representation was not official, there was no question that the College provided very important leadership in the deliberations of these councils and committees.

My report to the Board in November included some perspectives on the subjects of the special Summer Meeting.

1. Participation in College affairs by the members
      In my travels about the country, attending Regional Meetings, I encountered much membership interest in working more actively to implement College policies. I thought it would be desirable to obtain Governors' reactions to policies before they were adopted, although it was quite clear that the Governors were not seeking authority to establish policy.

2. The Governors' roles
      I favored local election of Governors by the Members and Fellows in their own Region. I also believed that making the election of Regents or at least a portion of the Board of Regents a prime responsibility of the Governors, would have a positive effect. In addition, all Governors should be encouraged to establish local Chapters, and it seemed desirable to set up several and test their applicability to increasing membership participation. I proposed that the Board authorize me to develop model bylaws suitable for such a legally viable organization.

3. Regents
      I reviewed the implications of establishing new positions of Chairman and Vice Chairman for the Board of Regents, removing from the President the responsibilities of a "Chairman of the Board". In most business organizations the Chairman of the Board works almost entirely on policy. Such a structure might improve the college governance. Of particular help would be the continuity introduced by the Chairman, who would hold office longer than one year at a time.

The Board of Regents, meeting in executive session, adopted the report of the Ad Hoc Committee on Administration. The Board accepted the recommendation to grant me an extension of three years as Executive Vice President, but would retain the option of reviewing my status annually after I reached age 65. It was moved, seconded and passed that a Search Committee be constituted by the President at least two years before the date established for my retirement.

## Community Services

The Community Services Committee, Dr. Maxwell G. Berry, Chairman, presented two items for recommended action; both were adopted by the Board:

1. Statement on Venereal Disease:

> The internist, as a clinician, as a teacher, and as an individual of stature in the community, has an important stake in the prevention, diagnosis, and treatment of venereal disease. Control of venereal disease is to teach the public to avoid infection, to recognize the symptoms of syphilis and gonorrhea, and to seek prompt treatment when the symptoms occur.

> Internists must not take part personally in these educational efforts, but they must also use their influence to spark other community-wide programs designed to stop the soaring incidence of venereal disease.

2. Delivery of Health Services:

   They recommend that the ACP endorse the concept of increasing utilization of intermediate level personnel in the delivery of health services.

Several other items under study in the Committee on Community Services were reviewed by the Board:

1. Model Management - Treatment Program

   Previously the Board had appointed a number of ACP study committees in the various subspecialties of internal medicine to develop minimum and maximum standards for delivery of care in various clinical conditions. These standards were then incorporated into the computer system at the San Joaquin Foundation for Medical Care. Progress was good, and it seemed likely the study would be helpful.

2. Survey of internists' activity

   Dr. Samuel P. Martin, Chairman of this study committee, reported that representatives at Health, Education and Welfare [HEW], with whom he had been meeting, were very much interested in the survey and he believed that federal funding might be available. The Committee needed to determine whether the ASIM was undertaking a similar type of survey, which included sending a questionnaire to internists as well as a representative sampling of physicians in family practice and in osteopathy. The Committee had reviewed the current questionnaire in detail and suggested revisions in several sections. The Committee hoped this project could be implemented early in 1973.

3. The place of the internist in primary care

   For a number of years the College had endorsed the principle that an internist was a physician well qualified to render primary care. However, until the survey of internists was completed, no data existed which documented how many internists actually provided primary care or how much primary care their practice included. The Committee, therefore, proposed that the study be expanded to include a new contract to survey the residents who were then in training, to ascertain how many of them intended to go into primary care.

4. Assistant to the Primary Care Physician (Physicians' Assistant)

Dr. Malcolm L. Peterson was appointed to serve on the Joint Review Committee for the Accreditation of Programs of Assistants to the Primary Care Physician which was sponsored by the ACP, ASIM, American Association for Family Practice [AAFP] and the American Academy of Pediatrics [AAP].

Dr. R. Carmichael Tilghman, Chairman of the Credentials Committee, reported that the attendance at Committee meetings of new Governors and Governors-Elect was instructive and was resulting in better decisions, particularly in evaluation of problematic cases. It was, however, causing time consuming reconsideration of cases, not because of undue influence by the Governors, but because the educational process resulted in Governors supplying new information to assist the committee to make more appropriate decisions relative to advancement to Fellowship. The committee had recently reversed some decisions in such cases and, although the additional review took time, the results were worthwhile.

Dr. John R. Graham, Chairman of the Fellowships and Scholarships Committee, recommended some policy changes regarding teaching and research scholarships which the Board approved. The policy stated that these scholarships should be reserved for young physicians who had been out of medical school from four to eight years and at that stage in their medical careers when additional support would facilitate further preparation toward teaching and research investigation. In addition, the Committee obtained Board approval to notify new scholarship appointees, that upon acceptance of the appointment, they would be invited to apply for participation in the College and a proposal for election to Membership would be submitted. The Board also approved instituting an Annual Teaching and Research Scholars Luncheon and Dinner during the Annual Session.

The report from the Finance Committee stating the increased cost of College operations because of the impact of federal income taxes for 1972, amounting to $842,000, caused concern. In order to keep the College solvent, meet all current obligations, and provide for future growth, the Finance Committee recommended an increase in dues. The Board approved the following rates: Masters, Fellows and Members, eleven or more years out of medical school $80; for those ten years or less out of medical school $40; for practicing physicians 65 years of age and over $40.

The Committee also recommended that registration fees be charged to members attending the Annual Session, but this motion was not approved.

The *Medical Knowledge Self-Assessment Program [MKSAP]* was a considerable success. Distributed in 1968, it resulted in subscriptions totaling 12,130, and netted an income of $126,251.

Dr. Richard Allyn, Chairman, brought several items for action to the Board of Regents from the Hospitals Committee.

1. The ACP should explore the possibility of conducting regional confer-

ences, convening program directors in charge of internal medicine programs in community hospitals. The purpose of the conference would be to exchange information to identify the best features in each type of program. The Board approved and directed the Committee to explore the possibilities.

2. The Hospitals Committee asked that ACP support the incorporation of psychiatry, office gynecology, and pediatrics into the training programs of general internal medicine, with the specific objective of developing wide spectrum training for the delivery of primary medical care. The Board endorsed this approach to training.

3. The Visiting Professors in Hospitals Program had received insufficient response and the committee recommended that it be discontinued.

4. The Committee also urged continued College representation at the national level in emergency care issues.

The Board approved application for official representation to the National Coordinating Council on Emergency Medical Services which was currently being formed. Dr. Douglas McGill served on the AMA Commission on Emergency Medical Care.

Later in the meeting, Dr. McGill reviewed the results of his first meeting as a representative on the AMA Commission on Emergency Medical Care. He explained that the College currently had little visibility in emergency care activities. ACP members were obviously involved, not only in critical care, but also in the use of emergency rooms as substitute offices. Dr. McGill also reviewed the current status of the delineation of hospital privileges. The Committee, which formulated this statement, thought that great care should be exercised in delineating too precisely the care of illness as differentiated from a more precise delineation of the privileges to do certain technical procedures. In a slightly briefer form, the statement was published in the *ACP Bulletin*.

5. The Regents approved the third joint conference of the American College of Physicians and the American Hospital Association.

The Board of Regents had previously adopted the policy statement, "Delineating Hospital Privileges for Medical Staff", which was published in the *ACP Bulletin* in July, 1972, written by Dr. Douglas McGill. The statement met with an enthusiastic reception and the Joint Commission on Accreditation of Hospitals had ordered 2,000 reprints for distribution at their workshops on Joint Commission on Accreditation of Hospitals [JCAH] standards.

The Medical Audit Feasibility Study was completed, and a final report was in process. In spite of some disappointing aspects of the study, College physicians conducting the study at hospitals in Reading and Allentown were enthusiastic about continuing the development of methods for medical audit. Methods had been revised since the original protocol was written, and significant audit activity was being carried out in both hospitals.

Dr. Lawrence E. Young, Chairman, reported that the International Medical

Activities Committee continued to struggle with the problem of how to offer Latin American scholars a chance to study in this country. Sources of revenue had to be found. Highly favorable reports were received on the postgraduate courses which had been given in Santiago, Chile, San Jose, Costa Rica, and Bogota, Columbia. The Committee expressed concern over the low registration which had forced cancellation of the International Congress of Internal Medicine scheduled for Boston in early September. United States physicians typically do not attend international conventions when they are held in the United States. The Committee, therefore, proposed that a joint meeting with this Society be sponsored at an Annual Session, comparable to that arranged with the Royal College of Physicians in London in 1968. The Board took no action.

Dr. Ralph A. Tompsett, Chairman of the Postgraduate Courses Committee, submitted a long term analysis of course activities. In 1965-66, the registration had 19 courses, 1,660 registrants and were over subscribed by 188 registrants. By 1971-72, there were 29 courses with 3,875 registrants, and 217 aspirants were not able to go to a course of their choice. Some change in the registration fees was suggested, and this was approved by the Board of Regents.

A plan for meetings of the *Annals* Editorial Board was submitted by Dr. Truman G. Schnabel Jr., Chairman of the Publications Committee. The new plan, which was approved, scheduled one annual meeting of the Editorial Board to be held during the Annual Session. Total subscriptions to the *Annals* was 58,333 in 1972. Five years previously the number had been 39,668. In spite of this increase in circulation, there was no comparable increment in the number of pages of advertising. Although there was some increased revenue because of higher page rates the lack of more advertising caused some concern. There was no change in the ratio of advertising pages to editorial pages; the number of editorial and news pages still represented 60 percent of the total pages in the journal.

Dr. Walter B. Frommeyer, Chairman of the Audio-Visual Techniques Committee, reported that progress with single-topic audio-visual films was good and six additional programs were in production, the six new topics were:

1. Nasogastric intubation
2. Emergency nasal packing
3. Abdominal paracentesis
4. Thoracentesis
5. Intermittent positive pressure breathing
6. Tonometry

### Patient Counseling Library

The Committee affirmed previous action approving the development of patient counseling films. Work would begin soon on films presenting "Esophagitis" and "Hypertension". The Committee had discovered considerable differences in the problems encountered in developing patient counseling films as compared to educational films for physicians, among them:

1. Patient counseling films would represent direct interference between the physician and his patient.
2. Much care must be given to content, addressing what a patient should know about a particular disease entity.
3. The College would, in essence, be entering into the practice of medicine.

Three levels of information for the patient were identified for inclusion:

1. How should patients do things correctly, (i.e., exercise, heat therapy, etc.)
2. General noncontroversial information (i.e., physiological mechanisms).
3. Specific information about diseases addressing the needs of individual patients. In this aspect, the College had to be very careful to avoid information that some physicians might not wish their patients to have.

The "objectives" of patient counseling films was a second question; two major objectives were identified:

1. The film should save the physician's time spent in counseling.
2. It should supplement the physician's counseling with basic physiologic or biologic information.

The Committee recommended the appointment of core curriculum committees to develop individual problems. The core chairman should be a person knowledgeable in the field under consideration, who knew the techniques of the specialty in considerable detail and had experience in teaching. A second member should be an internist who was not a specialist in that particular field, and there should be a third member who might or might not be a specialist in that subspecialty field.

In 1972, the Board of Regents was considering the development of an in-training examination for internists, and polled Associates of the College and internal medicine program directors, who responded positively to the plan.

At the November meeting, the Regents debated whether the examinations should be designed and administered jointly by the ACP and the ABIM, but concluded that it should be the responsibility of one body and that the ABIM was better suited to the task.

The ACP-APA Task Force, Dr. John R. Graham, Chairman, requested:

1. That the Educational Activities Committee study further its proposal to initiate a study to determine how effectively the teaching of emotional aspects of organic disease and the organic aspect of emotional disease were currently being taught in a sample of internships and residency training programs in the United States.
2. That a representative of the ACP Task Force be sent to a forthcoming conference on medical residencies. The Board approved and requested that the Executive Vice President provide the Task Force a list of psychiatrist members for selection.

The Council of Medical Specialty Societies [CMSS] presented an important status report. Dr. John A. Layne outlined its major developments:

1. The American Academy of Ophthalmology and Otolaryngology was elected to membership in 1972.
2. At several meetings, the Council had discussed the proposed LCGME and the proposal for the establishment of the CCME. Drs. Rosenow and Sodeman reviewed them for the Regents' information. The CMSS had also taken important steps on some matters requiring communication with the AMA.
   a. It recommended to the AMA that Current Procedural Terminology [CPT] be designed as a coding system, which would include definitions of the procedures and services that a primary care physician provides for his patients.
   b. The CMSS moved to inform its member organizations that the Secretary would duplicate and forward communications regarding CPT to the AMA, and maintain correspondence on the matter.
   c. However, the CMSS would not assume sole responsibility for the project, and would offer to coordinate its development with the AMA and the specialty societies.

Dr. Layne reported that an application of ASIM for membership in the CMSS had been denied. The Council also debated whether members representing certain specialties on the Council could be counted twice if they were also members of the ACS but voted to maintain its original policy against duplicating representation by membership in two societies.

## Medical Practice Committee

At the April, 1973 meeting of the Board of Regents, the President-Elect, Dr. Walter B. Frommeyer, Jr., reported a generally positive reaction to the issues of recertification and the dues increase among those he met at Regional Meetings.

At the conclusion of the meeting in November, 1972, the Board of Regents discharged the Advertising and Exhibits Committee, referring advertising functions to the Clinical Pharmacology Committee and exhibits functions to ACP Staff. They also combined the functions of the Committees on Community Services and the Hospitals Committee and named the new standing committee the Medical Practice Committee.

## Annual Session 1973

With the election of new candidates for membership at the 1973 Annual Session, Dr. Michael Tilghman, Secretary-General, reported that total College membership had increased to 22,593, of which 84 were Masters, 11,907 Fellows, 5,455 Members, 4,847 Associates, 43 Honorary Fellows, 72 Corresponding Fellows and 185 Affiliate Members. Associate Membership was gradually increasing.

He also reported that with the election of Masters at the current meeting, there would be over 100 Masters in the College. The Board had moved to increase the proportion of Masters in the membership several years previously when it was discovered that although the College had grown rapidly, the number of Masters was almost unchanged from 25 years previously. The new policy of electing more Masters permitted the recognition of qualified senior Fellows in a larger number of districts, and eventually would enable the election of at least one Master from almost every Region.

The Treasurer, Dr. William F. Kellow, announced that the College had engaged the services of A. G. Becker & Co. of Chicago and New York, to analyze the performance of the investment portfolio for the past five years and to continue analysis on an ongoing basis. This company provided a service based on an enormous amount of data from various investment portfolios including those held by many organizations similar to the College. Utilizing this service, the Investment Committee could monitor management of the investment portfolio by comparing its performance with that of similar organizations rather than to some arbitrary standard.

I reported one interesting side effect of the increase in dues. In previous practice, the College had always given members a chance to become Life Members under the old dues structure whenever the dues were increased. Following the recent increase, new Life Members increased by 800, contributing in one year a half-million dollars to the investment portfolio.

In my travels during the year, I had discussed chapter formation with many Governors. It became clear that in setting up any new organizational structure, serious efforts should be exerted to keep the Governors in a strong policy formulation role and to assure continued effective liaison between the Board of Governors and Board of Regents. Much of the detailed work of implementation in the local area should be done by local committees. Governors generally agreed that, if properly organized, the formation of chapters would make a Governor's workload lighter.

I stressed the importance of the newly formed CCME. This Council, formed in response to the findings of the Millis Commission Report of several years previously, was predictive both of the increasing coordination of medical education and the understanding of what is required to make all aspects operate properly. Although the College had no direct representation on any of these councils or committees, it was represented in bodies such as the ABMS, CMSS, AMA, AAMC and the American Hospital Association [AHA], and its Regents and Officers invariably would serve on the Council through these organizations.

The Headquarters Staff, I reported, was rapidly growing, having increased since 1960 from 29 to 96. A new Manager of Publications had been hired to help Dr. Huth, the *Annals* Editor, and Mr. Dauterich with the growing and time consuming publishing activities. Mr. Elmer Jones who was Conventions Manager since 1963 was appointed to this position.

In conclusion, I reviewed my activities and those of Dr. Calvin C. Kay, the Deputy Executive Vice President, in representing the College on other organizations. Dr. Kay was liaison for the College on the Committee on Stroke (which was an outgrowth of the President's Commission on Heart Disease and Stroke). He also served on the Commission on Professional Hospital Activities, and on a special committee of the Joint Commission on Accreditation of Hospitals which was administering the accreditation of facilities for the treatment of heart disease patients. I was continuing my work of the past four or five years as Chairman of the AMA Advisory Committee on Continuing Medical Education, serving on the LCGME as a representative of the College from the CMSS, and also serving as a member of the Advisory Committee on Medical Devices to the Food and Drug Administration [FDA].

### Progress in Recertification

In the year 1972-73 important steps were initiated to prepare for recertification. In October, 1972, a Joint Recertification Committee of the ABIM and ACP, chaired by Dr. Truman G. Schnabel, Jr., had designed a plan for recertification following discussion with the Board of Governors. At that meeting, the Board of Governors had expressed strong feelings that the time had not arrived for recertification, and in April, 1973, they requested that the Board of Regents reconsider its support for recertification which was approved in November, 1972. A special joint meeting of the Boards was convened on Monday, April 9, to resolve the differences of opinion between Governors and Regents. The Regents had deliberated at length about recertification and concluded that, since it was inevitable, the College should prepare for it and take leadership. Therefore, it would not withdraw its support, and in April, 1973, voted unanimously to accept the plan.

The timing of the first recertification examination was projected to coincide with the distribution of the *MKSAP III* in 1974. Questions could be selected from the *MKSAP*. It was hoped this would emphasize the voluntary nature of recertification rather than a punitive requirement. ABIM recognized that this procedure would reflect only cognitive areas of a physician's performance and it was anxious to develop other techniques to evaluate performance.

The final report presented at the Annual Session meeting of April, 1973, outlined 10 points which were listed in Appendix I of the Report:

1. The Committee reaffirmed its belief in the necessity for developing some mechanism by which clinical competence might be assured in physicians previously certified by the ABIM whether in the broad field of medicine or its subspecialties.
2. Whatever the mechanism of recertification, it should have both an evaluative and educational function.
3. The Committee believed that neither the present ABIM certifying examination nor the examinations in the subspecialties alone were satisfactory instruments for the recertification of clinical competence in general medicine or a subspecialty field.
4. The recertification process should not be punitive in character.
5. Whatever method of recertification might be adopted, a certain level of competence must be achieved and firm criteria should be established. It was felt that the College *MKSAP* could not wholly fulfill this function.

Despite the establishment of such criteria, the educational aspects of the program would assure ultimate recertification of the great majority of physicians being evaluated.

6. Physicians certified in the field of general internal medicine would be recertified in this broad area. Physicians certified in subspecialty areas would have the choice of recertification in only their subspecialty field or in the broad field of internal medicine or both.

7. The mechanism for recertification should consist of two components:
   a. An assessment of knowledge. ABIM in association with the ACP, should develop an educational program which would be followed by an examination based on the contents of the program. A physician would be required to achieve a set minimum level of performance on the examination following participation in the educational program.
   b. An assessment of performance. An assessment should be made of the performance of a physician both in the hospital and his office. This evaluation should include a study of the physician's records as well as direct observation of the individual's performance with patients. Such an evaluation should be carried out in accordance with guidelines and standards to be set by the ABIM.

8. Assessment of a physician's performance would be conducted on a regional basis under the general supervision of the ABIM. Physicians conducting the regional evaluations would be appointed by the Board, possibly with the aid of the ACP.

9. The ACP would be urged to develop the educational aspects of the program in conjunction with the ABIM.

10. The joint ABIM and ACP Ad Hoc Committee on Recertification should develop a pilot program for recertification for implementation within the next two years. This pilot program should concern itself solely with recertification in the field of general internal medicine.

Items (1) to (7a) were adopted by the Board of Regents. In addition, the Board passed the following motion regarding point (7b): "there should be an assessment of a physician's performance, and methods for this evaluation should be developed by a special committee of the College interacting with a committee of the ABIM. No current action should be taken regarding Items (8) and (9)."

In approving Item (10), the Board voted that emphasis should be placed on recertification in "the field of general internal medicine" rather than the subspecialties. In summary, the Regents adopted the points outlined in Appendix I in principle, with the following exception: that participation in educational programs should not be compulsory for recertification. They also specified that if the plan was changed in any way by the ABIM, the Board of Regents of the ACP should have an opportunity to review the changes.

## Cancer Detection Statement

Dr. Marvin Pollard, Chairman of the Cancer Committee, requested and received

Board support on a position regarding early detection of cancer:

The recent legislation which established the Commission on Cancer calls for specific activities toward early detection of the following: cancer of the breast, cervix, colon, pancreas, lung, and prostate. The members of the American College of Physicians are engaged in delivering primary care to many patients and, therefore, every effort should be made to provide them with all information necessary to detect these cancers at an early stage. This should be provided through publications, Annual Sessions, postgraduate courses and Regional Meetings of the College. Members of the ACP could be expected to exert leadership in their own communities to promote early detection of cancer.

a. The ACP advocates periodic physical examinations at intervals appropriate to the age and health of the individual patient, supplemented by appropriate laboratory procedures.

b. The ACP has not established standards for physical examinations that differ from those currently accepted and widely advocated in standard texts dealing with this question.

c. An adequate physical examination included as an integral component a cancer detection examination. Clearly, age, sex, history and key risk factors would alter the nature of a cancer detection examination (and thus, the content of an adequate physical examination).

d. The ACP recognized the need to provide not only preventive medical care, but total medical care to all persons regardless of ability to pay and supported all reasonable efforts, both public and private, to achieve this goal.

Dr. Robert G. Petersdorf, Chairman of the Educational Activities Committee, reported on the progress of *MKSAP III*. A new feature was the development of a Syllabus for each of the nine subspecialty areas. He also reported that part of *MKSAP III* would be employed in developing the recertification examination.

Dr. Petersdorf indicated that Annual Session attendance figures had been low for two successive Sessions held in Chicago, where inclement climate in April was a negative factor. Therefore, the committee decided that cities farther south in the middle part of the country should be considered for Annual Session sites.

In the 1972-73 academic year, Regional Meeting attendance had grown to 6,202 physicians attending 43 meetings. Postgraduate Course attendance was 3,404 physicians at 34 courses. However, 12-14 additional postgraduate courses to be presented in the current year would make it one of the highest in attendance.

Dr. John R. Graham, Chairman, reporting for the Fellowships and Scholarships Committee, made several recommendations which the Board approved in April, 1973.

1. The Committee recommends to the Board of Regents that the granting of funds for the second and third year of the Teaching and Research Scholarships be made contingent upon the awardee being proposed for membership in the College by January 15 of the first year of his/her scholarship.

2. The Committee recommends to the Board of Regents that if a Teaching and Research Scholar resigns, at the end of the first year the funds budgeted for that scholar may be used to support another candidate if a

suitable one is available for a period of not less than two years. In such a case, the funds allotted would be those ordinarily supplied for the first and second years of the scholarship.

3. The Committee recommends the appointment of Dr. William Lee, currently Chief Resident in Medicine at Columbia Presbyterian Hospital, as the first Eli Lilly Fellow in Medical Sciences, to pursue research and teaching in the field of liver diseases under the supervision of Dr. Roger Williams at the Liver Unit, Kings Cottage Hospital Medical School in London. This new scholarship was to be funded by the Eli Lilly Foundation in order to enable young scholars as a way of getting people to obtain education in Great Britain.

In the Finance Committee report, Dr. John Layne, Chairman, updated the Board on the issue of the payment of federal income taxes. The U.S. Treasury Department had adopted new regulations on previously established Congressional law taxing net income from advertising appearing in the journals of tax exempt organizations effective from 1968. From 1968 to 1972 the College had paid $801,550. In 1972, the College filed a refund claim for income taxes paid for the year 1968-69, amounting to $376,977, claiming that the regulations under which the taxes were imposed during this period were invalid.

In 1970, Congress passed a new law expressly taxing net advertising revenue. Only 1968 and 1969 were therefore subject to question about legal tax liability. However, regulations explaining how to compute the tax had still not been adopted. The amount of tax liability for 1970 to 1972, as a result, was also subject to change.

The International Medical Activities Committee, Dr. Lawrence E. Young, Chairman, submitted recommendations received from the Ad Hoc Committee on Post-Convention Tours. The Board confirmed that Post-Convention Tours would be continued and planning should be coordinated with the International Medical Activities Committee.

1. The Executive Vice President would continue to make arrangements for tours in consultation with the President, President-Elect and, (if a College Region existed in the area to be visited) the College Governor in that region. The International Medical Activities Committee would be kept informed of plans for tours.

2. Expenses of one official representative of the College and his/her spouse could be defrayed by the travel agency as a cost item related to the conduct of the tour.

For information, the Committee reported that the postgraduate course held in Caracas, Venezuela, was considered successful. Several new courses had been given, one in Lima, Peru, and the usual one in Santiago, Chile. One was also planned for Bogota, Columbia. I informed the Regents that I would be representing the College at the dedication of a new National Medical Center in Amman, Jordan.

## Primary Care Surveys

Dr. Richard Allyn, Chairman of the Medical Practice Committee, reported on several items:

1. Regarding the ACP survey on delivery patterns in internal medicine in conjunction with the Leonard Davis Institute of the University of Pennsylvania, sources of funding were still to be found. However, surveys of this kind were high on the priority list for federal limited funds grants. Dr. Samuel Martin and I met with Dr. Lybrand and his staff in Washington at the Division of Manpower Intelligence of the Bureau of Health Manpower Education on behalf of the College. We made it clear to Dr. Lybrand that the College would not object to cosponsorship, but would not approve any plan which did not delineate clearcut lines of authority. We explained that the College would prefer to act as the grantee, so that clear direction could be developed between the sponsoring groups and the Leonard Davis Institute.

2. In support of the San Joaquin Foundation Project, the College had appointed committees to set acceptable levels of management in nine subspecialty areas. Those data had been put into the San Joaquin Foundation computers. After prolonged discussion, the Medical Practice Committee expressed strong sentiments that as soon as possible, even before the proposed validation process, (part of the San Joaquin Foundation Project) the standards set by the nine subspecialty committees should be made available to other authorized groups. This was especially important because of current pressure from many medical societies which were considering establishment of Professional Services Review Organizations [PSRO].

The Publications Committee, Dr. Truman G. Schnabel, Jr., Chairman, heard a report from Dr. Edward Huth and Mr. Fred Dauterich, Jr., on the editorial and business affairs of the *Annals*. Subscriptions had increased from 57,000 in 1972 to 64,700 in 1973, despite an increase in fees. The January issue of the *Annals* was distributed to 64,692 of which 20,686 were members of the College. The number of pages of paid advertising was slightly fewer than in 1972. The revenues were slightly greater because of an increase in advertising rates.

The Scientific Program Committee's report reviewed the current Annual Session. Dr. Richard W. Vilter, Chairman, iterated the observations about attendance made by the Educational Activities Committee. Registration was below what had been expected. Poor weather affected attendance by physicians in the local Chicago area. The Committee expressed some concern about the selection of Annual Session sites and agreed that attendance might be improved by selecting areas that offered greater potential attraction. The Committee also recommended that future Annual Sessions be scheduled for four days, Monday through Thursday, rather than have them continue through Friday. The Board of Regents approved the New York meeting in 1974 and scheduled it for four days only. I reported that the College had been operating the Annual Session at an increasing loss each year and the Finance Committee was studying Annual Session expenses to develop a plan to make the Sessions more nearly self-supporting.

Concerning the 1973 program, the State of the Art Lectures were well attended and generally of superior calibre. Panels were also well attended. Workshops and Meet the Professor Sessions had all been sold out.

The television programs were not properly exploited. Some of the participating physicians did not accept direction very well from the professionals who operate the television equipment, and many of the programs presented were of a panel type and were not well suited for television. The committee would continue to study this problem.

The Committee on Administrative Structure of the College submitted its final report in April, 1973. Dr. John A. Layne, Chairman, presented the following recommendations:

1. Increase participation and interest of the membership in College activities:
   a. All Governors should be reminded that formation of a chapter was desired but not mandated, but it would provide the necessary structure to implement local activities. Headquarters would help with advice and legal counsel in writing Bylaws.
   b. Governors should be required to report annually any local activities.
   c. Local Credentials Committees should recommend the election of Members directly to the Board of Regents. Direct election to Fellowship and advancement to Fellowship would still be the responsibility of the central Credentials Committee. The Board of Regents rejected this proposal after reviewing the report of the Credentials Committee.
   d. The Regents accepted the proposal system of electing Governors which read as follows:

   Post cards (as currently sent to Masters, Fellows and Members for suggestions) should be returned directly to the local Nominating Committee which will forward two or more names to the central Nominating Committee. The central committee will then nominate a candidate whose name will be published in the *ACP Bulletin*. Subsequently, additional names may be presented upon petition of not less than 20 percent of the total members of that area (this can never be less than five members). A deadline for the receipt of such petitions will be announced in the *ACP Bulletin*. A ballot will then be prepared in those Regions where additional nominees have been presented by petition which will be distributed to all members in each separate jurisdictional area. Election will be determined by the posted vote of the members in that Region. In the absence of any petition, the nominee of the central Nominating Committee will be elected.

2. The Board of Governors
   a. The Board of Regents approved a motion to limit the of term of Governor to four years in addition to one year as Governor-Elect.
   b. The Board of Governors should be expanded to include subspecialties. The Regents, in approving this item, also directed the President to appoint an ad hoc committee to study and propose appropriate means to include subspecialties.

c. A motion was approved that the Board of Governors should have the right to review actions of the Board of Regents, but the Board of Regents would remain the policy making body.

d. A previously approved motion was overturned, that the Board of Governors, by a majority vote, should approve dues and assessments recommended by the Board of Regents. Originally approving this motion, the Regents rescinded the action after considering the recommendations of the Committee on Administrative Structure. The Board of Governors offered a further motion that it obligate itself to review changes in dues and assessments at its meetings, which was approved by the Board of Regents.

e. The Board of Governors should be empowered to elect some Governors to the Board of Regents. This motion was tabled for further study.

3. Board of Regents

The new positions of Chairman and Vice Chairman of the Board of Regents should be established. A motion to table this was defeated, and the Board returned this item to the Committee for further study.

4. The College as a whole

A motion was approved to establish a panel of consultants on graduate medical education; available upon request from hospitals to help with any problems in their residency programs. The hospital would bear the expense of such consultation. It was reported that the mechanisms to implement this were already in place.

b. In a final action, the Board affirmed as College policy a continuing commitment to address the sociologic aspects of health care delivery in all its aspects.

Reporting for the Council of Academic Societies [CAS], Dr. Richard Vilter, Chairman, reviewed several important developments. The Council had prepared a document entitled, "Structure and Functions of a Modern Medical School", which would be presented at the next assembly of the AAMC and to the House of Delegates of the AMA. The document position, essentially, was to eliminate the freestanding basic science medical school, requiring that any new school of basic medical science must be related functionally to a school of medicine with clinical programs.

The AAMC had also developed the following policy statement on professional standards review organizations:

> The AAMC believes that the development and implementation of norms and standards for assessing the quality of health care is a vital responsibility in medical schools and teaching hospitals. A major part of this responsibility is the incorporation of quality of care assessment in the clinical educational programs to develop in medical students a lifelong concern for quality in their practices. The AAMC, therefore, strongly recommends its member institutions to become intimately involved in the development and operation of peer standard review organizations.

Dr. Harrison J. Shull, Representative of the College on the AMA Section Council, reported the work of a Committee to Study the Modus Operandi of the

Scientific Sessions which presented the following recommendations to the AMA House of Delegates:

> After two years of study, we believe that the American Medical Association can achieve greater unity by:
>
> 1. Inviting the national medical specialty societies to play a more active and responsible role in planning and implementing the AMA Annual Convention scientific program; and
> 2. Giving these national medical specialty societies, whose specialties correspond to those comprising the AMA Scientific Sections the privilege of participating in the selection of the Section delegates and alternate delegates in the AMA House of Delegates and other Section officers.

> Your Committee is convinced that adoption of the following and their incorporation into the Bylaws of the AMA will:
>
> 1. Establish a mechanism for stimulating increased cooperation between the specialty medical societies and the AMA, thus forging a relationship that will bind specialty societies and the AMA closer together, generating a singleness of purpose which will benefit all of medicine.
> 2. Give more satisfactory representation in the House of Delegates to the specialty organizations.
> 3. Provide for an increase in experienced and competent manpower to assist the Council on Scientific Assembly in developing the Association's Annual Convention scientific program.
> 4. Generate stimulating and engaging interdisciplinary and specialty-oriented programs which will command the interest of greater numbers of practicing physicians.
> 5. Provide a direct and continuing liaison between a Section and its corresponding specialty societies.
> 6. Permit specialty societies direct access to the House of Delegates through their appointed delegates.
> 7. Give AMA Specialty Sections recognized status by identifying them directly with the specialty societies.

The JCAH requested the opinion of the Board of Regents on a recent resolution. In December, 1972, the Commissioners voted "to accept as a basic premise for further consideration, that the fundamental philosophy of the Joint Commission does not necessarily preclude a change in the composition of the Board and/or corporate membership provided such a change would result in the improvement of health and medical care." The Board of Regents concurred in this resolution of the Board of Commissioners, also stating that "the nature of the vote exercised by one of the College's Commissioners would be based on the representative's conviction of the justification of the action proposed".

A second resolution addressed the representation of consumers on the central policy body. Although the Regents considered the resolution reasonable, they also recognized that consumer representation mainly would serve to heighten the recipient's awareness of the services and to promote acceptability of JCAH services and policies. Consumer representation would not add knowledgeable judgment on the technical and professional considerations involved, and the Regents cautioned that consumer representation should not overbalance professional representation.

## Professional Standards Review Organizations

Some important new considerations for the Joint Commission had resulted from the enactment of US Public Law 92-603 in the fall of 1972. Three main parts of the law were reviewed by Dr. Layne:

1. The enacted law permitted the Secretary of HEW to adopt conditions for hospital participation in Medicare which could exceed the hospital accreditation standards of the Joint Commission following consultation with the Commission.
2. The new law also provided that the Secretary of HEW should conduct a sample validation of JCAH hospital accreditation decisions, with state agencies performing the inspection using a federally established random sample of recently surveyed hospitals. Comparison of the state agency's decisions with those of JCAH results would be performed periodically to test the validity of JCAH decisions for Medicare use.
3. The law also created a system of PSROs which were expected to be in full operation by January 1, 1976.

Dr. Layne pointed out that the use of clinical faculty from medical staffs had resulted in a high rate of acceptance of PSRO's and the number of medical staffs adopting the procedure increased monthly. Hospitals exhibiting an effective internal quality surveillance could be exempted from the regional PSRO, according to the federal law. It was the JCAH's objective to help all accredited hospitals achieve this exemption by 1976.

Dr. John Gamble made a special report on the College's involvement in PSROs. He reminded the Board about the program which had been approved in 1971, when the ACP had participated with the San Joaquin Foundation for Medical Care in establishing criteria for acceptable management of groups of diseases related to internal medicine. The project utilized computers for more effective review of the quality of patient care.

The intent of the PSRO Amendment to P.L. 92-63 was to permit health care providers for Medicare and Medicaid, specifically physicians, to determine the quality of medical care by true peer review on a local or regional basis. The criteria developed by the ACP were ideally suited for such application as guidelines for these organizations.

The involvement of foundations in health care delivery united individual practice patterns into a system for comprehensive health services delivery, but such systems were dependent upon effective peer review. Foundations had been the leaders in PSRO legislation. In order to obtain funding, the American Association of Foundations for Medical Care required a broad base of support. Support and backing from the specialty societies, particularly those that work with foundations to develop criteria of disease management, was necessary. The following resolution was submitted to the Board of Regents and approved.

Be it resolved that the Board of Regents of the American College of Physicians agrees that the PSRO Law provides an opportunity for the medical profession to monitor itself and thus give the public assurance of quality care and at the same time provide a means for education of its members. The proposal for an Institute for Professional Standards is essential for effective implementation by the medical profession of the goals of the PSRO Law. The American College of Physicians will take part in the formation of such an institute and participate in its activities, particularly with regard to those related to further development of criteria for quality and to education. The ACP will engage in other aspects related to the PSRO Law, as necessary or desirable, to assure the realization of goals i.e., education of our members and quality of care.

A significant report came to the College from the National Society for Medical Research [NSMR], an organization which the College supported by official representation. This Society was concerned with maintaining an adequate supply of animals for medical research and was in a position to monitor the rules which insured the humane care of animals. The meeting that year featured a presentation by Robert Berliner, MD, Associate Director of the National Institutes of Health [NIH], and by Dr. Dale F. Schwindaman, Doctor of Veterinary Medicine, who was the senior veterinarian of the Animal Care Staff of the USDA Animal and Plant Inspection Service. Dr. Berliner presented a factual and highly informative account of the current status of prospects for funding of biomedical research and education in the next several years. He also discussed the current position of the NIH regarding guidelines for human and animal experimentation. He indicated that the NIH expected to make compliance with its animal experimentation guidelines a more formal part of grant or contract arrangements.

Dr. Schwindaman dealt candidly with the problems of the USDA in implementing the Animal Welfare Act. He reported that there were more than 2,000 units carrying on research which were covered by these regulations. Some members of the Council stated that there were not enough veterinarians in the entire country to carry out such inspections, even if they were all employed full time in this activity.

The report of the Treasurer of NSMR made it clear that any relaxation of public education in connection with the human importance of humane experimentation on animals would be most unfortunate. However, if the types of changes in regulations which had been suggested by Dr. Schwindaman were to be put into effect it would unquestionably cost American medical research institutions many millions of dollars to comply. Not only would new cages be required for virtually every research facility which now complies fully with existing cage standards, but in order to house as many animals as before, floor space would have to be doubled, requiring any one institution to expend perhaps a million dollars in construction costs.

Dr. John C. Beck, Chairman of the ABIM, made a comprehensive report to the Board of Regents. The 1972 certifying examination represented a transitional period, and the current number of examinations for the year would not be representative of future activity.

Examinations in the subspecialty areas were being offered on a biennial basis. All subspecialties would be tested, including a new one; Medical Oncology. At the May, 1972 meeting the ABIM agreed to rename its test committees in the subspecialty areas as Subspecialty Test Committees and recognized that their terms of reference would include not only the development of an evaluation of materials for the Board, but also provide important input in describing the essentials and guidelines of subspecialty training and, in the future, accreditation activities.

He pointed out that the oral examination technique, traditional since the founding of the Board in 1936, had been phased out and there were very few examinees who were still eligible under the old rules. As a substitute for this phase-out of the oral examination, the Board was working very hard on a new program for the evaluation of the clinical skills of applicants to be certified. This evaluation would be performed by the training program directors with advice from ABIM committees charged with this responsibility.

He described some new programs which were in their final stages of development, including a plan to offer "in training" examinations for residents, in the form of an achievement test. The College had already demonstrated the great demand for such an examination by a survey of Associate Members and residency program directors.

Dr. Beck described a new Division of Evaluation which would be under the direction of Dr. George Webster. The division had already obtained extensive feedback from candidates who sat for the first ABIM examinations in the subspecialty areas. There was general consensus on the part of the examinees that the procedures were fair, challenging and relevant.

## Federal Support of Medical Schools

On April 13, 1973, the Board of Regents adopted the following policy statement entitled, "Federal Support of Medical Schools":

> The nation's medical schools face a severe financial crisis as a direct consequence of some budgetary actions taken by the Administration in its fiscal 1974 budget. These include:
> 1. Elimination of training grants, fellowships and career development awards;
> 2. Reduction in research grants in all areas except cancer and heart disease;
> 3. Reduction and eventual elimination of general research support grants;
> 4. Funding of capitation grants at levels far below those recommended by responsible advisory bodies;
> 5. Elimination of all construction funds for health-sciences facilities;
> 6. Elimination of Regional Medical Programs.
>
> These actions threaten the immediate fiscal solvency of virtually all medical and health science schools because they will abrogate support of faculty that is essential to the schools' teaching programs. Moreover, these actions come at a time when medical schools have increased the size of their classes in response to the increased need for health manpower. In the long term, these cuts will be detrimental to the generation of new biomedical knowledge that is essential to patient care, and to the development of the faculty that will need to do the teaching of medical students, interns, residents, and practicing physicians in the next twenty years.

## Part Five (1973-1974)

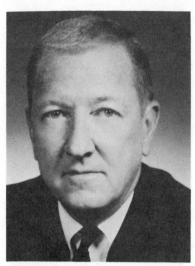

*Walter B. Frommeyer, Jr., MACP*

Born in 1916 in Cincinnati, Ohio, Walter B. Frommeyer, Jr., married Elizabeth Lee in 1944 and they had two daughters, Lee and Virginia. He died in Birmingham, Alabama, January 8, 1979.

Receiving his BA in 1939 from the University of Cincinnati, he also earned his MD degree there in 1942.

He served an internship and assistant residency in medicine at the Cincinnati General Hospital between 1942 and 1948, interrupting his training during World War II to serve in the U.S. Army Medical Corps from 1943 to 1946. Following a Research Fellowship at the Thorndike Memorial Laboratory at Harvard Medical School in 1948-49, he was appointed Assistant Professor of Medicine at Harvard in 1948.

In 1949, he began his long association with the University of Alabama College of Medicine as Instructor and progressed to the position of Professor of Medicine and Chairman of the Department of Medicine in 1957, in which he served to 1969. In 1968 he was appointed Distinguished Professor of Medicine and held this title until his death. He was Chief of Staff of University Hospital and The Hillman Clinic from 1957 to 1968, Director of the Blood Bank at the Jefferson-Hillman Hospital and Chief of Medical Service at the VA Hospital in Birmingham. He was also Associate Dean of the Medical School from 1954 to 1957. He was made Chairman of the Human Use Committee in 1971, Director of the Physicians' Assistant Program in 1972 and Director of the Student Health Service in 1972, serving in these positions until his death.

He was President of the Alabama Heart Association in 1958-59 and of the American Heart Association in 1968-69. A diplomate of the American Board of Internal Medicine in 1951, he served as its Vice Chairman in 1967-68, and as Chairman of its Subcommittee on Patient Management Problem Examination. He was a member of the Examining Panel for the American Board of Family Practice from 1970 to 1972.

His societal memberships included the Association of American Physicians, Association of Professors of Medicine, American College of Cardiology, American Association for Advancement of Sciences, American Federation for Clinical Research, American Medical Association, American Society of Internal Medicine, Southern Medical Association and the Southern Society for Clinical Investigation. The University of Cincinnati College of Medicine bestowed on him the Peter T. Kilgour Award, and his long service to the Heart Association merited him the Distinguished Service Award from the Alabama Heart Association. For his outstanding community service he was nominated Man of the Year for the Greater Birmingham Area and the Gold Heart Award of the American Heart Association in 1970.

Elected a Fellow of the American College of Physicians in 1955, he rapidly assumed a leadership role. Elected as Governor for Alabama from 1960 to 1966, he also served as Chairman of the Committee on Postgraduate Courses from 1964 to 1967, and Chairman of the Scientific Program Committee from 1967 to 1970. During his service as a Regent from 1966 to 1969, he was Chairman of the Committee on Educational Activities. He was then elected Vice President and in his 18th year as a Fellow of the College, he was elected President-Elect, assuming the Presidency in 1973-74. He received Mastership in 1974 and the Stengel Award in 1977.

Dr. Frommeyer contributed strong leadership in establishing and promoting acceptability of the recertification effort. He was equally committed to the development of Chapters in the College and to the development of audio-visual programs, such as the *Medical Skills Library* and the *Self-Learning Series.* He was consistently energetic; an incisive leader in his many activities.

The Board of Governors found it hard to accept the idea of recertification. At the special joint meeting of the Governors and Regents, Dr. Frommeyer demonstrated both fairness and firmness in his leadership. After a fairly long and not entirely pleasant discussion, he stood and said, "I've heard all of your arguments. You say the Board of Regents doesn't listen to the Governors. This is incorrect. We listen but don't agree. Recertification will be approved by the Board of Regents. What we need from the Board of Governors is the understanding and willingness to make it effective".

This directness was again portrayed at the first Board of Regents meeting over which he presided in April, 1973. "Gentlemen, he said, we have 24 agenda items to consider, and I figure if there are five minutes for each item, we'll be here for two and a half hours. If you talk longer we'll be late for lunch, so let's get working." With this introduction, he used the gavel with enough force to break the head into two pieces. Laughter and a relaxed atmosphere ensued and the Regents finished in time for lunch. Today, this gavel, a reminder of his forceful leadership, remains on display outside the Board Room with other objects of the College's traditions.

Forceful he was, but very easy to work with. He was always interested in what the Staff at Headquarters did, but trusted us implicitly in how we did it. He displayed good judgment about people when working on special programs, especially in developing the audio-visual programs.

In his work as Head of the Department of Medicine at Alabama and as a Regent he scheduled himself very rigidly. He never went out for dinners or banquets, but had an early dinner and usually retired by 9:00 p.m. He got up at 4:00 a.m. and worked in his office from 5:00 until 9:00 on letters, reports, and studies. From 9:00 to 5:00 he was unfailingly available to students, residents, and faculty. In the waves of nonchalance of the 1960's, medical students were showing an indifference to their personal appearance, so he always carried a few neckties in his pocket. Whenever a student showed for "rounds" without a tie, he lent the student one, with an admonishment never again to show up on his service without one. His wife once told me that one of the things he liked to do on Sunday mornings was to shine everyone's shoes. He felt it an effort that provided excellent returns.

His brother was a priest and once asked Wally to present a position on a ethical subject which at that time was unpopular with most physicians. He presented it, but did not push for it, showing great respect both for his brother and his colleagues, without great fuss or argument.

On one occasion, a Regent asked me to encourage Wally to come to the Regents' dinners. I convinced him that this would disconcert Wally; as long as he was doing an effective job as President, we should leave things as they were. The subject was never raised again. All the Regents seemed to understand his need for rest and accepted his early bedtimes. The service he gave unquestionably merited the Alfred Stengel Award, which he received in 1977.

Wally had a direct and practical sense of fairness. On one occasion a group of us were trying to board a bus at Convention Center in Philadephia to return to the hotels in center city and one of the doctors was berating the bus driver for not letting him on without a ticket. Wally, not very large in stature, sized up the situation and said to the doctor, "Stop picking on the bus driver, he's doing exactly what he's been told to do. What you can do is get off this bus now and go and buy a ticket. The rest of us are ready to leave". Sheepishly the man got off and everyone on the bus gave Wally a round of applause.

During Dr. Frommeyer's time as Chairman of the Scientific Program Committee, he and I developed a set of rules for the conduct of panel discussions. The main features of this plan prohibited the use of slides and eliminated the short introductory speeches usually made by each of the panel members. Panel chairmen were instructed to ask each panelist to send a list of questions he or she would be comfortable answering. Having previously selected from the list of questions, the Chairman would introduce the session by asking each panelist to respond to specific subject questions. Discussion and questions from the audience completed the exercise. This mode of presentation averted lengthy and non-specific panel delivery. It proved to be successful in heightening audience interest.

Over a number of years we had developed a set of instructions to mail to program participants. We included helpful suggestions such as how to use microphones, and prepare slides. We even sent out a sample slide for comparison with the size of lettering on their own slides.

I always cautioned participants that it was not possible to get more than 10 to 12 lines of type on a properly prepared slide. I was amused and discouraged when one of my friends quoted an academic colleague, "Rosenow's got a good idea about sending out those suggestions but he's wrong about slides, I can get 48 to 50 lines on a slide".

Dr. Frommeyer was kindly forgiving of Staff mistakes, and especially reassuring to persons who were more demanding of their own performance than they needed to be. He was more than forgiving, he was actively encouraging, as some of our Staff well remembered.

Dr. Thomas N. James, ACP Governor for Alabama, said of him at the time of his death in 1979,

> In everything he did, his personal traits of humility, dignity, integrity and compassion shone through . . . A man who was completely undaunted by committees and other necessary paraphernalia of administration, he made all meetings purposeful, sensible, courteous and maximally effective. While there was no doubt about who was in the Chair, one never felt less than a full participant in the proceedings. He could make people work together and combine their unselfish efforts for results from which all could take pride. It was a singular talent, maybe the very essence of true leadership, and it will be sorely missed.

# 1973-1974

> New York - First ACP Chapter. Recertification exam. *MKSAP III*. Nutrition Foundation Scholarships. ACP wins favorable decision in *Annals* advertising tax suit. P.L.92-603: PSRO. Private Initiative in PSRO. Medical Liability Commission. National Coordinating Council on Emergency Medical Care.

At the final meeting of the Board of Regents at the Annual Session, April 13, incoming President, Dr. Walter B. Frommeyer, Jr., presented his aspirations for the year.

> I believe that you should know what some of my objectives are during this all too brief period of a year as President of the ACP.
>
> 1. Organization of the College at the so-called 'grass roots' level, i.e., the establishment of a local functioning unit in each state or jurisdictional area of the College. This concept will take a major selling job on the part of each of us since the Governors do not desire this, in the main.
>
> Such local units, however, could and should result in much more active participation of our College members in the affairs of the College. This could also result in this Board of Regents and the Board of Governors learning more rapidly and more accurately what works in the field and what doesn't work.
>
> 2. The Board of Regents should get out of the business of what I call 'housekeeping matters'. This means that the Board must learn to recognize those matters which are functions of the staff and to recognize those matters which are proper functions of the Board. We must show our confidence in the abilities of the staff and let staff do what staff can do far better than any Board can ever expect to do in such matters.
>
> 3. This Board should concern itself with policy matters. In this way we can lead the Governors, as well as the membership, and thus the College, to greater heights of accomplishment.
>
> In these times of change, when change often occurs rapidly, this Board must make many policy decisions which must be wise and fair and, in addition, this Board must have the courage to be unpopular in relation to some of its decisions.

In this way the Board of Regents will provide the leadership which the Governors and the membership of the ACP look to this Board to provide for them.

This Board must also concern itself with the future so that the College can meet the future well prepared and well armed, i.e., we must develop a long-range plan. To that end I am appointing an ad hoc committee to develop such a plan and to report its final recommendations in November, 1973, after having input from the discussions at the Board Meeting in August of 1973.

4. My final objective is to heal the breach between the Board of Governors and the Board of Regents brought about recently by the Board of Regents policy decision in favor of recertification. To this end, when any of us is the official representative of the College at a Regional Meeting, it is imperative that we take up first the matter of recertification and carry out a detailed and clear discussion of it.

Material for such a presentation will be supplied to you by way of a copy of the material I am to write which is to appear in the *Annals* as well as in the *Bulletin* of the College.

At the following meeting in November, Dr. Frommeyer explained why a scheduled Summer meeting of the Regents was not held. Several committees which he had appointed had not had sufficient time to meet and had not been ready to report to a Summer session. Two of those committees were the Ad Hoc Committee on ABIM Qualifications, Dr. Julius Stolfi, Chairman, and the Ad Hoc Committee to Develop a Statement of ACP Policies and Plans for Implementation, Dr. Jack Myers, Chairman.

Dr. William F. Kellow, Treasurer, described the current financial base as being quite satisfactory. No progress was yet noted regarding the claim for refund of income taxes for 1968 and 1969. The engagement of A. G. Becker & Co. was showing positive results concerning the investment portfolio. Analysis showed that, in 1970, when the common stock holdings in the College portfolio showed a total return (income and capital gains and losses) of 3.79 percent, only 4 percent of the other funds included in the study performed better. But in the following year when the College portfolio's total return rose to 16.24 percent, 85 percent of the other funds performed better than the equities in the College's fund, illustrating in a dramatic way the importance of comparison of results with similar funds.

## MKSAP III

I announced in my Executive Vice President's report that the *Medical Knowledge Self-Assessment Program III* was published within two weeks of its projected date and already had 11,000 subscriptions. The work load of the Credentials Committee was increasing as membership grew. The Committee was reaching the realization that it must either meet more often, increase the size of the Committee or figure out some way to simplify the procedures for processing membership applications.

For the Board's information, I described the work of the AMA Advisory Committee on Continuing Medical Education, on which I had just completed 11 years service, occupying the position of Chairman for the past four years. This Committee had established the system of accrediting institutions that wanted to offer postgraduate education courses or other types of educational activities and had created the Physicians' Recognition Award to recognize postgraduate activities.

I also reviewed the background of Governors Conferences for the Board's information. Governors Conferences had been initiated six years previously; during this time, much attention was given to the question of increasing members' participation in College affairs at the local level, but at the most recent, the 6th Annual Governors Conference, strong resistance to developing local Chapters as a solution had been evident.

At this conference, the Governors also considered College involvement in Professional Standards Review Organizations [PSRO]. I had contributed the observation that the College could not get very involved in PSRO unless each Governor, individually, assumed the job of going to the State Medical Association and finding out what he could do to support PSRO. When PSRO districts are formed, the law stated that they must seek the help of specialty societies. Obviously, the local PSRO would call on the State Medical Association to ascertain who represents the specialty society in internal medicine. I emphasized that the College was not yet on that roster and should be. The College was far behind other societies in working with State Medical Associations. Twenty-four state associations had specialty sections. Six states were forming interspecialty councils on which they were inviting specialty societies to participate. Ten of the states provided for direct specialty society representation in their House of Delegates.

Action in these above areas was important to implement any ACP involvement in PSRO. Dr. Henry Simmons, the Governor for the Public Health Services in the College, recently had been given responsibility for national development of the PSRO mechanism and addressed the Governors Conference on the subject. He thought that PSRO legislation reflected dissatisfaction with medical care and noted that the PSRO system had been given to the profession to establish standards and to make them work. He stressed the crucial nature of educational feedback in the operation of these plans.

Dr. Stolfi, Chairman of the Ad Hoc Committee on American Board of Internal Medicine [ABIM] Qualifications, also addressed the 6th Governors Conference. The Governors were in substantial agreement with the Committee's views, some of which were as follows:

Shortening the medical school curriculum was viewed as unwise in light of the increasing mass of complex information to be taught. The Committee had some reservations about the proposal that the fourth year of medical school be composed entirely of electives. The Governors endorsed the Committee's view of firm basic science requirements. They were concerned generally about the apparent fall in the number of general internists, especially the thoroughly trained consultant-internist-diagnosticians of past years.

The Board of Governors took up the important subject of the formation of local chapters. Displaying no great warmth toward the idea during lengthy discussion, the Governors nevertheless agreed that it would be useful to try these in several areas and see how they might operate.

In November, an up-to-date report of *MKSAP III* and its relationship to recertification was submitted to the Board of Regents from the Educational Activities Committee, Dr. Robert J. Petersdorf, Chairman. In February there would be a meeting with the Chairman of the Test Committees to choose questions for the self-assessment program. Dr. Petersdorf and Dr. George Webster would then spend several days in Philadelphia choosing appropriate questions for the recertification examination. These questions would be submitted for approval to the Recertification Committee of ABIM.

The Fellowships and Scholarships Committee, Dr. John R. Graham, Chairman, reported the appointment of four teaching and research scholars.

Dr. Graham also conveyed that the Committee was pleased at the success of the campaign to enlist more past and present teaching research scholars as members of the College. Four previous scholars had become Fellows; one a Member; five had requested Membership applications. All teaching and research scholars currently in the program had become Members with the exception of the last three appointees, who had been notified that they were expected to apply for Membership by January 15, 1974.

Dr. Jack D. Myers, Chairman of the Finance Committee, pointed out that with the past year's increase in dues, the income attributable to general administration was projected to be $341,000, which meant an increase of approximately $270,000 over that period for 1972. The projected income for *Annals* for the year 1973 was estimated at $200,500, which was an increase. The postgraduate courses, because of the cancellation of four courses and an increase in operating expenses, had resulted in a net deficit of $12,400. The Board of Regents, therefore, approved a revised schedule of fees.

The Finance Committee continued to be concerned about the annual deficit of the Annual Session. Some members of the Committee thought that the time might be coming when even the members attending the Annual Session would have to pay a registration fee.

To date, no member of the College paid a registration fee. From a recent comprehensive study, the Committee projecting a deficit of $185,000 for the Chicago meeting in 1973, $21,000 higher than the previous Annual Session, estimated that without introducing membership fees, the deficit in 1974 could run as high as $232,400. The following fee scale was proposed: Masters, Fellows and Members, if graduated from medical school 11 years or more, $20; if graduated from medical school ten years or less, $10; Associate members would pay a registration fee of $5.

Estimating membership attendance at 3500, with an additional 500 Associates, in 1974 these rates would accrue approximately $62,500 in registration fees, reducing the estimated deficit to approximately $169,000. The Board wanted more time to consider this matter in conjunction with a variety of other changes being formulated relating to the Annual Session, such as fees and honoraria to speakers. It therefore disapproved the motion and the matter was deferred until November, 1974, when it approved a revised motion from the Finance Committee.

The very interesting analysis of the investment portfolio by the A. G. Becker Company was approved by the Board of Regents, and after discussion with the College's Investment Counsel, Drexel, Burnham & Lambert Company, the following investment policy was also approved by the Board of Regents:

> The investment objective should be a compound rate of return for the overall portfolio of seven to nine percent. Between 15 and 25 percent of the portfolio should be invested in fixed income securities including convertible debentures. Excluding the convertible securities, this portion should be expected to provide a return approximately that available from utility bonds. The common stock portion would be expected to contribute an 8-10 percent compound rate of return including yield and capital appreciation.

In order to operate under the suggested investment policy it would be necessary to adopt the principle of "total return" (income and capital appreciation together), with a portion of the total return being used for operations. Drexel, Burnham & Lambert recommended 50 percent at that time, the balance to be added to principle. This method left the investment advisor free to strive for return, either through high income, capital appreciation, or a combination of the two.

A new policy of the International Society of Internal Medicine indicated that the Society was going to have two types of membership. One type was an individual membership and the other a national society membership. The annual Society membership dues would be $10 per Society plus 10 cents for each of its active members. It was estimated that the total annual Society membership dues for the College would be approximately $2,000.

Dr. Richard Allyn, Chairman, reviewed the status of emergency medical care in a report for the Medical Practice Committee. He recommended that Governors consider appropriate places for residency training in emergency care relating to internal medicine. The Committee expressed concern that this critical portion of internal medicine training might be jeopardized through pre-emption by "emergency care" specialty groups. This recommendation was approved by the Board.

The Board also approved the recommendation of the Committee that the American College of Physicians appoint a liaison representative to the proficiency evaluation program of the College of American Pathologists. It also endorsed the Medic Alert Program and offered publicity in the *ACP Bulletin* for this organization.

Dr. Frommeyer conveyed the Report of the Audio-Visual Committee, noting some interesting developments in the patient counseling material. Dr. Alfred M. Sellers, Chairman of the Ad Hoc Core Curriculum Committee was writing the book on hypertension and had developed a questionnaire containing 30 questions that newly diagnosed hypertensive patients might ask. From these 30 questions, selections were made to be included as concepts in the film. Dr. Bernard V. Dryer, of MEDEX, described some design components, which reflected the underlying objectives of the project:

> A. We are not trying to make the patient into a "little doctor".

B. One of our primary goals is to save doctors' time.

C. We hope to modify the patient's behavior but are realistically modest in predicting our ability to reach this goal.

A multi-media approach was used, including a film as a high intensity, short duration learning stimulus and printed material as a long duration, low-intensity learning stimulus, to reinforce the the film and answer questions raised by it. The film was colorful and short, practical for office visit use. It was designed to accommodate a wide variety of patients, considering attention span, educational, regional, cultural and intellectual differences. To minimize the obstacles caused by variations in patterns of speech, emotional response to the subject of hypertension, age and sex, MEDEX suggested employing animation techniques.

Having considered the more realistic approach to films, that is, real people in real settings talking about their own problems in handling hypertension, the Committee concluded that while there is some value in this approach for assuring the patient, regional and individual differences can create resistance to the learning process. Animation films, therefore, had the best chance of setting the first attitudinal patterns. More factual films could follow, using the realistic approach. The first goal was to save doctors the time required to repeat the "message of hypertension," without replacing the doctor-patient intimacy of exchange for personalized details.

A second patient counseling film on "heartburn" was being developed. Work-in-progress on the *Medical Skills Library* included a film on manual positive pressure ventilation, as part of a series on emergency and elective airway management. Other films were scheduled on external cardiac compression and ventricular defibrillation.

Dr. Jack D. Myers, Chairman, reported that the activities of the Residency Review Committee in Internal Medicine [RRC-IM] were proceeding satisfactorily. Although a small number of unaffiliated community hospitals were still operating approved residencies, a growing number of them were becoming affiliated with academic health centers, conducting residency programs in cooperation with a university. The program to provide special consultants to training programs in difficulty, inaugurated by the College, had already made several consultants available with benefit to the programs. "The "Guide for Education In Internal Medicine" previously approved by the Board of Regents had been sent to the American Medical Association, which also approved it. The Guide's summary statement read as follows:

Graduate medical education in internal medicine requires a major commitment from administration, the chief of medicine, and the attending staff. Both in-patient and out-patient services must be well organized with a primary objective being education. Regularly scheduled, formal bedside teaching rounds by an attending staff dedicated to teaching is one of the keystones of a successful program. Although all programs must fulfill the requirements of the "Essentials," there is sufficient flexibility for diversity of approaches. It is not essential or even desirable that all hospital residencies should adopt exactly the same program or that they should offer a rigidly uniform sequence of experience. It is essential, however, that all hospitals participating in graduate training should be able to meet the fundamental essential requirements for an approved program and either alone or in collaboration should attain comparable results in the quality of training and the amount of experience obtained.

In response to the prevailing climate regarding consumer rights and specifically medical malpractice, a number of attempts to address the issues were occurring on the national medical scene.

The enactment of Public Law 92-603, in the Fall of 1972, created new responsibilities for the Joint Commission on Accreditation of Hospitals [JCAH], and focused on its Hospital Accreditation Program. In December, 1972, the question of consumer representation on the Board of Commissioners resulted in a position statement in which the ACP Board of Regents concurred in April, 1973:

> To accept, as a basic premise for further consideration, that the fundamental philosophy of the Joint Commission does not necessarily preclude a change in the composition of the Board and/or corporate membership, provided such a change would result in the improvement of health and medical care.

Dr. John Porterfield, Executive Director of JCAH, addressed a letter to the ACP Board of Regents, the substance of which was entered into the record. In part it stated:

> In view of the recent reaffirmation of the democratic principle of self-government, consumer representation on the central body is reasonable. It should be recognized, however, that consumer representation serves to provide awareness of the acceptability to the recipient of the services or policies to be considered, rather than a knowledgeable judgment on the technical and professional considerations involved. Consumer representation should not, therefore, overbalance professional representation.

## Medical Liability

The President's Commission on Medical Liability, convened in 1972, proposed that a National Commission on Medical Malpractice be created to address questions of malpractice and related issues. This led to several informal meetings of a variety of organizations interested in medical malpractice.

At a meeting at the AMA in late 1972, it was initially proposed that organizational representation should include physicians, hospitals, attorneys and insurance companies. Referring to the results of the survey on medical malpractice conducted by the ACP Group Insurance Administrators in 1971, I suggested that the inclusion of insurance companies could only be a complicating factor in the effort to address peer review effectively. The convened meeting agreed that such a Commission should have broadly based representation from medical societies and hospitals only.

The ACP Board of Regents voted to participate on the Medical Liability Commission in April, 1974. In November, 1974, the ACP representative reported that the Commission was comprised of the AMA, American Hospital Association [AHA], the American Osteopathic Association, the specialty societies represented on the Council of Medical Specialty Societies [CMSS] and the American Society of Internal Medicine [ASIM]. By November, the Commission numbered 24 representatives. The ACP appointed me as its Commissioner with Dr. Harrison Shull as alternate and approved $4,000 as ACP's assessment.

At its first meeting in September, 1973, the Commission approved the by-laws, elected officers and took the following actions:

1. Appointed a liaison committee to maintain communications with organizations concentrating efforts in the same field, such as the National Foundation for the Study of Health Sciences Liability.
2. Adopted a formula for determining additional membership assessments for the first fiscal year, based on the membership census of the supporting organization.
3. Accepted the AMA's offering of staff services and facilities through November, 1973.
4. Admitted the ASIM as a supporting member organization.
5. Adopted a resolution requesting supporting member organizations to take prompt action in malpractice prevention.

## ACP Chapters

Concluding the November Board of Regents meeting, Dr. Frommeyer elaborated on his statement of objectives in April and especially his reasoning about organizing the ACP into official Chapters. He was concerned about the breakdown in communications between the Governors and Regents over this matter and the Board of Governors' lack of enthusiasm for it. He referred to my report to the Board, which later appeared in the *ACP Bulletin* in December, in which I had described the difficulties our present structure presented in trying to implement College policy. In each PSRO area, for example, the law specified that the PSRO would seek the help of specialty societies. It was unlikely any PSROs would direct requests to College Headquarters, because of low Regional visibility. They would more likely consult those specialties that organize at the local level, which have thus high local visibility. The same article, he noted, reviewed the results of my recent poll of Governors at their request which sought to determine whether College policies were being implemented locally. Of six policy statements mailed with the questionnaire, response revealed that only three of the policies had been significantly implemented in any of the ACP regions. Dr. Frommeyer then enumerated the advantages of forming chapters:

1. Increased visability for the ACP, both locally and nationally.
2. More opportunity for involvement of many members in College activities. (At the moment, such involvement was primarily limited to Regional Meetings, which may be held as infrequently as every three to seven years in a given Governor's jurisdictional area, depending upon the conglomerate of states involved.)

3. An opportunity for members to implement ACP policies at the local level.
4. An opportunity for the College to participate actively with other constituted bodies, such as:
   a. Participation in State Medical Associations in
      (1) Organization and development of the annual scientific programs in internal medicine.
      (2) The opportunity for election of delegates from the ACP Chapter into the State Association's policy body and various committees.
   b. Playing an active role in voluntary health organizations and associations.
   c. Participation in state and local hospital organizations.
   d. Playing an active role in governmental agencies such as state and local health departments.
   e. Active official participation in other specialty societies such as:
      (1) The State Society of Internal Medicine. This could, and probably would, result in a better relationship between the State Society of Internal Medicine and the ACP.
      (2) The American Psychiatric Association [APA]
      (3) The American College of Surgeons [ACS]
      (4) The American Academy of Family Physicians [AAFP]
   f. Play an active role in PSRO's.
5. Chapters would also afford "grass roots" input into the Board of Regents policy formulation through recommendations discussed and proposed by the Board of Governors.
6. There could be local nomination of individuals for Governor. "What are the disadvantages of chapters?" Dr. Frommeyer asked rhetorically, "I think of none. This Board of Regents needs to take a strong stand on the matter of chapters."

## Annual Session 1974

By April, 1974, Dr. Frommeyer's report of the progress on two of his main objectives, namely, recertification and ACP chapter organization, was encouraging.

Recertification was a reality. He paid particular tribute to the tremendous leadership of Dr. Robert Petersdorf; it was because of the efforts of the members of his Educational Activities Committee and the phenomenal work of the test committees that the first goal was achieved. The Syllabus with its 481 references was being used by over 23,000 individual subscribers to *MKSAP III*. Estimates suggested that approximately 4,000 subscribers would take the ABIM recertification examination on October 26, 1974. He did not feel as optimistic about the second goal, but saw some progress. The first official Chapter with legal status was organized in New Mexico; eight others were in advanced planning stages.

Supplementing Dr. Frommeyer's report, my April progress report pointed out that in all areas to date, Governors who had polled their members had found a majority in favor of forming chapters. In his New York State Region, Dr. Jeremiah A. Barondess reported a sentiment of 20-1 in favor of a chapter. The apparent overriding local concern about the formation of chapters was how they would impinge on the local state Societies of Internal Medicine. Some fear of territorial infringement obviously existed. Chapter formation implied a potential for differences of opinion between the organizations, but some Governors believed that chapters would improve operations between ASIM and the College.

My spring report included the status of the *Annals* advertising tax suit; we won. The ACP attorneys noted hopefully that the College might recover nearly $500,000.

I reminded the Board of Regents that in the near future they must make some decision about family practice trainees and College membership. The existing Bylaws did not prohibit it, stating that anybody who is qualified by the ABIM or a "recognized specialty board acceptable to the Board of Regents" could become a member of the College. The Credentials Committee had encountered one instance at its last meeting in which the first applicant to the College from a family practice program actually quoted the College's Bylaws to that effect. The Committee planned to garner additional information about the training programs to present to the Board of Regents.

I was pleased to report that the survey of internists engaged in primary care had been funded by the Robert Wood Johnson Foundation and would be run by the University of Southern California. The project was in the pilot study stage. As a member of its advisory committee, I considered this study adequate to ACP's needs and advised against the College undertaking its own survey. In addition to studying internal medicine, the plan for this funded program included study of all specialties to determine who, and to what degree, each engaged in primary care. I closed with thanks to the Board of Regents for their encouraging letters and sentiments to my wife, Esther, who had sustained a right-sided hemiplegia in July of 1973.

### Agenda - Special Joint Boards Meeting

Dr. Frommeyer announced the agenda prepared by the Executive Committee for the combined meeting of the Board of Regents and the Board of Governors for the Summer of 1974. The meeting would replace for one year the Summer meeting of the Board of Regents and the Fall meeting of the Board of Governors. The agenda included:

1. The improvement of communication between the two Boards.
2. Definition of the roles and duties of the Governors as individuals.
3. The role of the Board of Governors as a body in policy development or in exerting influence on policy decisions.
4. The role of the Governors in implementing policies.
5. Exploration of the possibility to assign certain specific matters to the Board of Governors.
6. The role of the ACP at the local level.

Projected issues for the discussion of College policy were:

1. Family Medicine
2. Patient education about health
3. ASIM
4. National Health Insurance
5. Assessment of the effectiveness of current continuing education programs
6. PSRO

The Board of Regents approved several motions from the Executive Committee:

1. Both Executive Committees of the Regents and Governors recommended that the Liaison Committee of ACP/ASIM be asked to review the 1968 agreement and recommend either revisions or dissolution of the agreement, with the proviso that local Governors be permitted to retain the option to associate or cooperate with the local society in accordance with established College policies as proposed by the Board of Governors and approved by the Board of Regents in November, 1973.
2. The Executive Committee requested that Chapter formation be one of the items on the agenda for the joint conference.
3. The Executive Committee endorsed the idea of the College participating in the conference sponsored by the American Psychiatric Association.
4. The Board also approved the Committee's resolution that the College had no objection to including representation from the American Academy of Physicians' Assistants in the Joint Review Committee on Physicians' Assistants.

Dr. Jeremiah A. Barondess, Chairman of the Board of Governors, commented on the general attitudes of the Board toward several issues. The major area of concern at the March meeting related to the results of the Governors' efforts to increase local activities. A second issue of concern was the improvement of the flow of information from the Board of Regents to the Board of Governors. The Governors talked freely about chapters and, upon reflection, Dr. Barondess concluded that the effort was progressing quite well. Though not much action was evident until the model bylaws were distributed in June, 1973, by April, 1974, nine chapters were at varying stages of development. No Governor involved had experienced any unfavorable attitudes on the part of the membership. The Governors' reports reflected increased concern for enhancement of local activity. The need for a College presence in PSRO was discussed, a few of the Governors had appointed people to the local PSROs. Several Governors had set up review courses in local medical schools. Some had appointed representatives to County Society Emergency Care Committees in their Regions and to County Society Peer Review Committees. These physicians were specifically functioning as ACP representatives.

The Secretary-General reported that the total membership of the College was 26,588, of whom 103 were Masters, 12,345 Fellows, 6,796 Members, 7,033 Associates, 186 Affiliate Members, 80 Corresponding Fellows, and 45 were

Honorary Fellows. This report showed a significant increase in Associate Membership.

Dr. Robert G. Petersdorf reported that *MKSAP III* had 23,000 subscribers to date, of whom 4,000 had applied to take the ABIM recertification examination in October, 1974. The Educational Activities Committee was continuing its evaluation of attendance at the Annual Session. Approximately 4,000 physicians had registered for the current meeting in New York. Dr. Petersdorf announced that the meeting originally scheduled for Chicago in 1977 had been rescheduled for Dallas, Texas.

I suggested to the Committee that the fiscal problems relating to the Annual Session were probably attributable, in part, to the change in the type of program. Many more workshops and small group sessions like "Meet the Professor", though highly popular, required many more program participants, which increased our costs, but did not necessarily increase physician attendance at the Annual Session. The decline in attendance over the past two years, due to this and a number of other factors, increased the fiscal dilemma, but attendance might be improved by the change of meeting sites.

The Postgraduate Courses Committee report described cumulative registration patterns from 1965, when the total registration was 1,660 in 19 courses, through 1973, when 4,079 were registered in 36 courses.

Over 90 medical schools had purchased some or all of the twelve films available from the *Medical Skills Library,* I reported for the Audio-Visual Committee. Two new ones were in preparation, on "Tonometry" and "Manual Positive Pressure Ventilation." Films on "Ventricular Defibrillation" and "External Cardiac Compression" were in the planning stage. *Patient Counselling Films* on "Hypertension" and "Reflux Esophagitis" were in progress. The Audio-Visual Committee debated whether to continue the television programs at the Annual Session. The Roche Laboratories had supported the program for several years since Smith, Kline & French Co. had stopped doing television for the College. Coordinating the programming at the local level was a continuing difficult problem. Local speakers, generally unaware of the advantages of the Annual Session as a public forum, seldom gave much advance attention to constructing presentations that would be suitable for televising. The Committee, therefore, considered the advance development of taped programs for the Annual Session, and decided to explore it with Roche Laboratories.

Two additional Teaching and Research Scholarships were approved by the Board of Regents, to be supported by the Nutrition Foundation. The Committee on Fellowships and Scholarships would screen candidates for these scholarships. They would be appointed by the Board of Regents under specifications duplicating those which applied to regular Teaching and Research Scholarships.

The Board of Regents approved several items presented by the Medical Practice Committee:

1. Dr. Richard Allyn recommended endorsement of the AHA statement regarding microbiologic sampling in hospitals, in which the Medical Practice Committee concurred:

Microbiologic sampling procedures, if carried out when indicated in the investigation of specified epidemiologic problems, can be extremely helpful in the control of nosocomial infections. Much research remains to be done in order to define possible reservoirs within the hospital of many organisms associated with nosocomial infection. Routine microbiological sampling of the hospital environment, however, has not only provided data that are impossible to interpret but also has contributed little to hospital control.

2. The Medical Practice Committee had received a letter from Dr. Bertram Bell requesting the College's endorsement of the utilization of nurses trained as surrogate physicians in ambulatory care services. After study, the Committee recommended the following College position statement:

The ACP should not be involved in certifying registered nurses in the role of substitute physicians and continues to approve of registered nurses as very good physicians' assistants. The American College of Physicians encourages and will assist in the development of academic and training programs for preparing RN's to be physicians' assistants.

3. The AMA Commission on Emergency Care moved to establish an intersocietal coordinating council. The Medical Practice Committee recommended that the ACP endorse the establishment of the National Coordinating Council for Emergency Medical Services. The Board directed Dr. Douglas McGill to vote for the establishment of this Council at the next AMA Commission on Emergency Medical Care meeting.

4. The Board endorsed the Committee's recommendation regarding ASIM's "Review Evaluation Program for the Medical Laboratory".

5. The Committee reported also its continued support of the "Proficiency Evaluation Program" of the College of American Pathologists.

Dr. Robert Tally reported on the San Joaquin Foundation study, which was currently working on a retrospective analysis of ambulatory care. Specific criteria concerning justification for hospitalization and other under- and over-utilization observations were yet to be developed.

In addition to continued support of the JCAH position on the delineation of hospital privileges, Dr. McGill stated, the Medical Practice Committee recommended that every hospital medical staff have its own method of delineating privileges. Any such method should include methods for determining:

a. Initial evaluation of each member's experience and training.

b. The general type of privilege accorded to each physician.

c. The proper use of consultations.

d. Specific procedures which may be performed by each physician.

e. A method of review for annual delineation of privileges.

The Public and Professional Communications Committee, Dr. Edmund B. Flink, Chairman, requested action on two items.

1. The Board approved action to update and expand national publicity about

*MKSAP III;* specifically the educational aspects of the Syllabus and the Self-Assessment Examination.

2. The Committee, seriously concerned about the visibility of the internist, urged that the Board approve the concept and recommendation of procedures to accomplish better definitions of "internist" and "internal medicine."

The Publications Committee received approval of its nominations for replacements on the Editorial Board. Dr. Stuart O. Bondurant, Jr., Chairman, also recommended that a section of classified advertisements concerning fellowships opportunities, faculty positions, and other appropriate professional announcements be developed for the *Annals.* He specified a provision that the full cost should be borne by charges and that a written policy defining acceptable types of advertising be developed by the editor. This was approved. He reported an increase in *Annals* circulation of 20,000 in four years, and a very satisfactory financial status.

I reported that the *ACP Bulletin,* was showing the results of a continuing effort to make it more visually attractive and more meaningful in content. Emphasis was being placed on articles with socioeconomic content. Whenever possible photographs were used to illustrate articles. The graphics department considerably enhanced, intramurally, the art work capabilities.

Dr. Edward J. Huth, Editor of the *Annals,* reported some recent difficulties in meeting schedules because of Staff turnover. The number of manuscripts received in 1973 totaled 12,010, approximately the same number as for 1972. The ratio of those chosen was approximately one out of nine or ten. The quality of papers published was holding up quite well.

He reported that as consequence of one of his many outside editorial activities, membership on the Council of Biology Editors, he served as a consultant at the National Library of Medicine and in UNESCO's UNISIST Program.

Dr. Frommeyer attended a meeting of the ACP/ASIM Liaison Committee in Chicago, January 17, 1974. Members of both societies generally agreed that the original so-called "Phoenix Accord" of 1968 was no longer viable. The College was entering into activity in the socioeconomic area and the Society was gravitating toward activities in PSRO. Appointment of a joint task force on the subject of health manpower was suggested. Some members recommended that the Liaison Committee consider having task forces assigned to study certain subjects, bringing their recommendations to the Liaison Committee for joint consideration. One problem receiving a fair amount of discussion was the current inability to effectively evaluate the internist's performance. If an evaluation method could be devised, they agreed, simple cognitive tests would be unnecessary.

The Liaison Committee discussed the implications of chapter formation. Without arriving at definite conclusions, this meeting revealed some areas of mutual interest, and it seemed useful potentially to consider ways in which both societies could develop them.

## Private Initiative in PSRO

Dr. John R. Gamble, Chairman of the PSRO and Peer Review Committee, reported major developments in PSRO activity:

The American Association for Foundations for Medical Care initiated the formation of an institute for professional standards with three types of membership: Foundations for Medical Care members, specialty societies members, and general members. Its research and development activity was funded by the Kellogg Foundation and named Private Initiative in PSRO [PIPSRO].

Health, Education and Welfare [HEW] published a description of an institute which fit the original plan for the Institute of Professional Standards. A recently submitted proposal added to the original group the University of the Pacific and the School of Public Health, University of California, Berkeley, and Boston University and the Harvard School of Public Health. This institute's prime objective was to train people to do administrative work related to PSRO.

Other developments included:

1. The PSRO Regulations Committee prepared a statement for the ACP President to send to HEW, emphasizing that the College was taking a strong position against the regulations on preadmission criteria relating to Title 19 which were being established by the Social Security Administration.
2. The nine subcommittees for the San Joaquin Foundation Project were to be reconvened. It was recommended that the critical criteria required by the PSRO law be added to their duties.
3. The Committee recommended that a letter be sent to the Officers, Regents and Governors providing information about the Kellogg Grant and other information on PSRO.
4. Regional Meetings programs should include the subject of the College's role in PSRO. The Official College Representatives should be adequately informed about PSRO and be prepared to present such information at Regional Meetings.
5. Maximum publicity should be given to all College activities in PSRO. I indicated that the Executive Vice President's column in the February issue of the *ACP Bulletin* was devoted to College activities in PSRO. A page or an article on PSRO could appear every month in the *ACP Bulletin*. Such articles would include information about PIPSRO. The Kellogg Grant would contribute for publication this information about criteria development and related subjects.
6. A Committee to Develop Guidelines for PSRO's on Antibiotics was formed. Dr. Calvin F. Kay reported that a meeting was held in Philadelphia at which the following organizations were represented: the AAFP, ACP, ACS, American Academy of Pediatrics [AAP] and the Infectious Diseases Society of America. To implement the plan, Dr. Edward Kass, Chairman, would prepare a draft contract to the ACP Board of Regents for approval. The final

proposal would be submitted to HEW for implementation funds. This research study proposed to examine the experience in several hospitals in a defined area, by reviewing the hospital records on which the development of guidelines for the appropriate use of antibiotics in hospital practice would be based.

### Plans for Recertification and In-Training Examination

For a special ACP-ABIM Committee, Dr. Truman G. Schnabel, Jr., presented to the Regents the plans for recertification and in-service training examination, which they approved.

The Committee recommended the following six points be accepted as important to the recertification process, incorporating attempts to deal with the problems imposed by the difference between performance and competence.

1. That the physician's performance in practice meet standards set by a PSRO.
2. That a physician's performance be judged satisfactory by a local peer review group conducted by a section of medicine in the institution in which the physician practices.
3. That the character or profile of a physician's practice be determined for the purpose of weighing the recertification evaluation in accordance with the nature of his practice, considering his special interest as well as the types of patients he sees.
4. That the test of knowledge based on the Syllabus and the Medical Knowledge Self-Assessment Test be continued but that it be altered in the following two ways:
   a. That while the assessment of knowledge should be primarily directed toward recent advances in medicine it should also evaluate an individual's competence in well-accepted practices in medicine. The relevance of questions to his special interest and his practice profile could be determined in two ways: a) by decision of the examination committee, and b) by the candidate indicating which questions are considered relevant.
   b. That a Patient Management Problem Section be added to the assessment of knowledge as a further step in the assessment of a physician's competence, and further that by selection of the subject matter of the patient management problems, the examination might be tailored to the type of practice conducted by the physician being evaluated.
   c. That continued efforts be made to develop better ways of testing a physician's competence through the use of computerized or other written techniques, e.g., computer based examination - patient management problem (CBX-PMP).
   d. That the ACP, ABIM, AAP, American Board of Pediatrics [ABP], AAFP, and the American Board of Family Practice [ABFP], having much in common, work together in the development of better methods

of assuring a competent performance on the part of physicians in their organizations.

The Committee then requested endorsement of the following positions on the in-training examination, which the Board approved:

1. That the development of a separate new in-training examination each year was unrealistic.
2. That the College did not, therefore, wish to be involved in such an effort.
3. That the College would consider holding further discussion with the ABIM concerning the use of the self-assessment test as an in-training examination.

Dr. Robert G. Petersdorf addressed a joint meeting of the Boards of Regents and Governors on matters from the ABIM, first reviewing its procedures and composition.

Methods of electing the Board had remained essentially unchanged since it was established. The size had increased, now comprising 27 members. Board members were approved for nomination by the ACP and by the AMA Section on Internal Medicine. Holding five one-day meetings per year, the Board followed each meeting with clinical competence visits in the geographic area of the meeting. The Board was organized into the parent board, three subsidiary boards, six test committees and two conjoint boards. The subsidiary boards were in the fields of gastroenterology, pulmonary diseases and cardiology; test committees existed in hematology, endocrinology, infectious disease, rheumatology, nephrology and oncology; and conjoint boards were in allergy and immunology and in nuclear medicine. The certifying examination was given annually in June and in recent years had examined approximately 5,000 individuals per year. Subspecialty examinations were given biennially in October. A recertifying examination would be given for the first time in October, 1974.

The Board had instituted a second major program for the assessment of clinical competence, following the discontinuance of the oral examination. It had become clear that certain aspects of clinical competence, such as history taking, performance of physical examinations and evolvement of plans of management could no longer be tested. The program for assessment of clinical competence, therefore, was introduced, making it mandatory for program directors to appoint an evaluation committee which, jointly with the program director, would certify the clinical competence of candidates. Two research and development efforts were underway. The first was a computer-based examination, a project being carried out in collaboration with National Board of Medical Examiners. A second project, with the acronym MERIT was being carried on under the auspices of the University of the Pacific in San Francisco. This project was monitoring the practice of a group of internists. Dr. Schnabel also announced that Dr. Palmer Futcher, the Executive Director of the Board, had asked to be relieved of his duties in the Fall of 1975. Search plans for his successor were underway.

Chapter Four

# Unfinished Business: Primary Care

## 1974-1977

# IV. Unfinished Business: Primary Care

## Part One (1974-1975)

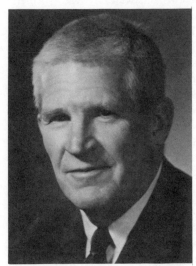

*Truman G. Schnabel, Jr., MACP*

Born in 1919 in Philadelphia, Pennsylvania, Truman G. Schnabel, Jr., married Mary Hyatt in 1947 and they have four children.

His BS degree was awarded by the Yale University Sheffield Scientific School in 1940 and he received his MD from the University of Pennsylvania in 1943. He completed his internship in medicine at the Hospital of the University of Pennsylvania in 1944. Interrupting his training, Dr. Schnabel served as Captain in the US Army Medical Corps from 1944 to 1946. On his return, he served his residencies in medicine at Massachusetts General Hospital in 1947-48 and at the Hospital of the University of Pennsylvania in 1948-49. In 1948, he was a Fellow of the American Heart Association and was a Markle Scholar in Medical Sciences from 1952 to 1957.

A specialist in cardiovascular disease and physiology, Dr. Schnabel devoted his professional life in those fields at the University of Pennsylvania. Appointed as an Instructor in 1950, he was successively an Assistant in Medicine, Assistant Professor, Associate Professor and from 1963 to 1973, Professor of Medicine. In 1973, the University honored him with appointment as full time G. Mahlon Kline Professor of Medicine, a chair he continues to hold to the present time.

On sabbatical in 1955-56, Dr. Schnabel studied with Professor Lars Werko at St. Erick's Hospital in Stockholm, Sweden. During his years with the University of Pennsylvania, he was Ward Chief at the Pennsylvania General Hospital from 1959 to 1973 and coordinated the University's Medical Service there from 1965 to 1971 and also at the VA Hospital in Philadelphia from 1973 to 1977. Since 1973, Dr. Schnabel has also served as Vice Chairman of the Department of Medicine.

Certified by the American Board of Internal Medicine in 1952, he has been a member of the ABIM and was its Secretary-Treasurer in 1971-72. He was a Member-at-Large on the National Board of Medical Examiners from 1967 to 1971, and was Assistant Secretary for Part III, from 1960 to 1968.

Dr. Schnabel's societal activities included governmental service on the Medical Education Advisory Committee of the Rehabilitation Services Administration, DHEW, from 1968 to 1971, and membership on the Clinical Research

Fellowships Review Committee of the NIH, Career Development Review Branch, Division of Research Grants, from 1966 to 1971. He is a member of the American Clinical and Climatological Association, serving as Vice President in 1968-69. He was President of the Inter-Urban Clinical Club in 1973-74. He is also a member of the American Federation for Clinical Research, American Society for Clinical Investigation, Association of American Physicians, American Physiological Society, and the Association of University Cardiologists.

Elected a Fellow of the American College of Physicians in 1947 and Master in 1975; he was Governor for Eastern Pennsylvania from 1962 to 1968; General Chairman of the 43rd Annual Session, Philadelphia, 1962; Regent, 1968 to 1973; President-Elect, 1973-74 and President, 1974-75.

During his Presidency, Dr. Schnabel made a great contribution by reviewing the entire organizational structure of the College with consulting help from the Massachusetts Institute of Technology. Presenting this review of the 1974 joint summer conference of the Board of Regents and the Board of Governors, his leadership set the College on a more stable course with improved relationships among its governing and policy bodies.

Dr. Schnabel's Presidential Address at the 1975 Annual Session introduced Sir Richard Livingston's "philosophy of the first rate" in his challenge to the ACP vocation:

> Change creates opportunity. Never before have there been so many opportunities for physicians to set the common good. Paradoxically, never have there been so many chances to literally destroy the human race. The challenge lies in the use of opportunities.

> Today, there is a desperate need: to dull the sharp cutting edge of medical technocracy with wisdom and compassion in its application; to balance the impersonal machine with your own personal touch.

> If you doubt we need more physicians skilled in the art of medicine as well as in scientific practice, you should listen to political leaders who are demanding increased numbers of physicians dedicated to providing broad and continuing care. There are countless new ways in which you may pass on your knowledge to those who follow you.

> Sir Richard Livingston, at a session of the First World Conference on Medical Education in 1953, introduced a philosophy of life which studied his purpose and gave it direction. Livingston called this philosophy the philosophy of the first rate. 'It means doing the very best that one can do and then trying to do better. For physicians, it is caring for those who seek help.' Livingston said, 'Never was a philosophy of life as necessary as in our age of divided purposes and paralyzing doubts about ultimate ends. Our civilization is fluid. Its future form still to seek and make. At present it is a curate's egg civilization. Some of it is excellent; some of it is fourth rate. Yet ours is an age of great vitality; of unlimited powers and possibilities too often frittered away or misused. We have the materials of a great civilization. All that is needed is to stamp it with the print of excellence.

Dr. Schnabel was always very proud of being a third generation physician. His grandfather, Edwin Daniel, who studied under William Osler as a member of the

1887 class at Penn, subsequently practiced in Bethlehem, PA. His father Truman G., Sr., who was a renowned Philadelphia internist, was Chief of the University of Pennsylvania Medical Service at the Philadelphia General Hospital, a former chairman of the American Board of Internal Medicine and a Vice President of ACP.

Dr. Schnabel, Jr., followed his father's traditions and was also, for 16 years, Chief of the Medical Service at the Philadelphia General Hospital.

One of Dr. Schnabel's hobbies is long distance running. On two occasions he ran in the Boston Marathon and had this to say, "I only beat one of the eight women the first time, but I fared better the second time, when I cut my time from four hours and thirty minutes to four hours and fifteen minutes." He has run in cities all over the world. In one year he clocked a total of 2,335 miles. I asked him about the possible benefits of running and he replied, "Most of us live a sedentary life. It should be interspersed with some kind of physical activity on a regular basis. If nothing else, physical activity teaches discipline and results in a sense of well being".

When my wife and I arrived in Philadelphia in September of 1959, I went to see Dr. Francis Wood, Head of the Department of Medicine at the University of Pennsylvania, about doing some volunteer teaching. After exploring my interests and available time, he advised me to see Dr. Schnabel, Head of the Penn Medical Service at the Philadelphia General Hospital. He agreed that I could take a service once or twice a year, making rounds with the intern and resident and the medical students. I continued this service for the next 17 years and soon discovered Dr. Schnabel was well respected and loved by all the residents and students. It was a stimulating experience, and one of many through which Dr. Schnabel and I became very close friends.

In 1962, he was the General Chairman for the Annual Session in Philadelphia. At the opening session, I was stunned to see that one of the lecturer's slides were melting, due to a crystallized lens in the art projector and because his slides had been made incorrectly. A friend of mine said not to worry about the slides, because he'd seen them before they bubbled and they were more interesting while they were melting.

When I had dealt with this unusual situation, and was leaving the room to get things in order for the next speaker, I met another old California friend limping into the room. He said he thought he'd broken his ankle getting off the bus. The phones from our first-aid room had not yet been connected, but Dr. Schnabel came along and said he'd send him over to the University Hospital. Later that afternoon Dr. Schnabel checked on his status, but could not find out what had happened to him. He had just disappeared. Dr. Schnabel later learned why. My friend had met a medical school classmate in the hallway at the hospital, who happened to be an orthopedist. Neglecting to initiate an admission record, the orthopedist promptly took him to the X-ray department and diagnosed a fractured ankle, reduced it and applied a splint.

During this Annual Session, the Schnabels were reluctant to share a suite at the hotel with us because they thought we would be too busy with friends, but later decided to join us in the suite. Because they had many Philadelphia friends visit them, Esther and I met a number of Philadelphians for the first time, who became our good friends.

We, of course, traveled a great deal together and had, mildly stated, some unique experiences. On our way to the 1975 Annual Session in San Francisco, we were grounded in a Chicago blizzard for 19 hours. We joined Dr. Wilbur, a former President of the College, and his group who were attending an AMA meeting at the Airport Hilton Hotel, for a makeshift dinner. In the overcrowded hotel, Esther and I shared a bedroom with the Schnabels, who slept on the mattress, while we slept on the box springs. Everyone claimed to have slept well, and the next day we were on our way again to San Francisco.

When the ACP and ASIM tried to merge, Dr. Schnabel was especially helpful in bringing people of opposite views together. I saw a lot of him also when we were beginning the Council of Medical Specialty Societies. He was later its Chairman. When the Liaison Committee on Graduate Medical Education was first created, he and I were among the few representatives who had ever participated in any type of residency training programs.

Dr. Schnabel was Chairman of the Council of Medical Specialty Societies in a most difficult year. A new executive, Richard Wilbur, had many new and good ideas but with all the cross currents of strong feelings and opinions, his ideas were not always easy to implement. In no small measure, Dr. Schnabel's kind and positive approach helped this organization over a particularly trying time.

As Chairman of the Liaison Committee on Graduate Medical Education, his steady guidance helped this organization to become a major force in graduate medical education.

He tried hard to convince the Board of Regents that graduates of the new training programs in family practice were worthy of membership in the College. Though he was disappointed that the Board did not agree, he became interested in the Board of Family Practice and was one of its members for five years.

# 1974-1975

Conference of Regents and Governors, Toronto. Steering Committee formed. *MKSAP IV* Courses. ABIM Conference on Primary Care. Internal Medicine Manpower Studies (Mendenhall/Tarlov). Federated Council of Internal Medicine. Intersociety Committee on Anti-microbial Usage. National Health Insurance. CCME: Foreign medical graduates.

## The Toronto Conference

The year 1974-75 was a significant one in the College's history. A complicated, but worthwhile, combined conference of the Board of Regents and the Board of Governors took place for the first time in Toronto, on June 16-17. Dr. E.B. Roberts, a consultant from the Massachusetts Institute of Technology's Sloan School of Management, worked with Dr. Schnabel and the executive office to develop the agenda and modus operandi of this conference.

In the introductory session of the conference Dr. Schnabel said it was clear that the College was formed in 1915 to foster the development of the internist, and to promote the discipline of internal medicine as a major specialty.

> In developing internists, the College has to play a major role in their education and does so in two ways: (1) by participating in the Internal Medicine Residency Review Committee's activities, which assures internists of the type of training essential for his future specialty and, (2) by developing a vast continuing medical education program that makes training available to the internist throughout his entire professional life.

The College had always wrestled with the problems of just how to find what an internist actually does and then to define his qualifications and delineate his actions and duties. An additional problem was how this delineation should be employed as a measure for determining qualifications for admission into the College, a society which clearly marked him as a specialist in internal medicine.

Since 1936, when College joined with the AMA Section on Medicine to form the American Board of Internal Medicine [ABIM], the Board had, through its certifying process, marked physicians as internists; therefore eligible for Fellowship in the ACP. Education had always been the College's primary mission; and through its educational programs, it has established the central role of internal medicine in relation to all its subspecialties. Dr. Schnabel observed that the College had increasingly become involved in activities other than the purely educational. In the past, it had usually declined such involvement and currently, although many of its educational activities were entwined with programs having vast social and economic implications, many of its members decried such an involvement and argued strongly against it.

But the world had changed since 1936. Medicine was no exception; it had also changed dramatically.

> Instead of dealing with patients on a one-to-one basis, a third party, the payor has become interposed; health has become a right and not a privilege; the philosophy that stresses ambulatory care as opposed to hospital care is being debated; the provider of care, the physician, has become more and more broad in his training; aided and abetted by an increasing number of assistants, while on the other hand he is being helped by a smaller number of subspecialists who are able to sort out difficult problems and maintain life in those critically ill or totaled disabled.

Dr. Schnabel asked the conference to explore how the College should respond to these changes and whether it was acting on these changes as it should.

Dr. Jeremiah A. Barondess, Chairman of the Board of Governors, emphasized a significant degree of unspoken agreement between the two Boards; the time seemed right to assess the College's goals and its internal and external ambitions. The current governance structure represented considerable enlargement and elaboration of the basic administrative arrangements of several previous decades. Fundamentally, this structure consisted of a strong central apparatus, the Board of Regents and the central administration, initiating and developing policies, with a peripheral effector arrangement, relying on individual Governors in their individual jurisdictions to implement those policies and promote membership matters.

He challenged the conference to consider whether the present governance structure was optimal; not just adequate, but optimal for present and projected areas of interest. He also asked whether the present role of our membership as consumers of the fruit of centrally conceived and developed policies needed to be changed; whether the College really wanted to decentralize to promote more input from the membership. This was one of the central issues in the divided reactions to the Chapter concept. Posing a third question, he asked whether the strength of the College would be enhanced if the Board of Governors assumed an input role in the development of policy. Governors bridged the distance between the membership and this central apparatus; a vital and unique position. Finally, he asserted that the increasing complexity of the climate in which the members practice and teach now included environmental and social factors in human health and a rapidly expanding interface between medicine and government and between the College and other organizations and bodies; all were parts of the rapidly expanding systemization of medicine.

E. B. Roberts, PhD, Professor of Management of The Sloan School of Management at the Massachusetts Institute of Technology, challenged the conference in his address, "Meeting Change In Today's Health Environment". Important changes were occurring in all professional fields, including medicine and its specialties. Organizations must make decisions for purposeful change or things would change for the worse.

Dr. Roberts perceived that fundamental to the College's future was the decision about what the "Core Mission" of the College had been and what it should be. Any changes in structure must, of necessity, be related to this "Core Mission". To be effective, the "Core Mission" must be what the College wanted it to be. The problems about the roles each body would play to make these decisions rested in the hands of the Board of Governors and the Board of Regents. In an extended period of questions, Dr. Roberts reiterated more strongly the points of his address.

Six workshops followed his address. The first, "Initiation and Development of American College of Physicians' Policy," was chaired by Drs. Jack D. Myers and William B. Spaulding. In summary, this workshop concluded that new mechanisms were needed to allow responses from the membership on major policy proposals.

1. The Board of Governors should have a stronger role in policy decision-making. In 1973, the Board of Governors had been given only the right to review decisions, after policies were made. Input from membership and the Board of Governors should be sought before policies were established.
2. The committees of the College should be structured with adequate tenure and continuity of membership to strengthen their role of presenting alternatives in developing policy.
3. Top leadership should have more continuity.

4. The use of periodic or continuing outside consultants probably would aid the College in the process of change. The College should strive to evaluate the effect of any current or new policies on the quality of medical care implemented by the College.

The second workshop, "Implementation of ACP Policies at the Local Level," was moderated by Drs. George W. Pedigo and William H. Bunn, Jr.

The advantages and disadvantages of chapter formation were discussed and some alternative suggestions to the formation of chapters were offered. The workshop also examined what Governors and Regents do as bodies and what Governors do as individuals. Some additional functions for Governors were defined, such as stimulating the scientific and professional advancement of local members, establishing very close liaison with the chairmen of the departments of medicine, stimulating active participation and sustaining interest of members by appointment to local committees.

The third workshop, "Implementation of ACP Policies at the National Level," was chaired by Drs. Walter B. Frommeyer, Jr. and Francis J. Sweeney, Jr., and reached the following conclusions:

1. Current mechanisms of policy implementation seemed satisfactory.
2. A feasibility study was suggested to test ACP policy development for possible impact on the Washington scene, utilizing local ACP members to inform Congressmen and delineating key questions that needed professional clarification.
3. The government doesn't really know what internal medicine is. The ACP is not recognized as speaking for internal medicine; but it must be able to influence people in Washington, on such issues as physician distribution, primary care, the accessibility, quality, and costs of care. If the ACP made policy decisions on issues of social importance, there would be a demand for more democracy in its actions, such as greater input from Governors and members.

The fourth workshop, "Interaction of the ACP With Government and the Public," was chaired by Drs. Stuart O. Bondurant and Robert M. Byrd.

After evaluating the College's role with other organizations in governmental interactions, this group concluded that the American College of Physicians should pursue a course of action to represent more directly the interests of the membership and to educate both government and the public as to the nature of the work done by College internists. It endorsed individual testimony before legislative committees. The College should also continue to offer its support to those organizations already existing whose interests and efforts parallel its own in regard to federal health legislation and regulation. The tradition of education of physicians for medical practice should be extended to health education for the public.

Drs. John R. Gamble and Thomas F. Frawley moderated the fifth workshop on "Interaction With Outside Organizations and Agencies".

Relationships of the College with specialty societies of internal medicine and with the American Academy of Family Physicians [AAFP] were considered important. The group reviewed extensively the relationship with the American Board of Family Physicians [ABFP] and the role of the internist as primary care physician and called for better definition. The American Society of Internal Medicine [ASIM] and the College, it suggested, should be complementary and not in opposition to one another. Although the primary principle— that the College's role should be in education and the ASIM's in socioeconomic matters— could be easily defined, jurisdictional borders were blurred. The "Phoenix accord" should be reexamined in light of the College's "Core Mission", and further liaison activity encouraged.

The final workshop, "Interaction between the Regents, Governors, ACP Committees and ACP Membership" was moderated by Drs. William F. Kellow and Robert M. Kark.

Consensus here was that our most important product was education. In the area of ACP-ASIM relations, the ASIM represented mainly the financial concerns of physicians. In common, both organizations placed emphasis on meeting the needs of society. Consideration should be given to maintaining a dialogue at the highest levels of the two societies, so that while each pursued its special interests, they could talk with one voice to society and government. In the area of ACP policy jurisdiction, the two governing bodies should continue as before, with Governors representing the voice of the membership, in an advisory relationship to the Board of Regents.

Dr. Schnabel thanked the Board of Regents and Board of Governors for their excellent review of these issues, saying, "I want the group discussions reported to everyone, not the Governors only". We must . . . plan to continue the momentum of this meeting". He reflected the general agreement that the Core Mission of the College really is, whatever else it is, education and scholarship.

> The flow of events in our society and our world indicates that education and scholarship, [to] which the College has always pointed for reaching individual members, should be sustained, and we should be cognizant of the fact that it is related, more than ever, to the quality of medical care. We do know something about some part of our mission and also that the mission should be broadened so that it includes the quality of medical care delivered to the public.

### Regents Review Conference

In his Presidential Report to the Board of Regents meeting in November, 1974, Dr. Schnabel reflected on the rapid growth of the College; 800 new members were admitted in 1972, 1,800 in 1973, and 2,000 during the current year. The College had already enlarged its scope of activities far beyond its former primary objective of merely educating its own members. As President, he quickly discovered that he had to speak out on issues, such as Professional Standards Review Organizations [PSROs] and the impact of medicine on inflation, for example. From discussions with officers in other organizations, he reached the disturbing conclusion that while the College seemed to be strong, visible and respected, individual general internal medicine practitioners were being given very little consideration in the country's burgeoning health system.

The new emphasis of family practice, paradoxically, stressed the importance of the discipline of internal medicine since it needed internists as teachers. Dr. Schnabel called upon the College to champion the cause of the internist as the premier primary care physician. He considered it imperative that the ASIM, the ACP, the ABIM, and the Association of Professors of Medicine [APM] work together to present internists as able primary care physicians. He believed that the College should accept well-trained family practitioners for membership, as the interests of family practitioners and general internists coincided closely and the educational programs of the College would be of great value to any physician engaged in primary care.

Surveying the results of the Regents' and Governors' Conference in Toronto in June, he noted that a broadened policy had been accepted conceptually, with direct implications for changes in operational structure. The first results were reflected in the formation of a Steering Committee, consisting of equally represented Governors and Regents. The essential governance changes were aimed at greatly increasing involvement by the membership.

The Treasurer, Dr. William F. Kellow, indicated a positive financial result from operations in 1974. The net operational income was expected to approximate $1,121,000, including $748,000 from the *Medical Knowledge Self-Assessment Program III [MKSAP III]* program. Since *MKSAP* was issued every three years, the Board had decided a year previously to spread the income from this program over three years. Therefore, $498,000 would be deferred to equalize the budget for the years 1975 and 1976. The College's legal advisors had no new actions to report regarding the claim for refund of advertising income taxes.

The A. G. Becker Company reported that investment results for the year ending in June, 1974, had been below average, although income had been rather high. Capital preservation in the current fair market and appreciation of capital during the bull markets had been poor. The Finance Committee and the Investment Committee were considering policies to assure that this would have no critical impact on the College's portfolio.

The committee appointed to prepare a statement on College policies and the newly appointed Steering Committee both had important results to present. The new Steering Committee recommendations were based on the joint meeting of the Board of Regents and Governors. In my judgment, I stated, primary care was going to be the arena of action in the next few years, and the College must take a leadership role in the promotion of internal medicine as a primary care specialty. Although the heads of departments of medicine gave strong support to the idea, the facts indicated that the largest number of professors in medical departments were subspecialists. Predictably there would be varying levels of understanding and interest in the promotion of internists as primary care physicians among faculties of medicine.

The Committee on Medical Services had studied the family practice movement and made reports at frequent intervals from 1965 to 1968. The College had gone on record as cooperating with the AMA Council on Medical Education and others in the formation of the ABFP. I suggested that each Regent should ask not whether admitting the newly trained and certified family physicians to College membership was good for ACP, but whether it was in the best public interest to admit them. The longer they continued their education, the better doctors they would be. The educational programs of the College would benefit them, and they were less likely to partake of these programs as nonmembers. I pointed out that the College had discovered years ago, when it decided to retain Members who did not achieve Fellowship, that few of those who had been dropped ever came to College meetings or courses. According to the present interpretation of membership criteria, the College admitted as Members those who had received their training in approved hospitals and had taken the ABIM examination, whether they passed or not.

I reported for the Audio-Visual Committee and the *Medical Skills Library* Subcommittee that the two patient counseling films on "Heartburn" and "High Blood Pressure" were progressing well. Additional topics being explored were diabetes mellitus, arthritis, ischemic heart disease, and duodenal ulcer. Preliminary analysis revealed that the potential buyers of the counseling films would be groups of individuals in practice and physicians in clinic-conjoint practice. This series was to be titled, *Patient Counseling Library*.

For the *Medical Skills Library* the following subjects were selected: IPPB (already in progress), emergency removal of superficial foreign bodies from the eye, gastric lavage, and venipuncture.

## Mastership Defined

Dr. Edmund B. Flinck, Chairman of the Awards, Masterships, Honorary and Corresponding Fellowships Committee, presented guidelines for the bestowal of Masterships to the College, stating:

> The award of Mastership . . . has traditionally been reserved for those Fellows of the College whose unique record of achievement embraces the highest standards of clinical performance, of outstanding qualities such as academic attainment, of universally recognized abilities of sustained leadership and traits of character which further distinguished that person.

Specific guidelines for selection of Masters were also approved by the Board:

1. The award of Mastership in itself stipulates that the candidate has either made major contributions to the College or has demonstrated unswerving interest in its affairs.

2. The physician candidate should be one who is sensitive to the fundamental human values of medical practice in its broadest sense. If a nonacademician, the candidate should have demonstrated these same qualities of being responsive to patients and to the career development of medical students, house officers and

junior faculty. He or she should be helpful to younger physicians and to the community, and these contributions should be national in their impact and so recognized by the medical community.

3. The College stands for upholding the highest principles of medicine. Candidates from a medical school setting should have shown through their long record of achievement that they are true clinicians who have practiced and taught comprehensive medicine in the fullest extent. Locally and nationally, the nominee should be known not only for clinical ability but for contributions as a clinical investigator through writings and other educational pursuits.

4. Although there should not be any specified age requirement, it is generally thought that the above mentioned attainments could not be achieved until the physician had demonstrated academic and human qualities over a span of time, that would assure maturity.

Because of traditional difficulties in differentiating between Honorary and Corresponding Fellows, the Committee recommended that the Corresponding Fellow category be dropped and that all current Corresponding Fellows be made Honorary Fellows. The Board agreed to discontinue the Corresponding Fellow category.

Dr. Charles H. Rammelkamp, Chairman of the Constitution and Bylaws Committee, requested a number of specific changes in the Bylaws, among which was an addition, designating that six members of the Board of Regents would be elected by the Board of Governors.

The qualifications for election to Membership and Fellowship were changed. In the future, candidates for Membership would be elected in the local area. Those to be elected directly or by advancement to Fellowship would continue to be proposed by the Credentials Committee and elected by the Board of Regents.

Dr. Lawrence T. Young, Chairman of the Educational Activities Committee, received approval to initiate development of *MKSAP IV,* projected for distribution in October, 1976. He stated that this would be coordinated with a second Recertification examination by the ABIM, scheduled in October, 1977. Dr. Young would serve as general chairman for *MKSAP IV.*

After a review of the audio-visual programs, the Committee wished to voice its opinion that those aids being developed by the College were serving a useful function. In the near future, the Department of Academic Affairs in the Association of American Medical Colleges [AAMC] and the National Library of Medicine's Educational Materials Project would be conducting studies on the usefulness and availability of audio-visual aids. Our Committee would meet in the near future with Dr. Robert Byrd of the Lister Hill National Center for the National Library of Medicine, Dr. James MacArthur of The University of Washington's Health Sciences Learning Center, and with Dr. William Spaulding and Dr. Edithe Levit, members of the Educational Activities Committee.

Dr. Jack D. Myers, Chairman, reviewed the Finance Committee's report of anticipated operating results. Projected net income from operations for 1974 was approximately $1,121,200, before appropriations to the Endowment and Building Funds and reservation of the two thirds income from *MKSAP III.* The projected net income increase of $769,800 over the $363,700 reported for 1973 was attributable to *MKSAP III,* which would earn for the College approximately $748,000 in 1974. A comparison of the total income from the previous *MKSAPs* showed a net income for Program I of $84,251, Program II, $148,995, and Program III, $748,914. Net income from the *Annals* was estimated to be $205,900, a decrease of approximately $9,200 from 1973. Advertising rates had been increased, resulting in fewer paid advertising pages, which accounted for this small difference. An increase in fees in 1973 resulted in a Postgraduate Courses net income of $27,640, offsetting the deficit of $10,254 from the previous year. The net deficit for the Annual Session was $192,421, an increase of $7,434 over the deficit of the 1973 Annual Session in Chicago. Considering this loss, the Finance Committee again recommended charging the members a registration fee for the San Francisco session in 1975, but the Board again delayed the decision.

Building Fund contributions showed that 11,496 Masters, Fellows and Members had contributed a total of $599,125. Very few still owed any outstanding assessments.

Adjustments in the College's medical coverage and life insurance plan were approved by the Board. These arose from the previous agreement that I would continue in office until age 68, subject to annual review and appointment. The provisions allowed for full coverage for employees working beyond age 65. My supplemental retirement benefits were also approved.

### Statements Approved: Primary Care, Emergency Care, Specialized Clinical Services

Dr. John R. Gamble reported two meetings of the Medical Practice Committee since the Annual Session and presented several items for action:

1. The Committee requested and received endorsement in principle of a document from the Residency Review Committee in Internal Medicine [RRC-IM] on primary medical care, which defined the internist as a primary care provider.
2. A revised document on Emergency Care written by Dr. Douglas B. McGill was reviewed and approved for publication in the *ACP Bulletin.*
3. The following statement on specialized clinical services in response to a communication from the Joint Commission on Accreditation of Hospitals [JCAH] was approved by the Board of Regents as a resolution of the American College of Physicians:

The Listing Program for Specialized Clinical Services of the JCAH has published a seven-volume catalogue of clinical facilities for stroke, heart disease, cancer and end-stage kidney disease based upon responses to questionnaires from hospitals. It had also developed and published criteria for categorizing hospitals into levels of capability for providing diagnosis and treatment of these disorders. It is now validating the questionnaire information and studying the feasibility of applying the criteria for categorized hospitals.

The Regents of the ACP recognize the potential value of this project for upgrading the quality of care, for cost containment in efficient utilization of facilities and personnel, in the assistance it provides in regional health planning and, hopefully, in reduction of morbidity and mortality in major diseases.

They also recognize that the adoption of categorization of hospitals in this manner as a potential basis for payment or nonpayment for services and/or for malpractice or other litigation poses a serious threat to essential human elements that must enter into medical decisions.

The Regents recommend to the JCAH that any categorization shall have the specific statement attached to all publications as follows:

The categorization of the clinical facilities described herein shall not be the basis for payment or nonpayment of fees for services, and should not provide the basis for malpractice or other litigation since essential human elements in medical care has not been and cannot be categorized by this or other known method.

Dr. Malcolm Peterson, reported that 53 schools had sought and received approval to organize programs for assistants to the primary care physician. There were at that time 1,000 graduates annually from these schools. Although the number of graduates was increasing, the rate was beginning to level off.

The Board agreed with the Medical Practice Committee on two general directions for its future activities: 1) the development of national policy statements on issues of importance in the area of health care delivery, especially in relation to other organizations working in the same area of primary care; and 2) increased attention to services to ACP members. It also approved addition of a staff person to assist the Committee.

Dr. Gamble, who was also Chairman of the PSRO and Peer Review Committee, noted that 91 Regions of the country were planning PSROs, and 11 conditional awards had been made to date.

The project, Private Initiative for PSRO [PIPSRO], funded by the Kellogg Foundation, had selected six sites for pilot study implementation. In compliance with the plan described, each of six PSRO districts selected by PIPSRO had agreed to abide by PSRO guidelines. The teams had been recruited, and separate function cost analyses would be performed for each district.

The AMA had received a $1 million contract to define criteria of care which was being administered through the Interspecialty Advisory Council. The Council involved a variety of groups in internal medicine including the College and ASIM. The ASIM and the College representatives were assigned to the Committee to draw up these criteria and to supervise their implementation where there were overlaps in internal medicine.

The JCAH was cooperating with the PSRO by writing into its regulations "that a hospital accredited by JCAH which does its utilization review, medical audit, etc., could be considered a delegate hospital." The Board of Commissioners would further strengthen this support with additional statements so that all PSRO requirements would be met.

Dr. Jack D. Myers presented the completed statement of ACP policies and the plan for implementation.

The document was published in the *ACP Bulletin* in January, 1975, and reprints were available for general distribution. The document covered the College's positions on educational policy and health care activities. Educational policy addressed efforts in continuing medical education and in recertification. Activities in graduate medical education in conjunction with the ABIM were set out in great detail. The College activities and relationships with the RCC-IM, the Coordinating Council on Medical Education [CCME], the Liaison Committee on Graduate Medical Education [LCGME], and the Council of Academic Societies [CAS] of the AAMC were included in detail. A position statement about financing of graduate medical education and approaches to setting policy for undergraduate medical education and allied health education were defined. In health care activities, the policy statement defined College positions on assessment of quality of medical care in internal medicine and on the organization of medical practice. In the latter statement, policy in matters of primary care, emergency and intensive care, prepaid medical care systems, and the organization and activities for internal medicine in the hospital were defined. Finally, the statement addressed the issues of manpower requirements and their financing, medical liability problems and public education regarding medical and health care.

### First Steering Committee Meets

The Steering Committee held its first meeting in September, 1974. It examined the Core Mission of the College and decided that its ultimate priority was quality medical care. The following statement was submitted and approved:

> The American College of Physicians is dedicated to maintaining and advancing the quality of patient care in internal medicine and allied specialties. The College accomplishes this through graduate and continuing education; by activities pertaining to the availability and effectiveness of physicians; and by concerning itself with matters of public policy as related to internal medicine.

The Steering Committee would consist of the President, President-Elect, three Regents, Chairman of the Board of Governors, Vice Chairman of the Board of Governors, and three Governors nominated by the Governors' Nominating Committee and elected by the full Board.

The Executive Committee of the Board of Regents was to continue with five members, the President, President-Elect, and the three Regents representing the Board of Regents on the new Steering Committee. The changes approved provided that the Governors' Nominating Committee would present six names to the Board of Governors for election to the Board of Regents. No more than two Regents would be elected in any one year until these six Regents had been elected by the Board of Governors. It was not necessary that the person elected by the Board of Governors be a sitting Governor during his term as a Regent. A recommendation that Governors be elected within the local jurisdiction by direct ballot was defeated, but action to elect Members locally was approved.

The Ad Hoc Committee on Medical Educational Opportunities for Minority Groups, appointed in April, 1971, by Dr. Hugh R. Butt, President, was charged to propose means of addressing the following concerns:

1. How ACP might help with medical education problems for all minority groups.
2. How to foster minority group participation in ACP affairs (e.g., officers, boards, committees, PG courses and regional activities.)
3. How to address the complex questions pertaining to delivery of good medical care among minorities.

In 1971, Dr. Butt related that some members of the College had questioned whether singling out minority groups of physicians for special consideration was in itself discriminatory and hence undesirable. However, the Committee was assured of the appropriateness of appointing such a committee by the overwhelmingly favorable response from the minorities themselves. The College, according to Dr. Butt, had been criticized openly in a few instances for failure to involve minorities in official activities.

The Committee first determined the number and educational status of the minorities, a most difficult task because of legal restrictions which prohibited questions on race, creed and color. In 1967, there were 4,800 members of the National Medical Association with 540 listed as internal medicine specialists, with approximately 110 of those board certified.

The Committee met frequently from 1971-1975, accomplishing a number of positive actions.

1. Questionnaires to Governors revealed that there were about 100 black physicians in the ACP and 134 representing other minorities.
2. The Postgraduate Committee scheduled courses at Meharry Medical School and Howard Medical School. Dr. Jack Myers served as visiting professor to Meharry. The course at Howard, however, was cancelled due to inadequate registration.
3. The ACP was in an excellent position to offer advice and help to department heads at Howard and Meharry and, on occasion, was requested to assist in searching for faculty members.
4. Activities in Puerto Rico and other Carribbean countries were referred to the International Medical Activities Committee.
5. Through the auspices of Dr. Chester Cassel, Governor for Florida, ACP members became quite active in encouraging qualified Cuban refugee physicians to participate in ACP activities. More than 10 of these became members of ACP.
6. Dr. W. Lester Henry had been elected to Board of Regents. Another black physician, Dr. Alvin Thompson, was elected Governor for Washington.
7. Attempts to establish an ongoing liaison with the National Medical Association did not bear fruit, but several meetings were held with Drs. Carl Meischenheim and Everett Rhoades, who were representatives of the Indian Health Service, which the College encouraged to publish material in the *Annals*. The Committee also suggested that Indian Health Service hospitals be informed about the advisory consultation services offered by the College for the development of approved training programs in internal medicine.

8. The committee was discharged in April, 1975, and continued work in these issues were referred to appropriate standing committees of the College.

## ABIM Conference on Primary Care

The American Board of Internal Medicine held a special Conference on Primary Care in Big Sky, Montana, which was followed by a meeting of representatives from the ACP, ASIM, ABIM and APM. They met informally and proposed that a federation for internal medicine be established, to act as a spokesman for internal medicine. Structure would be loosely construed with each of the organizations probably naming three representatives to such a federation, meeting as necessary to make statements in behalf of internal medicine. After approval by the four bodies, further meetings would be held. The Board of Regents approved the idea in principle, which later resulted in a very significant move, the official formation of the Federated Council for Internal Medicine [FCIM].

In a report from the ABIM, Dr. Sol J. Farber, Chairman, submitted some interesting figures on the pass rate for candidates taking the examination. Of 5,200 candidates who took the examination in 1974, 55.7 percent passed, a total of 2,900. Of American graduates who were first takers, 84 percent passed, of foreign medical graduates who were first takers only 37 percent passed. This phenomenon was generally true in all specialties. In a recent statement, the American Board of Medical Specialties [ABMS] reported that for seven years foreign medical graduates had about a 50 percent chance of passing.

Dr. Farber discussed in some detail the position of ABIM on the primary care issue. The Board considered general internal medicine to be a prime component of primary care. Ambulatory care should be included in the training of physicians in internal medicine. Such subjects as dermatology, office gynecology, psychiatry, nonoperative orthopedics should be considered in the training of the primary care physician.

The ABIM had recently reorganized itself to establish two councils, one on general internal medicine and the other on subspecialty medicine. In addition, the Board would now have officially elected representatives from the ACP, the ASIM, and the APM. In a recent report of the ABMS, it was noted that about 60,000 or 17 percent of all physicians in the United States considered themselves to be internists. This was through an AMA questionnaire. Interestingly, among all interns and residents who were then on duty, 22 percent were in internal medicine, showing a close parallel between the number in training as internists and those in practice who identified themselves as internists. In contrast, the study showed that 55,000 in practice considered themselves family practitioners, but only 1,000 interns and residents were training in family practice. By 1978, however, the study predicted that there might be 10,000 in training in family practice. It was obvious that internists were replacing themselves in the population of physicians but that family practitioners were not. Finally, Dr. Farber presented the ABIM's white paper, ''Position on Primary Care of the Board of

Internal Medicine Training and Certifying the Primary Care Physician,'' issued September 11, 1974.

Responding to the position paper, the Board of Regents passed the following resolution:

Recognizing the role of the ABIM in setting standards of training to qualify for the certifying examination in internal medicine and in the accreditation of residencies in internal medicine, the Board resolves that:

1. The ABIM will continue to certify excellent primary care physicians.
2. Residencies in internal medicine must include specific training for the provision of primary care internal medicine without compromising proven excellence.
3. The ABIM believes that the teaching and practice of general internal medicine are the core and the principal function of departments of internal medicine. Attractive facilities for ambulatory care and an environment that emphasizes the need for and the development of internists for primary care should be available.
4. Recognizing the public need for excellent primary care physicians in general internal medicine, the ABIM advocates the prompt establishment and funding of a substantial number of new residency positions of high quality in internal medicine.
5. Experience with ambulatory patients and with disciplines such as dermatology, office gynecology, musculoskeletal medicine, otolaryngology, and psychiatry should be assured.
6. In order to provide continued validation of the Board's current and future assessment procedures, the ABIM will participate with other organizations examining the quality and type of care which internists deliver.

The Board also passed a resolution to accept in principle the position of the Residency Review Document Committee on Primary Medical Care: "The Internist as a Primary Care Provider". In part, the statement presented to the Board of Governors and the Board of Regents read:

The American College of Physicians fully recognizes and endorses the concept that a genuine national need exists for increased numbers of physicians trained and prepared to provide primary care.

The present-day internists devote a major share of their time to primary care and are a significant force in meeting the current demands for this type of medical practitioner. They often combine this particular type of professional effort with the offering of specialty professional competence in a wide variety of medical subspecialties. This dual role of the internist has been of critical importance in meeting our current national health needs and should be continued.

In the future, increased numbers of physicians skilled in the delivery of primary care will depend essentially on training programs in internal medicine and pediatrics as well as in family practice.

The statement also included perspectives on first contact, a one-to-one personal relationship, continuity of care, and comprehensiveness in primary care:

A personal relationship implies that the internist or any physician providing primary care is recognized as the patient's personal physician by both the patient and the physician. Through the mediation of the personal physician, access must be on both an outpatient and in-hospital basis.

Probably the main ingredient (given appropriate training in primary medical care) is continuity of treatment. It facilitates sound relationships, and builds patient confidence.

The type of problem encountered in primary care will range from the simple to the complex. Usually the patient is ambulatory, but at times may require more specialized services and treatment only available in the hospital. In such cases, the physician providing primary care still remains the patient's physician of record. To provide such comprehensive care, certain specialized training is necessary.

Residency training programs in internal medicine should have adequate amounts of training in the ambulatory as well as in the hospital setting. Training may also include appropriate education in fields such as pediatrics, psychiatry, dermatology, office gynecology, otolaryngology, ophthalmology, and nonoperative orthopedics.

## JCAH Future Policy and Evaluation

Dr. John A. Layne reported that in November, 1974, the JCAH was to have a special meeting to discuss exclusively future policy and evaluation of past activities. He reviewed as background for the Board of Regents a sketch of the Joint Commissions' major activities in the previous ten years.

The Hospital Accreditation Program had been almost completely revised. Surveys were being done more frequently, were longer, and the more detailed information obtained was systematically reviewed. In 1970, the first overall revision of the standards in 19 years was completed. The major emphasis of accreditation had moved to focus on the quality of professional services in hospitals. Medical and other professional staff programs for its enhancement were required for continued accreditation.

Accreditation programs in special categories had been established for long-term care facilities, facilities and services for developmentally disabled and mentally retarded in a variety of psychiatric facilities. Each was self-supporting and guided by the national organizations.

As an outgrowth of highly successful professional educational programs dealing with standards, methods of retrospective evaluation studies of patient care as well as concurrent monitoring of the quality and appropriateness of care were being designed.

These activities were now being sustained on a budget that had grown from half a million dollars a year to $6.6 million, and the staff had grown from 20 to 250. Significantly, throughout that decade the annual financial support of member organizations, including the College, had remained substantially level and the Board of Commissioners continued their endeavor to assure that all new or expanded activities would be self-supporting. The special meeting was particularly timely to the question of private sector participation in national programs which was being challenged. The future of voluntary professional accreditation was in some jeopardy of government encroachment.

Having begun as an internal effort within the health professions, accreditation was intended primarily to provide objective perspective and guidance in meeting professionally developed standards. Originally, it meant reasonable conformance to minimum standards and evidence of progress toward further improvement. Within the health field, however, accreditation began to be used as an index of acceptability by arbiters of educational qualification and by private insurers. Third parties had since become more predominantly public, and with awakened consumer concern it was not surprising that accreditation had become, paradoxically, synonomous with warranty of full conformance with national standards. The need for the Commission to review its policies and programs in detail was compelling.

## Annual Session 1975

In his final report as President to the Board of Regents in San Francisco, April, 1975, Dr. Schnabel surveyed with satisfaction the results of the Toronto meeting. It inaugurated a new era in relations between the Regents and Governors, best exemplified by the new Steering Committee, which he believed would become the most important committee in the College structure. He also noted that the first recertification examination in medicine became a reality, from which both the College and internal medicine in general had profited. The Federated Council for Internal Medicine had also become a reality and was already a strong single voice for internal medicine. He spoke with hope that it would become the vehicle for closer cooperation between the College and the ASIM in the coming years.

In his last report as President-Elect, Dr. Robert G. Petersdorf presented his goals for his presidential year. He planned to expand the educational efforts in the use of audio-visual techniques to make continued learning readily available and convenient to both practicing and academic physician at home through programs sponsored by the College. Sophisticated programs of audio-visual materials could be letting the internist pace himself to his own learning style.

His second objective emphasized ways in which the College could be related in a more meaningful way to the subspecialty societies. No single society currently represented the subspecialty areas. The College could become a unifying force and should explore these possibilities. He announced that a search process would be initiated to find my replacement as the Executive Vice President.

Presenting my own perspectives on the Toronto meeting and the appointment of a Steering Committee, I viewed the events as a kind of "water shed" period in the College's history. This activity had real potential for smoothing out the information lag between Regents and Governors. I applauded the efforts in recertification; the next *Medical Knowledge Self-Assessment Program* would certainly include many more people because many had been convinced that the College was making recertification possible for any of those who wished to do it.

Progress in the search for a physician to staff the work of the Medical Practice Committee was slow, handicapping the Committee. I recommended, therefore, that selection of a physician for this Committee should be done after the new

Executive Vice President was appointed. In the meantime, other staffing would be provided for this Committee. The College was becoming a real leader in the health care area, e.g., the PSRO activities, etc. Through this type of activity, a great increase in local participation by the members was evident. I had reported to the Board of Governors on the previous day that two Chapters had already been formed and 15 other areas were studying the matter.

I announced the historic occasion on which, in Florida, a Governor of the College, for the first time, had been elected by a mail vote of the membership. Recalling changes in the Bylaws at the 1974 Annual Session, I mentioned the section concerning election of Governors which specified that local nominations from the canvas of the constituent membership should be forwarded to the central Nominating Committee, which would select one candidate, whose name would be published in the *ACP Bulletin*. In the absence of any subsequent nomination that candidate would be declared elected. However, if additional candidates were nominated by petition of 10 percent of the total membership, a ballot would be prepared and circulated to the members of that region. This is what occurred in Florida.

In matters of primary care, I believed the College had shown real leadership in dealing with the contemporary significance of these issues. We had made great strides, enhancing the visibility of internal medicine as a discipline devoted to primary care. Without the College's efforts and the support of the ABIM and the Residency Review Committee in Internal Medicine and others, government funding would gravitate increasingly toward family practice, considering it the principal or only group delivery primary care. I reminded the Board of Regents that the College could not rest on those efforts. The problem of the relationship of internal medicine practitioners and those in family practice would continue.

Finally, I reflected my concerns about the number of intertwining organizations springing up in the American medical field. This phenomenon hadn't always helped the effort to develop a unified voice. We were currently supporting the Council of Medical Specialty Societies, the only route by which the College could have even indirect representation on such other super organizations as the Coordinating Council on Medical Education. CCME had five directly represented groups, American Hospital Association [AHA], AAMC, American Medical Association [AMA], ABMS and the Council of Medical Specialty Societies [CMSS]. The College was also represented in the same way on the LCGME. Difficulties in getting all of these rather independent bodies to work actively in unison were common. Complete concurrence from all the parent organizations on every issue was next to impossible. In the present transitional stage, ineffectiveness were apparent.

In conclusion, I indicated that the new addition to the College headquarters was very helpful in providing room for expansion. About one third of two vacant floors had been opened up. There was no question that Staff support for new programs would quickly take up the six floors in a very few years. I also reminded the Board that the College currently owned eight houses near the College on the adjoining street, purchased several years before to provide for expansion. I was pleased to note incidentally that the physicians in Holland had purchased almost 400 of the *MKSAP III* programs. I had been invited to talk to several hospitals and medical centers in Holland on my way to the meeting of the Royal Australasian College in Sydney, where I gave an address on the maintenance of standards in internal medicine.

## Local Elections of Governors

The new procedures for electing Governors locally, referred to in my report to the Board, were presented by the Steering Committee to the Board of Governors and in November, 1974, recommended to the Board of Regents for approval. The plan provided for the following:

In each jurisdictional area, a Nominating Committee is appointed by the Governor, which will include appropriate representatives from both the academic and practicing communities where applicable, to nominate at least two candidates for Governor-Elect or, if necessary, for Governor. The names of these candidates will be forwarded to the Central Nominating Committee. The Central Nominating Committee will review all nominees to insure adequate representation.

The Central Committee will name two candidates, at least one of those submitted by the Local Nominating Committee, for each jurisdictional area. The names of these two candidates will then be published in the *ACP Bulletin*. Additional candidates may be named by petition of not less than 10 percent of the total membership of that area, but not less than five (5) members. A ballot will then be prepared in each region and will be submitted to all constituent members in that region for election by mail vote.

In the absence of any subsequent nominations, a suitably prepared curriculum vitae and the names of the candidates will be printed on a ballot. This will be mailed to all members in each area for a mail vote.

The ballots will be returned to the headquarters, where the votes will be counted, and the names of the elected governors published in the *ACP Bulletin*.

The Board approved the full proposal and presented it to the membership at the Annual Business Meeting on April 10, 1975. It was approved and incorporated into the Bylaws.

The Secretary-General, Dr. Richard W. Vilter, reported that the total membership of the College stood at 30,488, of which 126 were Masters, 12,934 Fellows, 7,831 Members, 9,272 Associates, 203 Affiliate Members, and 122 were Honorary Fellows.

The Steering Committee, hearing the progress report of the primary care study underway at the University of Southern California [USC] agreed that this study should replace the program previously initiated by the ACP. The study methods were very similar to what the College had proposed and the program at USC was adequately funded by the Johnson Foundation. The US Bureau of Health Services would probably participate in the statistical analyses.

Activities of the Audio-Visual Committee had led to some interesting new developments and the Board of Regents directed the the Committee to develop a plan of action aimed at the use of audio-visual techniques to supplement the educational goals of the College. The College was invited to join the Public Service Satellite Consortium [PSSC], and the Board accepted this invitation for further study. The Committee had heard from Robert Byrd, of the Lister Hill Center, a detailed discussion about potential governmental uses of satellite communications, which suggested important implications for their use in medical education.

James McArthur, of the University of Washington's Health Sciences Learning Resource Center, described to the Committee in detail some short courses directed to the practicing physicians, which they had developed in hematology, utilizing a combination of slides, tapes and written material.

The Joint Committee on Accreditation of Training Programs for Assistants to the Primary Care Physician was the subject of a request for action presented by the Medical Practice Committee.

The Joint Committee requested the support of the ACP to form a generic commission to include all physicians' assistants programs. Primary care physicians' assistants represented the largest of three groups, the others being the surgical and the OB-GYN physicians' assistants. The commission would establish criteria applicable to all assistants in any discipline.

## Delineating Hospital Privileges by the Medical Staff

The Medical Practice Committee also presented the final draft of the position paper on "Delineating Hospital Privileges by the Medical Staff," which the Board approved for publication in the *ACP Bulletin*. It appeared in the June, 1975 issue.

Dr. Gamble, the Committee's Chairman, reviewed the progress of the PIPSRO Project. Seven sites had been selected; two were conditional, and five had yet to receive conditional status. The Institute of Professional Standards had been formed in a contract with Boston University to develop a curriculum for training people in PSRO activities, and a pilot training program was scheduled in San Francisco.

Dr. Calvin Kay, ACP Deputy Executive Vice President, attended a meeting of the Inter-Society Committee on Anti-microbial Usage [ISCAMU]. The Health, Education and Welfare [HEW] contract awarded to the College to develop norms for antibiotic usage in hospitals was going well. Twenty hospitals were now participating in the field study. Dr. Kay had also attended meetings of the Commission on Professional and Hospital Activities [CPHA], which was currently developing guidelines for quality assessment, and methods of concurrent review and retrieval of patient care data.

Dr. Kay also advised the Board of Regents that the Core Library for Internists should be updated.

Dr. Richard Allyn reported that a training program in cardiopulmonary resuscitation was encountering great success. In Illinois, the program was training about 200 instructors to teach about 100,000 people in CPR.

For the CMSS, Dr. Frommeyer presented the following resolution concerning "Veto Power" on the CCME:

Whereas the presence of the veto power cripples the effective function of the CCME, thereby depriving medicine of an essential and an expected voice in matters of medical education and whereas, lack of this unified voice is detrimental to the best interest of the public and and the profession, now, therefore, be it

RESOLVED, that the CMSS request the CCME to speak and act for medicine in matters of medical education and be it further

RESOLVED, that when unanimity of opinion or thought is lacking among the five parent bodies then the CCME would indicate the division and proceed in behalf of the majority and be it

RESOLVED, that this resolution of CMSS be distributed to the other parent bodies of the CCME and to the LCGME.

In March, 1975, the CCME/LCGME Committee on the Impact of National Health Insurance on Medical Education and Financing of Medical Education issued its recommendations for approval by the parent organizations. In summary, the report presented the following positions:

1. The cost of approved programs of graduate medical education and teaching institutions shall be included in the overall cost of doing business. The cost of graduate medical education shall not be divided into cost for service, cost for education, and cost for teaching.
2. Graduate medical education shall be provided for within health insurance premiums.
3. All individuals involved in graduate medical education shall be considered part of the medical staff of the teaching institution.
4. The manner in which residents are paid shall be left to local options.
5. Any national health insurance system should provide support for research and development of programs in graduate medical education.
6. A national health insurance system should supply support for modification of programs in medical education.
7. Any system of national health insurance should provide for ambulatory patient care.

Recommendations (1) through (6) applied to education in ambulatory care, taking the position that reimbursement for ambulatory health care must include the additional cost of graduate medical education.

The Board of Regents referred the recommendations to the ACP Steering Committee for study prior to approving the Report.

The CMSS presented a position paper from its Committee on Physician Distribution as proposed by the CCME on the Health Manpower Act of 1974. Two options were available to the CCME and its five parent organizations:

1. Opposition to Title XIV of the Bill in its entirety on the grounds that

    A. Significant changes are already taking place and the choice of specialty by students and an increasing number are selecting specialties in fields of primary care.

B. There is a significant shift currently taking place in the location of training positions geographically and from large university affiliated hospitals to other types of hospitals.

C. A quota system for first year positions determined in legislation of a restrictive nature would adversely affect the changes that are currently underway without legislation.

D. The current state of knowledge of factors influencing the availability and distribution of medical services is limited. Accurate assignment of positions by region and specialization would not be reliable under these conditions.

E. The most important factors in determining services would be methods of payment and the nature of benefits under an insurance plan, and those were not yet determined.

2. Option II proposed that the language of Title XIV of HR-17084 be modified to fit the actual circumstances of residency choice by students in currently approved residencies and to provide for changes that are now occurring in student choices, in location and in numbers of positions offered in various residency programs. Removal of the 125 percent limit on total positions would alter the time frame and allow the CCME, if selected as the agency, to assign residency positions to take all known factors into consideration in making the assignments.

## Federated Council for Internal Medicine

The new FCIM presented to the Board of Regents for its concurrence the following statement of its purpose and objectives:

The Federated Council for Internal Medicine is a federation of organizations which are dedicated to improving the high standards of health care which internists have brought to American medicine, and to promoting the active participation of internists in all comprehensive efforts to better the provision of health services in the United States. The Council formulates policies that reflect the consensus of the member organizations. These policies are concerned with the training, qualifications, and continuing education of internists and their participation in the professional, social, economic, and legislative aspects of health care.

The Federated Council's objective is to facilitate and encourage the implementation of its policies through interaction with the medical and other health professions, professional societies, legislative bodies, governmental agencies and the general public. The membership of the Council would be made up of three voting members and one nonvoting staff member, if available, from the American College of Physicians, The American Board of Internal Medicine, The Association of Professors of Medicine and the American Society of Internal Medicine.

The Board of Regents directed Dr. Schnabel, as ACP Representative to FCIM, to convey its endorsement of the intent as read.

# Part Two (1975-1976)

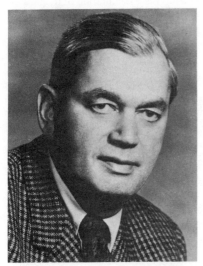

*Robert G. Petersdorf, MACP*

Dr. Robert G. Petersdorf was born in 1926 in Berlin, Germany. In 1951 he married Patricia Horton Qua and they have two sons, Stephen and John.

He received his BA from Brown University in 1948; his MD from Yale University in 1952. He served his internship and assistant residency at the Grace-New Haven Community Hospital from 1952 to 1954. From 1954-1957, he was a Senior Assistant Resident in Medicine at Peter Bent Brigham Hospital in Boston, a Research Fellow in Medicine at Johns Hopkins Hospital, and a Fellow of the National Foundation for Infantile Paralysis. He returned to the University Service, Grace-New Haven Community Hospital as Chief Resident in Medicine in 1957-58, and was appointed an Instructor in Medicine at Yale. Following a tenure as Assistant Professor of Medicine at Johns Hopkins University, he moved to Seattle, Washington where he was first an Associate Professor of Medicine, then Professor and Chairman of the Department of Medicine at the University of Washington from 1964 to 1979. His publications numbered more than 300 papers during his tenure at the University of Washington.

Certified by the American Board of Internal Medicine in 1959, he was a member of that Board from 1968 to 1977, becoming the Chairman-Elect in 1975 and Chairman in 1976-77. He was also Chairman of the Committee on Recertification.

He held membership in the following medical societies: American Association of Immunologists; American Clinical and Climatological Association; American Federation for Clinical Research; American Medical Association; American Society for Clinical Investigation; American Society for Microbiology; American Society for Nephrology and was on the Founders Committee; Association of American Medical Colleges of which he was Chairman; Association of American Physicians (President 1976-77); Association of Professors of Medicine (President, 1970-71); Infectious Diseases Society of America; Kings County Medical Society; National Academy of Sciences, Institute of Medicine, a member since 1973; North Pacific Society of Internal Medicine (Honorary Member); Seattle Academy of Internal Medicine (President, 1966-67); Society for Experimental Biology in Medicine; Southern Society for Clinical Investigation; Washington State Medical Association; Western Society for Clinical Research (President, 1970-71).

He became a Fellow of the ACP in 1962 and was a member of the Scientific

Program Committee from 1966 to 1972, Chairman from 1970-1972. He was a Regent from 1968 to 1974, President-Elect 1974-75; and President, 1975-76; he was made a Master of the College in 1976. During his Presidential year, he was Chairman of the Search Committee which recommended the appointment of Dr. Robert H. Moser to succeed Dr. Edward C. Rosenow, Jr., on his retirement as Executive Vice President.

Very active in the Association of American Medical Colleges, Dr. Petersdorf was named Chairman of the Council of Academic Societies in 1972-73 and Chairman of the Assembly in 1977-78.

He was the ninth most senior member of the Association of Professors of Medicine. Only three members of the ACP Board of Regents were more senior, Drs. Richard Vilter, Edmund Flink and Theodore Woodward.

He was President of the Peter Bent Brigham Hospital and Women's Hospital, in Boston, 1979-1981. Since 1981, he has been Dean of the School of Medicine and Vice Chancellor of Health Sciences at the University of California in San Diego. He is an editor of Harrison's *Principles of Internal Medicine* and served frequently as a visiting professor at other medical schools.

Dr. Petersdorf was Consultant to the U.S. Public Health Service Hospital in Seattle. He also served as a consultant to the Surgeon General of the U.S. Army and the U.S. Public Health Services. His versatile activities currently include Membership on the Board of Directors of the American Hospital Supply Corporation and he is also on the Medical Advisory Council of Merck, Sharp, and Dohme International. His many intersocietal connections were associated with his important duties in the American College of Physicians. The Association of American Medical Colleges, and the Association of Professors of Medicine, and many other organizations have permitted him to assume a major leadership role in the shaping of medicine and medical education in the United States over the past 15 years.

His enthusiastic support of the Federated Council of Internal Medicine helped to make this organization a reality and to move it from the outset in a practical and useful direction. He and Dr. Truman Schnabel both tried to elicit more recognition of family practice from the Board of Regents. Although they failed, the pressure of the issue resulted in more support to gain recognition for internal medicine as a primary care specialty.

Every now and then a person comes along who is such a natural leader that the number of offices held is staggering. If such a person is capable of doing a good job in all of those official positions simultaneously, then he becomes a tremendously effective integrating force. This has certainly been true of Dr. Petersdorf. He has not only held many positions at once, but did a thorough job with each one.

Such forceful and dedicated leadership can have personal disadvantages, however; Dr. Petersdorf, in a conversation with me in 1982, referred to himself as an insomniac, hardly ever getting more than five or six hours of sleep a night.

An important quality of leadership is understanding and flexibility. He was expert in compromise and exerted a strong influence in resolving differences so a group could move ahead. A good and witty speaker and raconteur, he was much in demand.

This Presidential year was an important turning point for the College, since a successor for the position of Executive Vice President had to be found. Dr. Petersdorf led a very thoughtful committee, originally appointed by Dr. Schnabel, to a successful conclusion in April of 1976. The decision was preceded by careful study, not only of the relationships between the Board of Governors and Regents, but also how they related to the administration.

I had very much enjoyed about 18 years of serving the College, but realized and even suggested the time for my retirement. In the last few months of my tenure I was concerned that the transition be as smooth as possible. It was particularly important for the Staff to know who was in charge until April, 1977, the designated date set for the change of administration. Dr. Petersdorf was very helpful and a good advisor in planning for the change.

On leaving office, Dr. Petersdorf reflected that he continued to be concerned about the College's current stance on a number of issues. In a conversation in 1981 he emphasized the following:

1. The College, he said, should be in the front line of defending the place of the general internist. This was far more important than showing concern for the subspecialists, of which he thought there were too many.
2. He was disappointed that the audio-visual program jointly sponsored by the College and the University of Washington's Health Sciences Center, called the *Self-Learning Series,* had been discontinued.
3. He thought the Federated Council of Internal Medicine was performing a useful function. The formation of the Association of Program Directors in Internal Medicine [APDIM] was important and he was happy that he had given it his support at its beginning.

His feelings about the ACP having a Washington Office were a bit mixed. Though conceding that internal medicine must be active in Washington, he wasn't sure of the efficacy of the ACP, ASIM and the Federated Council of Internal Medicine each having separate operations there. This potentially could cause confusion among the legislators and others in the government.

## 1975-1976

Dr. Robert H. Moser, FACP, new Executive Vice President-Designate. *A-V Self-Learning Series.* Rosenthal Awards. *MKSAP IV* Courses. Subspecialty Society Liaison Committee. CCME/LCGME: ACP representation. ABIM Councils: General Internal Medicine; Subspecialty Medicine. Annual Session (Bicentennial) with RCP-Edinburgh (250th Anniversary, Faculty of Medicine). AMA PRA Credit for Recertification. Declaration of Tokyo. JCAH "All-or-None" Accreditation Policy.

When Dr. Robert G. Petersdorf assumed the Presidency in April, 1975, he received the unfinished agenda of three major developments of recent years. Expansion of educational resources through experimentation with audio-visual programs was in full stride in cooperation with the University of Washington's Health Sciences Teaching and Learning Center. Lectures on tape and microfiche were in development to be made available by the 1976 Annual Session.

The organization of the Federated Council for Internal Medicine [FCIM] was in detailed definitional stages and serious efforts to establish liaison with subspecialty societies were underway.

The impact of College policy and structural changes of the past year would become strongly apparent as the implementation phase progressed. In the midst of this transition, Dr. Petersdorf also confronted the impending retirement of the Executive Vice President and the urgent task of the Search Committee to find a suitable successor by April of 1976.

Dr. Petersdorf's report to the Board of Regents in November of 1975 reviewed the implications of these developments and reflected much progress.

The Search Committee for an Executive Vice President had reviewed a large number of candidates, and Dr. Petersdorf was confident that a successor could be named by the time the Annual Session convened in 1976. The Committee hoped to conclude the process in time for the new officer to be available in the College offices to work with me toward the end of 1976 and through the first few months of 1977.

### FCIM Debates Policy Formation

The FCIM had met several times. Happily, the represented organizations expressed a high degree of agreement on most subjects. With so much overlapping and cross-over representation of the leadership in the other three organizations, there was good reason to believe that these four groups might work very well together. Initially, the representatives were concerned that the FCIM would experience difficulty, if every position they discussed had to go back to the parent organizations for approval. Getting approval through such an organizational structure as that of the American Society of Internal Medicine [ASIM] for example, might be a slow and difficult process.

The Council, therefore, proposed a policy that any policy decision taken by FCIM should be approved by the parent bodies, but the Council could endorse, without prior approval from the other parent organizations, positions already adopted by one of the constituent groups. This was an essential posture in the interest of shaping an organization unhampered by the possibility of being tied up by a single veto. Examples called to mind were the operation of the UN Security Council and, in the field of medicine, the Coordinating Council for Medical Education [CCME].

Dr. Petersdorf reminded the Board that the ASIM already had a part-time employee in Washington acting to keep abreast of legislative developments, arranging for testimony before committees and helping the society to make contacts with Congressional staff people. For the College to engage in similar activity at the same time, he believed, would be unnecessarily duplicative and expensive, and also might endanger the very foundation on which FCIM was built, namely the efforts to speak for internal medicine with a single voice.

Actions already implemented seemed to be working quite well. The decision to interface with the government under the auspices of ASIM did not mean, he stressed, that each organization should not relate to the government on individual issues as it deemed necessary, especially those subjects on which FCIM could not reach a consensus. The represented organizations should recognize that consensus through FCIM would not always be possible on certain important global issues such as health manpower, health planning or national health insurance. The leadership in internal medicine should expect that it would not always be able to formulate a single position that would represent the interests of an entire specialty.

Liaison with the specialty societies was beginning to look very promising. Dr. Petersdorf had already proposed a meeting with the presidents of all the sub-specialty societies to be held at the Annual Session in 1976. Dr. Petersdorf's personal professional involvement in the many organizations listed in his biographical profile was a significant individual contribution to the increasing cross fertilization of multi-societal efforts and ideas. He had just been made Chairman-Elect of the American Board of Internal Medicine [ABIM] and would take office as Chairman in July, 1976.

The impact of changing directions of the College on regional activity was reflected in the report of the President-Elect, Dr. Jack D. Myers. Interest in Chapter formation was gaining ground among the membership. But the ACP's ventures into socioeconomic policy issues was not readily understood or accepted among ASIM component societies, nor were the purposes of the formation of the FCIM as clear to them as among their national leadership. Dr. Myers was certain however, that successful implementation of FCIM goals would do a great deal to solve many organizational misunderstandings at local levels.

My Executive Vice President's report announced the success of the first recertification examination given in this country. Other societies held some doubts that their respective Boards would approve a need for recertification. The ACP venture was breaking new ground as it had with self-assessment programs. The College had fulfilled its pledge to the members by not only promoting a mechanism for recertification, but also for making it an integral part of educational opportunities for internists to fulfill a variety of requirements demanded by state medical associations and societies. In twelve states, the State Medical Associations were currently requiring specific levels of postgraduate education to maintain membership, and in eight states postgraduate education requirements were necessary for licensure. Six specialty societies had also adopted educational requirements for continued membership.

I expressed my concern that the College evolve appropriate modes to more effectively exert influence through the Council of Medical Specialty Societies [CMSS] in crucial intersocietal organizations, such as the Medical Liability Commission, AMA, Association of American Medical Colleges [AAMC] and FCIM. The College was a very strong organization and in each instance had had to contend with some dilution of its influence in the process of cooperating with these and other interlocking organizations. Intersocietal and cooperative policy development had become an accepted modus operandi in the United States, and the College must simply do its best to work through these means in whatever way it could.

The accelerating trend in Chapter formation, I enthusiastically reported, had resulted in formal chapters in New Mexico, Illinois, Montana, Michigan and Connecticut. Others underway were in Washington, Texas, Puerto Rico, Hawaii, Oklahoma, North Carolina, Ohio, Downstate New York II and, recently Upstate New York. In Oklahoma, an interesting experiment was being studied. The Oklahoma Society of Internal Medicine and the ACP membership might set up an organization in parallel Chapters with a common Board of Directors, although members would retain their individual societal memberships.

I reminded the Board that a final challenge to the College was beginning to surface in the United States: Total health resources were finite and someone would soon be faced with making important priority decisions about how these limited resources should be distributed, such as setting up criteria for patient selections for renal dialysis and open heart surgery.

Dr. Neal Elgee, Chairman of the Audio-Visual Committee, reviewed details of the new ACP audio-visual project, titled *Physician's Self-Learning Series,* being developed at the University of Washington Health Sciences Learning and Research Center. These programs were designed to use, to their fullest advantage, microfiche applications and multimedia self-instructional techniques.

Staff and faculty of the Center, together with the resources of the College assured multidisciplinary approach to content and the best possible results with these materials. The topics selected by the Committee had to meet the following criteria:

1. The subject must deal with a problem that is common in primary care practice.
2. The problem must be treatable or manageable.
3. The unit must be within the purview of the primary care physician and contribute to making the internist capable of integrated care.
4. The media must be appropriately used.

The Rosenthal Foundation had recently approached the Awards, Masterships and Honorary Fellowships Committee to fund two new awards. The proposed awards criteria would be: 1) for innovative approaches in the delivery of health care which are likely to increase its clinical and/or economic effectiveness; 2) work which gives promise of soon making notable contributions to improve clinical care in an area of medicine other than cardiovascular disease or cancer. Dr. Truman Schnabel, the Committee's Chairman, said the proposal would be explored further with the Foundation for a later report to the Board of Regents. The Awards Committee, in addition to the regular Masterships Awards, nominated Dr. Edward C. Rosenow, Jr., to receive a Mastership and also the Alfred Stengel Award at the next Annual Session.

## MKSAP IV

A report by Dr. Lawrence E. Young, Chairman of the Educational Activities Committee, expressed a strong hope that *Medical Knowledge Self-Assessment IV [MKSAP IV]* might reach 40,000 participants, a highly probable goal. He described new features of the *MKSAP IV* as follows:

1. Expansion from nine to ten subspecialty areas, separating allergy and immunology from infectious diseases.
2. Fifty percent larger Syllabus with fewer references to be cited.
3. Patient Management Problems, self-scoring examination, with pictorial atlas and a critique on each problem.
4. Early issuance of summary scores for each subspecialty area with comparison to the medium score of all responses.
5. Answers with critiques and references.

### First MKSAP Courses

In connection with this program, 25 separate five-day courses were scheduled from late August to mid-October of 1977 at strategic locations throughout the country, to be coordinated by the Postgraduate Courses Committee. Further supporting the program, annotated bibliographies for each of the ten subspecialties would be published in the *Annals* from January through November, 1976. Reprints of the cumulative annotated bibliographies would then be made available for distribution. The ABIM Recertification Examination was scheduled for October, 1977, to coincide with the conclusion of the *MKSAP* program.

The objectives and selection procedures of the Fellowships and Scholarships program were thoroughly studied by that Committee, reported Dr. Daniel S. Ellis, its Chairman. More information regarding candidates and their proposed study projects was clearly needed. The committee understood that the main objective in awarding Fellowships was to provide support for promising individuals, enabling them to carry out independent study to develop expertise as teachers or in productive research. The intent of the stipends was to support the aims of the individual in deciding on the ultimate course of his or her career, free of the burden of departmental duties or practice that would otherwise be necessary for financial support. Although the College would, in effect, be supporting departments of medicine by its support of departmental members, this was manifestly not the primary aim of the program.

The Committee urged more publicity and increased visibility of the Teaching and Research Scholars through the College's publications and other medical journals. The history of the scholarships should also be featured periodically and formal recognition should, in some way, be included in the Convocation. The exceptional work of these scholars was little known and the College had the means at hand to recognize it more appropriately.

## National Health Insurance

The Medical Practice Committee, Dr. John R. Gamble, Chairman, presented to the Board of Regents a statement on National Health Insurance [NHI] which was approved and published in the *ACP Bulletin* in December, 1975. The essentials of the College's position on this complex subject were reflected in a portion of the Prologue:

> Medical care is only one component among many affecting the "quality of life" and the maintenance of physical well-being. In promoting "health", NHI can directly address only a few issues. The insurance program should protect the individual against the extreme economic cost of catastrophic illness and contribute to the improvement of the quality and availability of health care services. It should stimulate innovation, experimentation and diversity.

The summary report of the 1974-75 Postgraduate Courses Committee presented by Dr. Varner J. Johns, Jr., Chairman, showed a total of 4,830 physicians in attendance at 38 courses. Of the 40 courses scheduled, two were cancelled because of insufficient registration. From the 1975-76 list of 45 courses, as of October 7, two had been cancelled because of insufficient registration.

The 24 *MKSAP IV* Courses scheduled for the late Summer consumed much of the Postgraduate Courses Committee's attention in 1975. These would be held in 24 cities, each course having a capacity to accommodate 250 to 500 registrants. The format of each course would include a three-hour preliminary review for each of the ten subspecialty areas and a 90-minute evening session with registrants divided into six groups. Concentrated in five days, two subspecialties per day would be covered in three hour sessions, with three faculty members per session. In the evening, three smaller group sessions would be conducted on each of these two subspecialty areas. The three faculty members, fully conversant with the Syllabus, would select questions from *MKSAP IV* for discussion in depth.

The Committee stressed the importance of uniformity in presenting the courses across the country because many people would be preparing for the Recertification Examination. When selecting questions from *MKSAP IV,* the faculty members should consider the following questions:

Why is the question significant?
Which of the answer options is, in his or her opinion, the correct or appropriate one?
Why are the other options not the best answer?

The faculty member should be expected to present evidence in support of the selected opinion. The College would furnish each course director with a slide of each of the 800 questions and a slide of each illustration or figure in the Syllabus and question books.

The Steering Committee had met twice since the April, 1975 meeting of the Board of Regents. Specialty society relationships were a large item on its agenda throughout the summer months.

The CMSS had issued a position paper on the impact of National Health Insurance on medical education and the financing of medical education. In most respects it was in conformance with the ACP's position taken in April, 1975, which generally approved the program.

The Steering Committee's Subcommittee to Establish Liaison with Subspecialty Societies in Internal Medicine was proceeding by several steps, reported Dr. Jeremiah A. Barondess, Chairman, to bring about closer working arrangements with the professional associations and societies representing the subspecialties.

One initial effort recommended, which would have impact, was to increase subspecialty society formal participation in the Annual Session programs. A jointly sponsored week-long workshop in a major subspecialty area was also recommended, directed toward the general internist. The call for abstracts for various parts of the Annual Session program should be especially directed to the subspecialty societies.

The College should also study the possibility of offering secretarial and other office functional support for specific subspecialty society endeavors.

The increasing complexity of intersocietal activity had led the President, Dr. Petersdorf, to appoint a Coordinating Committee with other societies in April, 1975, which was charged:

1. To clarify the various lines of authority with these organizations in which the College is directly or indirectly represented;
2. To determine how we can best intercommunicate and integrate our policies and points of view;
3. To discuss important issues which are before the College so that representatives to the other organizations would have the benefit of the free discussion of the Committee.

## CCME Representation Charted

In November, Dr. Jack D. Myers, Chairman, presented to the Board an excellent informational review about the operational interrelationships of the relevant societies and support organizations. He circulated a document which I had prepared showing that, at that time, the College had formal and direct representation in the ABIM, Joint Commission on Accreditation of Hospitals [JCAH], Residency Review Committee in Internal Medicine, [RRC-IM], ACP/APA Task Force, AMA Section Council on Internal Medicine, FCIM, AAMC's Council of Academic Societies, AMA Interspecialty Council, Joint Review Committee on Educational Programs for the Assistant to the Primary Care Physician, and the CMSS.

On the AMA Interspecialty Council and the Section Council on Internal Medicine, the ACP held divided responsibilities with the ASIM.

Dr. Myers then charted the relationships of some of the relevant organizations to the Coordinating Council on Medical Education, to explain the role of the ACP and its mode of influencing the policy decisions of the CCME.

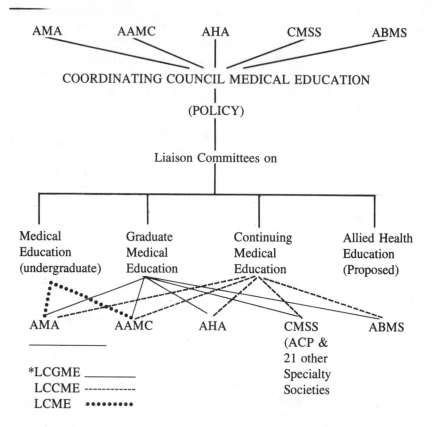

An in-depth discussion regarding specific organizations and subjects followed, particularly for the benefit of those representatives who would attend the Section Council on Internal Medicine within a few days.

The College's responsibility for approval of new members on the ABIM was regarded as extremely important. It was also noted that ACP Regents were no longer routinely appointed to the Board of the JCAH, which affected lines of communications about the Commission's activities.

National Health Insurance was a matter of great importance to the ACP and the College should develop a policy statement, particularly concurring with the CCME position that the cost of facilities for graduate medical education should be included in NHI as part of the "cost of doing business". The CCME's recommendations were currently being reviewed by the Council on Medical Specialty Societies, which would ask for an opinion from the ACP.

The National Health Planning and Resource Development Act of 1974, though its impact was more regional than national, should be brought to the attention of ACP Governors.

The Regents concluded that the AMA was in a much better position to deal with professional liability problems than any individual specialty society. The Medical Liability Commission, on which the ACP was represented, played a useful role in addressing long-range activity, but was not in a position to deal with immediate problems.

The CCME was in the center of the complex issues on health manpower legislation and had developed white papers dealing with primary care and foreign medical graduates. The "Rogers Bill", currently before Congress, named the CCME as the agency to determine the number of residencies by specialty and geographic distribution. With the AMA opposed to CCME participation, and the AAMC, AHA, and the American Board of Medical Specialties [ABMS] favoring it, it was important that the College influence a proper position for the CMSS, which was currently ambivalent.

The CCME's current position on primary care defined general internal medicine, general pediatrics and family practice as appropriate disciplines, with obstetrics and gynecology still under consideration. It also agreed that 50 percent or more of medical school graduates should be engaged in primary care. Both the ACP and other organizations concerned with primary care were consistently hampered in policy making by lack of adequate data. The College's involvement in current research promised some hope for solutions in addressing manpower problems.

### Foreign Medical Graduates

The subject of foreign medical graduates was certain to be a major topic of discussion at the meeting of the Section Council. An Invitational Conference of Foreign Medical Graduates [FMGs] held in April, 1975, was reviewed by Dr. Julius Stolfi for the Board's information. The conference was interested in two groups of FMGs:

1. The US citizen admitted to foreign medical schools.
2. FMGs applying for postgraduate training in the US

Many of those in the first group attempted to return home after their second year through the COTRANS route or by avoiding internship and social service requirements in Europe or Mexico by entering a "Fifth Pathway Program."

Foreign medical graduates taking postgraduate training in the US often lacked sufficient command of language and customs essential to effective training. They also frequently posed problems that destroyed the intent of the Fulbright Hayes Act. A significant number were not returning to their country of origin, but finding ways to immigrate permanently to the US and even managing to circumvent the provision to specify their intent to practice here in an area where there is a "shortage of physicians". The conference brought the complex issues involved into sharper focus and Dr. Stolfi offered some detailed recommendations to the Board of Regents, in summary:

1. The College should urge the Department of Labor and Immigration to change the law which grants "professionals in short supply" preferential status in order to discourage permanent migration of FMGs to the United States.

2. The law should continue to permit a true exchange visitor program to function.

3. Premedical advisors should be informed about the status of medical education in the United States and urge that they present the facts concerning difficulties of going abroad for medical education to those who failed to gain admission into medical schools in the United States.

4. The US should require the country of origin or the involved institution in the United States to orientate FMGs in the ways of Americans and teach them English language and American customs.

5. Another survey of the foreign medical schools which enroll US citizens should be done.

6. A single admissions test should be established for those applying for the Fifth Pathway Program.

7. Encouragement should be given to a unified state licensing examination (FLEX).

8. The fact that only a medical school can grant the MD degree should be re-affirmed.

9. FMGs must be actively encouraged to return to their country of origin.

10. Incentives must be devised to attract US graduates to medically under-served areas.

11. If all these measures fail, new methods of delivering health services to regions in need must be established. The models in Newfoundland, Canada, employing mobile units, air ambulances, telecommunication systems or nurse practitioners were worth studying.

The Steering Committee took no official action but accepted the report. They felt there was no objection to recommendations of the CMSS contained in this report.

The Residency Review Committee of the Liaison Committee on Graduate Medical Education [LCGME] presented some problems with the quality of reviews, according to several members with actual experience on the Review Committee. The review process was largely financed by the AMA, who controlled the secretarial and field staff. Recommendations that subspecialty fellowships be included in review of graduate medical education had not yet been acted on. However, for the first time, fees were to be charged to institutions that were reviewed. This was to start on July 1, 1976. This would reduce the AMA's financial contribution by 50 percent, which should have some impact. LCGME had already taken a position on fellowship reviews and ABIM's role in evaluation of residents in graduate programs should be expanded to include a larger role in residency review programs.

Emergency medicine proponents were pressing for specialty recognition and application to the ABMS for such recognition could be anticipated. The Coordinating Committee, Dr. Myers stated, recommended that the College oppose the establishment of emergency medicine as a specialty or subspecialty in medicine.

At a recent ABMS meeting, strong sentiment that uniform policies regarding recertification, especially its frequency, should be established, suggesting that the CMSS was in a position to expedite effective policies to insure continuing competence on a periodic basis.

Dr. Petersdorf described the deficiencies of the system which illustrated the importance of the newly formed FCIM. Need for a comprehensive health manpower study in internal medicine was complicated by the fact that fellowship training did not require accreditation by the RRC-IM. Hence, although it was not difficult to determine the number of internists or the number of internal medicine residencies, no organization had adequate data about what was going on in fellowship training. Having no data, it was impossible to ascertain the impact of training and what Fellows actually do in practice. The Association of Professors of Medicine [APM], at its recent meeting, passed a resolution agreeing to a moratorium on increasing the size of subspecialty training programs, except in unusual circumstances. This was not easy to accomplish.

A study was made by the APM which sought answers to two questions: 1) Who is in the "pipeline", that is, in training? 2) Identifying a cohort who had finished training in 1971, what happens to such Fellows and what they are doing? Another part of the study, already endorsed by the ACP Board of Regents studied " Who actually renders primary care?"

This study (later called the "Mendenhall Study", which was funded by the US Bureau of Manpower and the Robert Wood Johnson Foundation,) was to be extended, using a log diary technique by including the subspecialties of internal medicine. The Federated Council and its component organizations pitched in immediately, helping to fund the portion of the research pertaining to what happens to the Fellows in training and the recently graduated cohort.

## ABIM Councils on General and Specialty Internal Medicine

Dr. Palmer Futcher retired from the ABIM on October 1, 1975. Dr. Sol J. Farber, Chairman of the Board, announced that Dr. John A. Benson, Jr. would assume the newly created position of President of the American Board of Internal Medicine. Dr. Benson, from the faculty of the University of Oregon Medical School and head of the Division of Gastroenterology in the Department of Medicine, had been a member of the ABIM and had contributed much to the progress of the Board, serving as the Secretary-Treasurer and a member of the Executive Committee.

Dr. Benson's arrival coincided with the recent reorganization of the Board, which now would have two councils, comprising the Board of Governors. The Council on General Internal Medicine would receive special emphasis to further the importance of general internal medicine in teaching and training qualifications for certification. The Council on Subspecialty Medicine would be concerned with developing guidelines for training in the subspecialties. The composition of the Board of Governors also included four members-at-large, one each elected from nominations by the AMA, ACP, APM and the ASIM.

Dr. Jeremiah A. Barondess, Chairman, evaluated the work of the ACP/APA Task Force over the previous six years. A number of contributions could be viewed with satisfaction. A result of mutual programming activities, for example, was the reinstitution of the internship in psychiatric training programs. The influence of the Task Force was apparent, also, in the recent emphasis on psychiatric training in internal medicine programs.

The Task Force, however, had been more successful in introducing psychiatric subjects into ACP courses than getting medical subjects scheduled at the Annual Session of the Psychiatric Association. The American Psychiatric Association [APA] members continued to express concern over the general separation of psychiatry from medicine. Departments of Medicine were lagging significantly behind departments of family practice in encouraging psychiatric education and training, and, conversely, cooperation to introduce more internal medicine into psychiatric training was lagging. Improvements in these areas, Dr. Barondess said, required the continuing cooperation and influence of the Task Force, but he recommended that efforts continue on an ad hoc basis. Current areas of cooperation could certainly continue without the formal convening of a joint task force.

A comprehensive report on activities of the Council of Academic Societies [CAS] was given by Dr. Richard W. Vilter, ACP Representative. A bill, sponsored by the AAMC, recommended that one half of federal capitation grants be provided without specific requirements in recognition of the fact that basic support of medical education is, in part, a federal responsibility. In order to qualify for capitation, medical schools would be required to initiate programs responding to public concerns regarding health manpower in several areas.

A recent bill passed by the House of Representatives, H.R. 5546, restricted the option of capitation to a choice of two, either increasing first or third year enrollment by five or ten percent or developing a plan for remote site training for undergraduate medical students. The Council representatives questioned whether capitation was really worth the effort involved in obtaining it. It would be hard for state schools to turn it down and twenty-seven private schools now get state support. State legislators would be unsympathetic if capitation was turned down.

The CAS and the Council of Deans issued formal opinions regarding the President's Biomedical Research Panel and presented testimony to members of this panel. They emphasized concern about the instability of research funding, the need for support of research training programs, basic biomedical research and for increased participation of the research community in the planning of future biomedical and behavioral research initiatives.

In biomedical research training, the Administrative Board of the CAS reaffirmed a 1974 position of the American Society for Clinical Investigation's Committee on National Policy. This position stressed that the institutional grant should be the key element in biomedical research training programs of the National Institutes of Health [NIH], with individual fellowships serving as a useful supplement to fulfill special needs.

## Annual Session 1976

At the Annual Session in Philadelphia, April, 1976, the College welcomed the Royal College of Physicians of Edinburgh to celebrate with us the Bicentennial of the United States. The Edinburgh College presented a quaich to the ACP, especially engraved to honor simultaneously the Bicentennial of the United States and the 250th Anniversary of the founding of the Faculty of Medicine of the University of Edinburgh. The Royal College of Physicians of Edinburgh also presented the College with a complimentary copy of its recently published history in anticipation of the Royal College's 300th Anniversary in 1981.

Dr. Robert G. Petersdorf, in his final presidential address to the Board of Regents emphasized his continuing concern in two critical areas of concern commanding the College's attention:

The relationship of the ACP, in respect to medicine's position vis-a-vis the federal government, had made real progress through the FCIM, and these efforts must continue. The immediate success of these efforts was evident in the fact that internal medicine was included as a primary care specialty in recent health manpower legislation.

His second concern, already expressed by others, especially in the report of the Executive Vice President, was the lack of direct ACP representation on such coordinating educational bodies as the CCME and the LCGME. Internal medicine was only able to influence educational policy decisions by indirect representation through the CMSS. Dr. Petersdorf pointed out, however, that the Council was weighted in favor of general surgery and its related specialty fields. Representation is established proportional to the existence of primary boards. Most surgical specialties are represented by primary boards, while internal medicine is represented by only one board and three-and-a-half recognized subspecialty boards.

The operation of the ABMS presented the same disparity in numerical representation. However, representation on the CCME and its LCGME presented a better balance through the ABIM. Though still outweighed by the surgeons, ABIM had won adequate representation on the ABMS by appealing on the basis of its large number of certificants.

Financial support for CCME was based on the number of certificants of each of the Boards.

> The College must continue [Dr. Petersdorf said,] its persistent and determined espousal of the general internist as the best primary care physician for adults. The increased emphasis on subspecialties must not negate the emphasis on internists as primary care physicians. Proponents of family practice had gained enormous momentum in legislatures, both state and national, in selling family medicine as the principal primary care specialty. Through the FCIM, legislation that excluded pediatricians and internists must be strongly countered.

Dr. Myers, President-Elect, expressed hopes that the new Steering Committee of the College would make it easier to comprehend some of these issues. On the CCME and the LCGME progress would always be difficult as long as there was the "security council" veto arrangement, now present in both of these organizations. Both were also hampered by the lack of a separate adequate staff structure which made them less than efficient in their operation. The AMA furnished the support for the secretariat, and Dr. Myers submitted that some method must be devised to create a staff structure independent of one represented organization.

Turning to the internal affairs of the College, the reports of the Secretary General and the Treasurer presented an encouraging picture. The total membership of the College, reported Dr. Richard W. Vilter, was now 33,073 of which 140 were Masters; 13,326 Fellows; 9,058 Members; 10,229 Associates; 196 Affiliate Members, and 124 Honorary Fellows.

The Treasurer, Dr. Edward J. Stemmler, announced a positive balance in operations and a sound financial status at the end of 1975, in spite of governmental and inflationary factors. In addition to the inevitable inflationary rise in costs, the decline in revenue from pharmaceutical advertising, and the gratis distribution of the *ACP Directory* to all members were proving to be very costly. Furthermore, new regulations issued by the Internal Revenue Service applicable to the allocation of membership dues to the *Annals* and the *ACP Bulletin* substantially increased the amount of payable tax. Considering all of these things, a positive balance was most gratifying.

Dr. Stemmler had good news regarding the suit against the federal government for a refund of taxes for 1968-69. The United States Court of Claims heard the case in December and had found in the ACP's favor, which would result in a refund of approximately $377,000, plus interest less the legal fees. Unofficially, the government did not plan to appeal the decision. The Investment Portfolio was responding well in the changing market conditions. The A.G. Becker Company who monitored the performance of Drexel, Burnham & Lambert, ACP's Investment Counsel, indicated that, related to 3,000 other endowment funds, the College's investment performance had improved significantly during the past year. The College's performance was, in fact, in the top seven percent.

I added some executive notes to the officer's reports, announcing that the CMSS had appointed a Search Committee to recruit a permanent staff, and in the meantime, had hired an assistant. This assistant, Mr. Jack Carow, had been on the staff of the American College of Surgeons [ACS].

In College affairs, I noted that the Credentials Committee was working on a new problem since the discontinuance of a Corresponding Fellow class. Rather than assigning the task to the Awards Committee, the Credentials Committee was exploring the possibility of establishing credentials which would permit election of noncitizens from foreign countries to direct Fellowship. The election of candidates to direct Fellowship also presented another problem. Some who had recently completed their training program and who were in academic centers had been directly elected. Others who were their contemporaries but who were elected to Membership were expressing irritation and unhappiness, which was a source of considerable embarrassment and problems to the Governors. I suggested that postponing direct elections to Fellowship until a later date, and making all candidates who were just out of training Members for two years, might ease the problem. By doing this a person still could be advanced to Fellowship faster than under the existing rules.

I advised the Board that some problems had developed in the contract with ROCOM, the educational arm of Hoffman-LaRoche which put out the *Medical Skills Library*. ROCOM had been unable to promote the publications enough to make them profitable. Everyone agreed that the program was excellent in quality, so the Audio-Visual Committee was negotiating with ROCOM to develop other promotional arrangements. The Public Service Satellite Consortium [PSSC], of which I was a member, was exploring ventures in transmission of educational material. I predicted that it would soon be possible to run continuing medical education courses at weekly intervals similar to those being presented by medical schools in local areas.

One of the College's Associates at the University of Pennsylvania had written a letter indicating that currently there were at least twenty-four identifiable general internal medicine track programs for training physicians in primary care. I finally announced my intention, upon retirement, to write a history of the College, as requested earlier by the Board. This history would update events since the publication of *Gateway of Honor* in 1962, in a year-to-year chronicle.

The Educational Activities Committee Chairman, Dr. Lawrence E. Young, recommended that the American College of Physicians send to each state licensing board for medical practice an opinion of the College that recertification by the ABIM should be accepted as fulfillment of state requirements for continuing medical education and relicensure. A press release announcing this position statement was issued at the Annual Session. The main points of this release were:

1. that the first recertifying examination in internal medicine had been taken in October, 1974, by 3,000 previously certified internists;
2. a full description of the examination was delineated;
3. the recertifying examination administered by the ABIM had been planned to have close relationship to the *MKSAP* of ACP in 1977 as it had been in 1974.

The release further described the process, stating that nearly all of the internists who planned to take the 1977 recertifying examination were expected to obtain and to study intensively the *MKSAP IV*. A Syllabus with annotated references and precise explanations of recent advances in internal medicine would be distributed in 1976. The second part of the self-assessment program would consist of booklets with a total of approximately 800 Multiple Choice Questions [MCQ] and ten Patient Management Problems [PMP]. These would be distributed in May.

## AMA Category I Credit for MKSAP

In addition, most participants in the ACP Program were expected to attend one of the five-day ACP Postgraduate Courses to be given in 23 cities across the country. These would be taught by highly qualified teachers and would deal systematically with the self-assessment program. Since those who passed the recertifying examination were previously certified internists, their recertification by the ABIM should, in the opinion of ACP, be accepted by State Licensing Boards as fulfillment of the state requirements for continuing medical education and re-licensure. The AMA, incidentally, had already allowed 100 hours of credit for Category I of the Physicians' Recognition Award to those who completed the *MKSAP*. The AMA did not give additional credit for completion of recertification, regarding it as an examination, rather than an educational program.

Dr. Stolfi reported for the Finance Committee that since the original installation of the computer center in April, 1972, the College's computer usage had grown to an operational level requiring a higher performance system which would be more efficient and economical in processing the additional applications being developed. More sophisticated equipment requirements typically follow successful computer operations as additional applications are supported by computers, justifying their cost. This expenditure was approved by the Board of Regents.

The net income of the *Annals* for the year 1975 was $173,590, a decrease of $98,518 which reflected a continuation of the downward trend in advertising revenues and rising publications costs. The number of subscribers, on the other hand, continued to increase with the January, 1975 issue, having 73,221 paid subscribers including members, an increase of 5 percent over the previous year. In order to stabilize the continuing decline in revenues, the Board of Regents approved a raise in advertising rates and also approved the budget for increased classified advertising. In the revised budget for 1976, after taking into account the effect of the new IRS regulations on allocating subscriptions to membership, the projected subscription income was estimated at $1,149,000; net advertising income at $841,000; classified advertising at $11,000, for a total of $2,041,000. Offset by expenses of $1,997,300, net income before taxes was projected at $43,700.

Revisions in the insurance plan were recommended by the Insurance Committee, Dr. Daniel S. Ellis, Chairman. The Board adopted a change in the high limit accidental death and dismemberment group insurance plan; increasing benefits by 25 percent, and also made substantial changes in the major hospital expense insurance plan, both with no increase in premiums. A recommendation to preclude the presentation of any other insurance programs at Regional Meetings of the College was tabled. Discussion of the recommendation clarified that it would be unpleasant to enforce, since Regional Meetings were commonly joint meetings with the local Society of Internal Medicine.

## Declaration of Tokyo

The International Medical Activities Committee, Dr. Theodore E. Woodward, Chairman, asked the Board of Regents for approval of the World Medical Association's "Declaration of Tokyo". This declaration articulated guidelines for medical doctors concerning torture and other cruel, inhumane or degrading treatment or punishment in relation to detention inprisonment. The document was approved and published in the *ACP Bulletin* in June, 1976.

The activities of the Medical Practice Committee, reported Dr. John R. Gamble, Chairman, included important investigations on issues being considered for future ACP policy statements, and called attention to the following decisions after review:

1. The Committee had studied the Federal Trade Commission's position on physician advertising, in which it had decided not to become involved.
2. An ad hoc committee was formed to work on establishing "Guidelines for the Use of New Diagnostic Techniques in Internal Medicine".
3. The Committee recommended that the position paper, "Public Education and Its Role in the Office Practice of Internists" be referred to the Committee on Public and and Professional Communications.

Dr. Gamble also reported that the Private Initiative in Professional Standards Review Organization [PIPSRO] project's current contract was due to terminate in June, 1976.

Dr. Varner J. Johns, Jr., enthusiastically reported the results of the Postgraduate Courses Committee's request that the Board of Regents ask the AMA to allow credit toward Category I of their Physicians Recognition Award to those physicians who completed *MKSAP IV* for computer scoring.

The Publications Committee, asked for approval of two *Annals* appointments: Dr. Paul C. Davidson was approved as the new Associate Editor, and Dr. Huth was appointed to the Editorial Board. Dr. Stuart O. Bondurant, Chairman, then asked for consideration of an adjustment in subscription price to maintain the financial balance of the *Annals*. The Board approved an increase in the subscription rates to $25 for a regular subscription and $12.50 for house officers and students.

Of statistical interest in 1975, *Annals* had published 692 main articles, 486 case studies and communications, 164 letters, included in a total of 1,573 pages of editorial content. The number of subscribers to the *Annals* continued to grow but the rate of growth had fallen sharply. This fact generated extensive discussion in the Committee, which reached the consensus that it would be useful to undertake College-wide analyses of current and projected educational programs in order to assure more effective interaction of all programs with the *Annals*.

In reviewing my plan to compile the information for the eventual writing of the history of the College, I indicated to the Committee that I would need additional help. I appointed Ms. Pearl Ott to the position of Archivist, with the assigned duty to review the Board minutes by subject and make copies of pertinent material for each of the subject areas to be included in my writing. Mr. Mark Christmyer then replaced Ms. Ott as the Associate Editor of the *ACP Bulletin*.

### Steering Committee Reviews FCIM Statements

In January, 1976, the Steering Committee reviewed the policy statements approved by the FCIM at its meeting in December, 1975. The College's published position on National Health Insurance was received favorably. ASIM had also published a statement which urged the inclusion of coverage for catastrophic illness. Without the inclusion of this position in the joint statement, ASIM could not endorse it, while the other members of FCIM could not agree to inclusion of the following clause in the ASIM statement: '' The finance from general revenues would supplement reallocation of current federal health program expenditures''. The Board of Regents, in April, 1976, sustained the reservations about including catastrophic coverage in any statement receiving College support. Such a position in a national health insurance plan would tend to emphasize subspecialty medicine at the expense of primary care medicine. The Board referred the statement to the Medical Practice Committee, directing it to explore the statement with ASIM in detail.

The ASIM's policy statement on "Learning and Using New Techniques" was endorsed by the FCIM. The Board of Regents also referred this statement to the Medical Practice Committee for study.

Following a report from Dr. Stolfi about the meeting of the Interspecialty Council of the AMA, the Steering Committee took action to reaffirm the ACP position that the appropriate specialty organizations should have direct representation in the AMA House of Delegates, commensurate with the number of the AMA members among their membership.

On the Steering Committee's recommendation, the Board approved accepting the invitation to participate in the formation and continuation of the Council on Clinical Classification of Diseases, and financial support for ACP representation. Preparation of the 9th edition of the *International Classification of Diseases (ICD-9)* was nearing conclusion after several years of work.

The Committee advised that taking the recertification examination should not be promoted as prerequisite to purchasing *MKSAP IV*, although it should be suggested that the recertification program would be a useful conclusion. This was a necessary posture, inasmuch as the College did not officially "recertify" anybody. To avoid confusion, the Board of Regents agreed that no certificate would be given for completing the *MKSAP IV* Program.

A letter from Dr. Irving Wright, a former President, requested support of a resolution from the Geriatrics National Advisory Council urging the promotion of interdisciplinary programs in geriatrics. The Steering Committee suggested that the Geriatric National Advisory Council should address medical schools directly, stating that the College hesitated to suggest to medical schools what they should do in their curriculum.

The Steering Committee studied the reorganization of JCAH, which was now structured in four main divisions: Hospital Accreditation Program, Quality Review Center, Office of the Director, and the Office of Administrative Services. The Accreditation Program now included five Accreditation Councils: Long-Term Facilities, Facilities for Mental Retardation, Psychiatric Facilities, Ambulatory Health Care, and Occupational Safety and Health.

Some Commissioners wished to have the Hospital Accreditation Program charged to be a separate council, and JCAH sought the advice of the parent bodies. It was observed that such a council would be represented by the same parent bodies and the Board, with duplication of functions. After debate, the Board of Regents rejected a motion to support formation of a Council.

The ACP was taking public positions on many general medical issues. The Steering Committee urged the development of mechanisms for addressing these issues as they emerged.

1. It recommended that Governors be encouraged to report emerging issues in their localities and if the subjects seemed appropriate, that the President appoint ad hoc committees to review and prepare statements for potential ACP support.
2. It recommended specifically an ad hoc committee to respond to the issue of the "statutory determination of death", presented in a letter from Mr. Stephen Donohue to Dr. Barondess relating to a recent New York State public hearing. This item was placed on the agenda for the Board of Governors' meeting in April, 1976.

### FCIM "Statement on Primary Care"

The Board heard information on the progress of projects in primary care:

1. The "Statement on Primary Care", prepared by FCIM, would soon be published in the *ACP Bulletin*. The ABIM would send reprints from the *ACP Bulletin* to all Internal Medicine Program Directors. It would also be distributed to a list of people in Washington.
2. The survey of internal medicine was progressing very well. The three parts of the program included the "Mendenhall Study", which employed a log-type diary maintained by participating physicians. The study expanded to include not only what physicians do in primary care, but also how much primary care is done by those practicing in the subspecialties of internal medicine.
3. An additional study under FCIM auspices was being conducted by Dr. Alvin Tarlov, at the University of Chicago. This study concentrated on determining the extent of primary care offerings in training programs for internal medicine.

At the recent FCIM meeting, Mr. William Ramsey, ASIM Executive Director, and ACP's Dr. Stuart Bondurant also called attention to another challenge to general internal medicine in the primary care field: In 14 states, family practice programs had been mandated as a line item in the medical school budgets. Dr. Bondurant reported that the family practice group had been pressing for this in New York for five or six years. The programs had been funded at the rate of 9 million dollars per year for two years and internal medicine was not included in the funded mandate. A conference on primary care was to be held in the Institute of Medicine at the end of the week of January 9.

The Steering Committee concluded its report by recommending that in recognition of my 17-plus years of distinguished service to the College, the Board approve plans for a portrait of me, to be hung in an appropriate place in College

Headquarters. The Finance Committee recommended approval of adequate funds. The portrait would be painted in the coming year and formally presented at my retirement. A Portrait Committee was appointed consisting of Dr. Schnabel, Chairman, Dr. Stemmler and Mr. Fred Dauterich. The artist chosen was Nelson Shanks of New Hope, Pennsylvania.

Because of the important role of the internist in cancer education, prevention, diagnosis and management, the Committee to Determine Patterns of Care in Cancer, Dr. Vilter, Chairman, urged that the Board of Regents recognize the need for the ACP to provide information and advice concerning these areas to agencies dealing with cancer planning. In the diagnosis and care of patients with cancer, resources of excellence should be available to general internists in clinical pathology and laboratory medicine; diagnostic radiology; therapeutic radiology; surgical specialties related to cancer; blood bank and blood component therapy; and diagnostic and therapeutic nuclear medicine.

The internist should also have access to other internists with special training in oncology or related fields appropriate to the needs of the patient. The internist's responsibility extends beyond curative measures, and must include continuing care and rehabilitation of the patient with cancer.

The American College of Physicians should have a permanent cancer committee to work with public and private groups making policy decisions regarding cancer training, continuing education, prevention, diagnostic care, restoration and rehabilitation. The ad hoc committee was discharged with thanks, having completed its task.

### Subspecialty Societies Meet

At the Annual Session on April 5, 1976, the Committee on Relations With Subspecialty Societies met with representatives of nine subspecialty societies: The American Heart Association; The American Association for the Study of Liver Diseases; The American College of Cardiology; The American Gastroenterological Association; The American Rheumatism Association; The American Society of Nephrology; The American Society of Hematology; The American Society of Clinical Oncology; and the Infectious Disease Society of America.

A sentiment advocating more unity among the societies was clearly expressed in the assembly. Dr. Barondess, Chairman of the Committee, recommended that the Board of Regents approve hosting a one-day invitational conference at ACP Headquarters for representatives of the major subspecialty societies, specifically on the subject of manpower issues in internal medicine. The agenda should include residency review, activities of the ABIM in relation to manpower questions, review of the manpower study sponsored by FCIM and the APM, and activities in family practice.

The plan was approved and the Committee acted immediately to develop the program. A tour of College Headquarters was included. The conference would seek to address expansion of interaction both in ACP and in subspecialty society programs. The Committee also considered the possible need for a secretariat, for which the College might offer support. A list of resources bearing on secretariat functions at the College was suggested for presentation to one subspecialty society of modest size for reaction and comment. The number of the committee was increased to five members.

The expanded scope of programs of the JCAH to include accreditation for four other forms of health related services increased the number of full time staff and the volume of work for the ACP. Dr. Ellis, ACP Representative to the JCAH, reported that the present work load of members of the Commission amounted to 18-22 working days a year. The Director of the Commission, Dr. John Porterfield would retire in 1977, and the Search Committee was actively interviewing candidates for his replacement. Accreditation issues under study at the Joint Commission currently included:

1. Privileges of nonradiologists in performing specific limited diagnostic and therapy monitoring studies.
2. Standards of hospital medical records.
3. Periodic health evaluation of medical staff members.
4. Physician participation in hospital governing bodies.
5. Limits on private practitioners in teaching hospitals.
6. Extent of application of a standard requiring delineation of clinical privileges of other professional hospital staff.

In addition, the JCAH requested action by the Board of Regents on the following matters:

1. The JCAH requested support for repeal of the second portion of the "all or none" policy, which currently stated that a hospital with more than one accreditable program must meet approval in all of its programs or would receive no approval at all.

For example, a new ambulatory care program, not yet meeting the standards of the ambulatory council, would result in disapproval of the hospital which had always been accredited. Accreditation would be withheld until the ambulatory care program could be approved.

The "all or none" rule had caused a tremendous furor within the Board and within its accreditation councils. The rule, therefore, had been suspended, awaiting further input and decisions. However, this action resulted in adverse outcomes in the opposite direction. Some of the councils began offering accreditation for small programs within a facility and some of these accredited programs were using the "all or none" policy to pressure the parent institution to reorder the priorities within the institution.

Many of the Commissioners believed strongly that the Hospital Accreditation Program, being the most significant of the JCAH programs, should not be compromised by the "all or none" principle. The other accreditation programs were voluntary evaluation programs and should operate independently of hospital accreditation. Some of the accrediting councils were unhappy with this position and threatened to withdraw if the "all of none" rule was repealed. The Board of Regents supported repeal of the "all or none" principle.

2. Admission of podiatrists to the medical staffs of hospitals was a problematic item on the JCAH Board agenda.

The Podiatric Association was strongly pushing for eligibility with full admission privileges. Present JCAH standards declared them ineligible, but allowed hospital privileges under supervision of appropriate medical staff. Some states had recently passed laws declaring podiatrists eligible for medical staff membership.

Podiatrists were considering class action suits in areas where they were denied hospital staff membership. A proposal within the JCAH to accept their eligibility had not yet been acted on and parent organizations were asked for guidance. Any JCAH ruling contrary to state laws would inevitably make it subject to class action suits. The Board of Regents responded with the position that membership of podiatrists on hospital staffs should be a matter of local option.

At the April, 1976 Annual Session, on recommendation from the Ad Hoc Search Committee, the Board of Regents approved and announced the appointment of Dr. Robert H. Moser, FACP, of Haiku, Hawaii, as Executive Vice President-Designate.

Members of the committee were commended for their efforts in the year-long search. Dr. Petersdorf chaired the committee, which consisted of Drs. Jack D. Myers, President-Elect; Truman G. Schnabel, Jr., Immediate Past President; Maxwell G. Berry, Vice President; Jeremiah A. Barondess, Immediate Past Chairman of the Board of Governors; and Bryan Williams, Chairman of the Board of Governors.

### Robert H. Moser (FACP), Executive Vice President-Designate

The College membership was informed in the May, 1976 issue of the *ACP Bulletin* that Dr. Moser would assume his new duties in April, 1977, and would be present at the College by January 1, to work with me in transition. Describing the Executive Vice President-Designate as having a strong background in the practice of internal medicine, the article conveyed a picture of wide-ranging expertise and concern in medical affairs:

> The ACP Executive Vice President-Designate has broad experience in internal medicine over a 16-year period (1953-1969) in the military service—serving as Chief of the Departments of Medicine at such institutions as Walter Reed General Hospital (1968-69); Brooke General Hospital (1967-68); William Beaumont General Hospital (1965-1967) and at US Army hospitals in Salzburg, Austria, and Wurzburg, Germany (1953-1956). He was also Assistant Chief of the Department of Medicine, Director of Education, and Hematologist at the Tripler General Hospital (1960-1964).

> While at Walter Reed, he was a member of the medical team that cared for President Eisenhower during the last year of his life. At the time of his European tour of duty, he was appointed physician-in-charge of medical services at the 1955 "Big Four" Foreign Ministers meeting in Geneva.

> Dr. Moser joined the Maui Medical Group in 1969, where he says he considers himself an internist-cardiologist in a "small town" environment. Maui is a com-

munity of 50,000 population, an island 90 miles southeast of Honolulu.

The Hawaiian internist returned to the Mainland for a period (October, 1973 to May, 1974) to serve as the Editor in Chief of the *Journal of the American Medical Association* and Director of the AMA's Division of Scientific Publications.

Dr. Moser is a native of Trenton, New Jersey, and attended Loyola College in Baltimore, Maryland. He received his medical degree from Georgetown University in Washington, DC in 1948. This was followed by graduate training as a civilian physician at the District of Columbia General Hospital and the Georgetown University Hospital and as a military physician at Brooke General Hospital, where he was a Fellow in Cardiology. Later (1959-60), Dr. Moser took a Fellowship in Hematology at the University of Utah (Salt Lake County) Hospital.

During the early days of the American Manned Spacecraft Program (1959-1968), Dr. Moser was one of the original medical flight controllers (monitoring orbiting astronauts during the Mercury Program from a base in Hawaii). As a consultant in internal medicine to the Gemini Program, he did pre- and post-flight physical examinations on the astronauts.

Since 1958, Dr. Moser has held faculty appointments at five medical schools. He was Clinical Associate Professor of Medicine at Baylor University College of Medicine (1958-59) and Clinical Professor of Medicine at Georgetown University School of Medicine (1968-69). He is now Clinical Professor of Medicine at the University of Hawaii School of Medicine (1969- ); Clinical Professor of Medicine at the University of Washington School of Medicine (1970- ) and Clinical Professor of Medicine at the Abraham Lincoln School of Medicine, University of Illinois, (1974- ).

The new ACP official became a Fellow of the American College of Physicians in 1961. He was certified by the American Board of Internal Medicine in 1955—and passed the recertification examination in 1974. He is also a Fellow of the American College of Cardiology and a member of such organizations as Alpha Omega Alpha, the American Osler Society, the American Society of Clinical Pharmacology and Therapeutics, and the Council of Biology Editors.

Dr. Moser is married to the former Stella Margot Neeson. They have two sons: 27-year-old Steven Michael, a newly-graduated MD who is in an internal medicine graduate program at the University of Illinois in Chicago; and 24-year-old Jonathan Evan, an aspiring television producer in Hawaii.*

*ACP Bulletin 17:5, (May) 1976, pp. 12, 19.*

## Part Three (1976-1977)

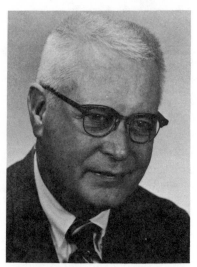

*Jack Duane Myers, MACP*

Born in New Brighton, Pennsylvania in 1913, Dr. Jack Duane Myers married Jessica Helen Lewis in 1946. They had five children, John, Jessica, Elizabeth, Margaret, and Judith (deceased).

He received his BA and MD degrees from Stanford University, in 1933 and 1937 respectively. He took residency training in internal medicine at the Stanford University Hospital and at the Peter Bent Brigham Hospital in Boston. An Associate Professor in Medicine at Emory University in 1946-47, he was then appointed Instructor and later Associate Professor in Medicine at Duke University School of Medicine from 1947 to 1955. He moved to the University of Pittsburgh in 1955, where he served as Professor and Chairman of the Department of Medicine until 1970, at which time the University conferred upon him the highly-respected title of University Professor of Medicine.

Dr. Myers served as Secretary-Treasurer of the American Board of Internal Medicine from 1964 to 1967, and as its Chairman from 1967 to 1970. He was also Chairman of the National Board of Medical Examiners from 1971 to 1975; Chairman of General Medicine Study Section, National Institutes of Arthritis and Metabolic Diseases, from 1963 to 1965; and member of its Advisory Council, 1970-1974. He served in the U.S. Army Medical Corps and rose from Captain to Lieutenant Colonel between 1942 and 1945.

He is a member of the Association of American Physicians, American Physiological Society, American Society for Clinical Investigation (Secretary, 1954-1957), and the Institute of Medicine, National Academy of Sciences.

In the American College of Physicians, he was a Regent from 1971 to 1978, President-Elect, 1975-76 and President in 1976-77, when he was made a Master of the College.

As an investigator he contributed significantly to understanding splanchnic circulation and its effect on metabolism. He has studied renal function of the dog fish at the Mount Desert Biological Laboratories. For some years he has been a pioneer in working on a computerized system of medical information retrieval [INTERNIST/CADUCEUS] to assist clinicians.

Having a keen interest in medical education, Dr. Myers has been a member and Chairman of the Liaison Committee on Graduate Medical Education and of the Coordinating Council on Medical Education. He also has been a member and Chairman of the Residency Review Committee in Internal Medicine.

Recognized as a superb clinician and teacher, he has always been revered and respected by his students and viewed by most as a prominent medical statesman.

Dr. Myers and I attended the Conference on Primary Care sponsored by the ABIM in the mountains of Montana. One evening, on our way to a barbecue, a young worker fell off a bus and injured his knee. Among that august bevy of highly specialized Board members, the reaction was "Where's Jack?" Dr. Myers immediately took charge of the problem in a first class clinical way.

In 1975 Dr. Myers was chairman of the ad hoc committee charged to prepare the statement entitled "ACP Policies and Plans for Implementation," which was a natural follow-up to the special joint meeting of the Board of Regents and Governors held in Toronto in the Summer of 1974. His grasp of the essential directions of the organization and leadership of the Committee attested to the potential leadership he subsequently demonstrated as President.

I saw a lot of Jack as we traveled to many meetings of the Residence Review Committee in Internal Medicine and the LCGME He always represented the ABIM on these bodies, while I represented the ACP or the Council of Medical Specialty Societies. He was a patient listener, but also a driving force in settling difficult matters. Though he might differ strongly with others on medical issues, such differences never affected his friendships. While the course of opinion did not always go his way, he maintained an innate respect for other peoples' opinions and received their respect in return.

On one occasion, he wanted to write an editorial on the Federal Trade Commission. The ACP had received a subpoena relating to the FTC investigation of several medical organizations including the AMA. The investigation sought to determine whether the AMA and other named societies were acting to prevent the increase of physician manpower. At the time, Jack and I were in Colorado Springs for the Regional Meeting; I told him our attorneys had called and did not want any of our officers to publish anything on the record, because at the moment we had not been charged with anything specific. Jack agreed not to, but added that he would like to write an editorial on the subject at some time.

For a number of years, Dr. Myers has been working on a computerized medical decision-making information retrieval system of a free access type. Promising to be, in time, a most useful part of medical care, his system differs from most others in that the physician enters only real data as he records them in his examination, his history, and in the results of laboratory and x-ray procedures. The computer analyzes the data at each point of diagnostic entry and may ask the physician additional questions. When enough data are available, the computer makes a diagnosis or suggests differential diagnoses. In this way the computer becomes a sort of consultant to the clinician.

For almost all known diseases, Dr. Myers and his staff have assigned certain strength values to each symptom or sign. With these values available, it will become possible for physicians to assimilate many more data than they can in the ordinary way of analyzing diagnostic problems. He and his colleagues are also working on developing similar programs for pediatrics. He is a very exciting and interesting person to work with, and it was a great pleasure to have spent the time I did with him through the years.

In 1982, when I asked him what he thought had been his biggest contribution to the College, he replied,

> Well let's look at the setting. This was your last year [1976-1977] and I felt the internal workings of the College were going along very well. Because of the various positions I held, I was in a good spot to help materially in the integration of College influence in some of the multi-organization representative bodies, e.g., Council of Medical Specialty Societies, the Coordinating Council for Medical Education, the Residency Review Committee in Internal Medicine, the Liaison Committee on Graduate Medicine Education, and the Federated Council of Internal Medicine.

As the events of 1976-77 attest, Dr. Myers did, indeed, contribute strong influence to the progress of ACP's position in multi-organizational activity.

A few excerpts from his interesting President's editorial page in the *ACP Bulletin* reveal his valuable perspectives:

> [May, 1976] "ACP must show increasing concern about the accreditation programs in internal medicine. Current methods leave much to be desired—It is almost certain we will need more general internists."

> [June, 1976] "One major factor in determining the increase in costs of medical care is the practice, almost universal among 3rd party payors including government, of paying without question for procedures. This encourages the use of procedures. This should be changed. There is not enough recognition for basic office or bedside patient work-ups. Another factor in increasing costs is the intensive and expensive care of illness for which there is little expectation of significant improvement. Another factor facing internists is the problem of financing graduate medical education especially if there are to be increasing numbers of training programs for general internists."

# 1976-1977

Dr. Rosenow retires; address to Board of Regents: "Unfinished Business". Council of Subspecialty Societies. ABIM Clinical Competence Program. Audio-Cassette Program. Medical Necessity Project. JCAH/SSA suit on confidential information. Annotated Bibliography, *MKSAP IV;* Library for Internists II. H.R. 2222: House Staff as "Employees".

In his President's report in November, 1976, Dr. Jack Myers surveyed the national scene in medical education and health practice. He predicted the demise of the Coordinating Council on Medical Education [CCME] and the Liaison Committee on Graduate Medical Education [LCGME] if the "security council" veto arrangement were not resolved. Unanimity was important, but if one parent organization could veto any action of the Council, both organizations would be rendered ineffective. Some solutions must also be found regarding the College's relationships with the CCME and LCGME.

He believed that relationships with the Council of Medical Specialty Societies [CMSS] should improve, since Dr. Richard Wilbur, an ACP Fellow and a capable administrator, had been appointed as the Executive Director. Relationships within the Federated Council for Internal Medicine [FCIM] were good and it gave the College an effective, although indirect, window to the Washington scene.

The Treasurer, Dr. Edward J. Stemmler, reported a quite satisfactory financial status, with major factors reflecting the improvement. Interest was being received from the government on taxes refunded, income from the new *Self-Learning Series* was promising, and increasing investment income and savings had accrued because the membership directory was not published that year.

Offsetting the favorable picture, however, was the continuing decline in net revenues from the *Annals of Internal Medicine*. The amount of tax refunded was $532,118, of which $154,623 represented interest gain. The legal cost of pursuing this claim was $50,500. Claims for refunds were also filed for federal income taxes paid for 1970 through 1975, totalling $780,000. Since the initiation of the first claim, however, Congress had enacted a new law, effective 1970, which essentially approved the regulations previously adopted by the IRS. For this reason, success with additional claims was doubtful.

The portfolio analysis by the A.G. Becker Company showed that the College had been much more successful in its investments in recent years and ranked in the top 6 percent of similar funds for the year ending June 30, 1976, and in the top 26 percent for the four years ending in June 30, 1976.

In my Executive Vice President's report, I confirmed the status of the *Self-Learning Series,* which showed a positive balance and was making good progress. Negotiations to terminate the College's contract for the *Medical Skills Library* with ROCOM were very amicable, and ROCOM had delivered to the College over $600,000 of inventory on the program. The College was obligated to develop to the stage of reproduction four more subjects for which ROCOM had already paid Dr. Bernard Dryer. The only cost to the College was to make a master print of these subjects. If the College was successful in selling the *Medical Skills Library,* then these additions could be produced.

Later in the meeting, Dr. Neil J. Elgee, Chairman of the Audio-Visual Committee, reported that the *Self-Learning Series* had 1,500 subscribers and the new subjects were in preparation. The Committee had inventoried $600,000 worth of print and film materials which ROCOM would deliver to the ACP. The cost of commercial storage was considerable and the material would be stored at the Headquarters while intensive efforts to develop new marketing were being made to continue and expand the sale of these materials.

I was pleased to report to the Board that 14 chapters were officially incorporated and 27 others were actively discussing Chapter formation. I attended the Regional Meeting in Puerto Rico which had recently celebrated, the incorporation of its Chapter, and was honored when the local members passed a resolution making me an Honorary Charter Member of their Chapter.

On the national scene in internal medicine, I believed the creation of the FCIM was one of the best things that had happened in the efforts to coordinate the voices of internal medicine. One apparent problem, however, should be addressed. Because of the popular perception of the ACP as an academically oriented society, some members of FCIM thought that many physicians would have difficulty recognizing the FCIM as representing the practicing internist. The College representatives, at that time, were mostly academic physicians, promoting the impression that American Society of Internal Medicine [ASIM] was the only organization representing practitioners. While, in fact, the College's membership included many more practitioners than ASIM, it was nevertheless true that the practicing physicians of ACP were not visable in the composition of FCIM at that time. While FCIM encouraged much better interactions between the ACP and ASIM, I ventured the opinion to the Board of Regents that it would still be worthwhile to keep exploring, from time to time, an amicable merger of the ACP and ASIM.

On a personal note, I informed the Board that Mrs. Rosenow and I had recently represented the College at a meeting in Colombia, which 140 physicians attended. We also traveled to Mexico and then to Helisinki with other members to the International Congress of Internal Medicine. On another recent trip, I had been made a Fellow of the Royal College of Physicians of Ireland.

Associate membership, Fellowship eligibility, and the constitutional status of the Steering Committee were subjects commanding the attention of the Bylaws Committee. Dr. Charles H. Rammelkamp, Jr., Chairman, reported that several changes were required in the Bylaws concerning Associate membership. Associates were defined as medical graduates who have been accepted for training in internal medicine or a closely related specialty. Except in special circumstances, appointment as an Associate would not be admissible when the physician had passed the point of eligibility for Board examination, whether or not the candidate was still in training. Since Associateship did not constitute a claim on regular membership and normal termination was approximately 18 months after eligibility for the Board examination, any Associate continuing in training would be granted a maximum extension of not more than two years to the normal termination date, whether or not examinations of the American Board of Internal Medicine [ABIM] had been taken.

The Committee also recommended that eligibility for Fellowship be changed to provide that candidates should have been graduated from medical school at least ten years before being proposed, rather than the eight years stipulated in the current Bylaws. The Bylaws were also changed to define the constitution of the Steering Committee.

Dr. Richard Vilter reported the Credentials Committee's recommendation that noncitizens may be elected Members of the College without evidence of intent to become citizens of the US, Canada, Mexico or a Central American Republic. He also announced that of 1,082 candidates for membership, 96 were recommended for direct election to Fellowship and 966 were elected to Membership. Of the 230 candidates for Fellowship, 179 were recommended for advancement.

Dr. Ralph R. Tompsett, Chairman of the Educational Activities Committee, reported a proposal received from the Audio Digest Foundation, which had for years been recording the College Annual Session panel discussions. These recordings represented about 25 percent of Audio Digest tapes. Audio Digest proposed to tape other parts of the Annual Session programs, assuming the entire cost of production. Any profits from this program would be split; 60 percent to the ACP and 40 percent to Audio Digest. It was suggested that the name be changed from "Postgraduate Courses" so that there would not be confusion with the College's regular postgraduate courses. The Board of Regents accepted the proposal, and for the next two years received a net contribution from the program of $38,000. The project was later known as the Audio-Cassette Program.

The Audio Digest Foundation also contributed to the College's Scholarship Program. Dr. Daniel Ellis, Chairman of Fellowships and Scholarships, received Board approval for the recommendation to establish the George C. Griffith Memorial Traveling Scholarship, to be funded by the Foundation's $10,000 contribution.

The Finance Committee asked the Board to reconsider its actions in April regarding dues and fees, at the request of the Steering Committee. The previous action eliminated the reduction in dues for Members and Fellows during the first ten years out of medical school. The Steering Committee noted that several factors had not been considered in the previous action. For example, under the action taken, an Associate who became a Member would have a very large increase in dues, from $15 (many times paid for by the chief of his program) to $80 a year plus an initation fee of $25.

On becoming a Member, the Associate also encountered the increased costs of the *MKSAP* and postgraduate courses. Agreeing with the Steering Committee, the Finance Committee recommended that reduced dues rate be changed from ten years to eight years out of medical school, which would be closer to the time of eligibility for Membership.

The Finance Committee again brought to the Board the growing necessity to charge the membership registration fees for the Annual Session. Discussed for several years, and tabled again in 1975, the Board at last approved the introduction of membership registration fees. Members would be charged $20, while registration for nonmembers would be $100, Associates would pay no fee, but non-Associate residents and interns would pay $15, which could be credited to annual dues if the individual became an Associate.

In April, Mr. Fred Dauterich, Director of Administration and Finance, was directed by the Board to revise the Pension Plan and Trust Agreement. Working with both legal counsel actuaries to redefine the plan to comply with the Employment Retirement Income Security Act of 1974, the administration presented an acceptable draft from legal counsel in November, 1976.

The College's entry into major health care policy issues was increasing the work of the Medical Practice Committee. Dr. John R. Gamble, Chairman, brought several items to the attention of the Steering Committee and the Board:

1. An ACP statement on procedural evaulation research was needed. After much study, the Committee decided that some form of peer review was essential, if the College were to continue to involve itself in funding health services research. They recommended to the Board that all health services research propo-

sals be submitted to qualified experts for adequate and impartial peer review. Members of the Medical Practice Committee could be utilized as reviewers.

2. The Committee recommended ACP endorsement of a separate Department of Health in the Federal Government and support for the concept of a functionally reorganized Department of Health.

3. A proposed national Medical Necessity Project, sponsored by National Blue Shield, was approved by the Steering Committee and the Board approved its implementation. Participating medical organizations would comprise a resource panel to evaluate the relative merits of new diagnostic procedures and identify procedures of dubious value, procedures redundant when performed in combination with other services, and procedures unlikely to yield additional information through repetition.

4. The Committee proposed that a conference be held to demonstrate how general principles and methodologies of social marketing could be applied to specific areas. A subcommittee was appointed, composed of Drs. Sam Martin and Henry Simmons and Mr. Isaak Kruger to explore the feasibility of using the Intersociety Committee on Antimicrobial Usage [ISCAMU] findings as an appropriate topic.

5. Social Security regulations relating to confidentially of records were posing problems for the Joint Committee on Accreditaton of Hospitals [JCAH].

The JCAH asked for College support for a proposed change in these social security regulations. Over the previous few years, Health, Education and Welfare [HEW] had conducted a validation study of hospitals that had been accredited by JCAH and released confidential information publicly. An out-of-court settlement was made in which HEW agreed they would not do this in the future. The regulations that appeared in the Federal Register served to clarify this problem and JCAH very much approved of these interpretations. The Steering Committee approved this, and a letter would be sent to the HEW Commissioner of Social Security.

6. Adopted by the National Academy of Sciences on the Committee's recommendation, the Board of Regents endorsed a resolution entitled "An Affirmation of Freedom of Inquiry and Expression".

## Governors' Conference

From a meeting of the Steering Committee held on September 21, 1976, following the Governors' Conference in New Orleans, the Board of Regents received a number of recommendations from the Governors.

1. A separate jurisdictional area for Alaska was approved by the Board of Regents.

2. The Governors suggested that the College become active in development of criteria for diagnostic and therapeutic procedures. This was referred to the Medical Practice Committee.

3. The Board of Governors asked the Regents to oppose the 1976 Congressional amendments to the Health Maintenance Organization [HMO] law that

would restrict the availability of services and quality of medical care, supporting the position of the AMA House of Delegates.

4. The Governors' Conference also debated the question of a specialty board for emergency care. Both the Board of Governors and the Steering Committee opposed the establishment of a freestanding board. However, they did consider the possibility of establishing a conjoint board representing the several specialty boards concerned. At the Steering Committee meeting, the President appointed a study committee, consisting of Drs. James A. Clifton, Chairman, Brian Williams and Robert G. Petersdorf, to prepare a statement for presentation to the Regents in November. In part, the approved statement read as follows:

> The American College of Physicians opposes the formation of a primary specialty board in emergency medicine. . . . . The practice of a type of general medicine localized to a specific area of a hospital does not warrant the formation of a separate specialty board with the attendant additional fragmentation of medical care, increasing costs to hospitals and thence to the public, and the creation of more jurisdictional areas within hospitals.

> Emergency room medicine potentially encompasses the broadest range of all clinical practice. The physician undertaking such practice must be trained in all areas of medicine, a task that is difficult to complete and one that will require significant input from the training program from all of the currently recognized specialties.

> There is an identifiable body of knowledge only in the pragmatic sense, and few, if any, fundamental contributions to medical knowledge will derive from this field. Emergency care must necessarily be provided by internists, surgeons, pediatricians and others in recognized specialties.

> The College is strong in its position that emergency internal medicine must remain a part of the graduate educational programs in internal medicine. In order to conduct this training effectively, departments of internal medicine must utilize and, to an appropriate degree, control administratively emergency medical services. It would be harmful if emergency facilities fell under the exclusive administration of another medical specialty. Surgeons, pediatricians and others can make the same case.

> Currently physicians practicing in emergency rooms have their professional backgrounds in a number of disciplines - family practice, internal medicine, and surgery probably are most heavily represented. It is appropriate that physicians from such diverse backgrounds group themselves into a specialty society in order to facilitate exchange of ideas and to assist in bringing recognition to their particular mode of practice. Many other groups of physicians have done the same and one has only to consult the listing of specialty society meetings in the *Journal of the American Medical Association* to appreciate the number of such societies in American medicine. The AMA officially recognizes some three score specialty activities, but in only one-third of these has it been deemed appropriate to establish specialty boards.

> The American College of Physicians welcomes the emergence of a group of physicians interested in emergency room practice and is ready to assist the American College of Emergency Physicians [ACEP] in its educational programs in any way possible. The College, however, does not equate the need for a specialty society with a need for a specialty board and urges the Liaison Committee on Specialty Boards to keep this differentiation in clear focus as it considers this petition.

5. Graduate Medical Education was the subject of a statement endorsed by the FCIM. Published in the *ACP Bulletin* in October, 1976, the statement, entitled "Training More Primary Care Internists," was presented to the Board of Governors and Steering Committee for comment, and was later approved by the Board of Regents. The statement began:

> The most urgent need for professional manpower today in the United States is for physicians who will provide primary care.
>
> This need is estimated to be 168,000 by 1980. In 1974 there were only 133,198 (47,572 internists; 52,141 were family physicians and general practitioners; 16,302 were pediatricians and 17,183 were obstetricians and gynecologists).

The statement also presented the sobering fact that although 120,000 internal medicine residents were in training in the past year only 3,000 were in their final year of training, and many of these would become subspecialists. The Federated Council was disturbed by this obvious shortfall in primary care manpower, and proposed several possible solutions:

a. Existing approved residencies have the best opportunity to help by assuring the quality of training and distributing resources over all three years of the program. The ACP offers a consultative service for faltering residencies, and the Residency Review Committee in Internal Medicine [RRC-IM] submits suggestions in its reports.

b. A student matching for a first year practice should be assured, upon satisfactory service, of being able to complete three years in a given program.

c. The number of training positions in internal medicine simply must be increased . . . Over 80 percent of residents in internal medicine learn in university affiliated hospitals. It remains, [the statement doubly emphasized,] for training program directors to extend those resources in any manner feasible in local situations. [Modes suggested were extension of affiliations with community hospitals, group practice training, increase of positions in internal medicine from unwanted "flexible" R-1 positions, and developing stipends from practice fees earned by chief residents that are consistent with existing regulations.]

Having committed the College to do everything possible to increase the number of residencies in internal medicine and increase the primary care manpower, the Board then turned its attention to the other end of the spectrum: subspecialty medicine.

## Council of Subspecialty Societies

In October, 1976, 13 major subspecialty societies met together and were represented by their senior officers. These societies were: American Association for Clinical Immunology and Allergy, American Association for the Study of Liver Diseases, American College of Cardiology, American College of Chest Physicians, American Gastroenterological Association, American Heart Association,

American Rheumatism Association, American Society of Hematology, American Society of Nephrology, American Thoracic Society, Endocrine Society, Infectious Disease Society of America and the National Kidney Foundation.

Highest on the docket was the subject of manpower. The agenda included a review of current manpower studies by Drs. Alvin T. Tarlov and Robert C. Mendenhall. Dr. Wallace N. Jensen, representing the RRC-IM, depicted the problems of balancing training slots between general internal medicine and the subspecialties. This problem of balance in relation to primary care issues extended into the activities of the ABIM, which was represented at the conference by Dr. John A. Benson, Jr. After Dr. Myers surveyed the implications of the Institute of Medicine's manpower study, he reviewed the recent work of the FCIM and the impact which internal medicine and its subspecialties could expect from the work of the CCME.

The delegations then reviewed, with Dr. Jeremiah A. Barondess moderating, the possible options for mutual aid in programming and education and potential ways of structuring ACP-specialty society relationships to facilitate further development.

The conference was especially informative on many manpower issues about which the subspecialty societies had widely varying degrees of knowledge. It demonstrated the great potential usefulness of such meetings for development of areas in which the College and the societies could be of help to each other. It clarified some of the organizational structure of regulatory and educational bodies in medicine. It underscored the potential value of an ACP effort to serve as the umbrella organization for the societies. The delegations agreed that another meeting should be held in 1977 at the Annual Session.

Following Dr. Barondess' report, the Board agreed that an ad hoc committee should be appointed to work toward the development of an official council of subspecialties as an activity of the College and to organize the next meeting in 1977.

The growing pressures to address manpower and health care delivery needs was strongly affecting the work of the ABIM. The Board, noted Dr. Robert G. Petersdorf, its Chairman, had been criticized for being heavily weighted with academicians. In a recent restructuring, a significant number of practicing internists had been added to the Board, including ten practicing physicians from widely distributed parts of the country. The functions of the ABIM had been revised to focus on the following activities:

1. At the most recent general certifying examination, of 7,802 candidates examined, 51.4 percent passed, but among the first takers, the graduates of US and Canadian schools had a passing rate of 79.6 percent.

2. Subspecialty examinations included 2,241 candidates. In the last cycle of all nine subspecialty examinations, 5,028 candidates had been examined.

3. In October, 1977, the Board gave its second recertifying examination. The Patient Management Problems were more difficult than those used on the self-assessment test. However, the candidates were not required to answer all PMP's, but were free to choose those most pertinent to their practice.

4. The Clinical Competence Program, which replaced the old oral examinations, required a thorough evaluation of the candidates by the program director. This decentralized approach demanded rigorous standards, and the Board was asking the program directors to stiffen their requirements by recommending that each candidate be evaluated in person by members of the faculty. Particular attention should be given to history, physical examination, and case synthesis. Since 1973, members of the Board have made site visits to over 300 residency programs to help with this in-house evaluation program. The entire program would be completed in 1977.

5. Computer evaluation methods were in experimental stages. Dr. Petersdorf announced that the Board would include two computer programs. One, called "Merit," was in development under a contract with the University of the Pacific, being directed by Drs. William Harless and John Gamble. The procedure would permit the candidate to work up a case step-by-step, using the computer from the beginning. The second computer program, "CBX", was jointly sponsored by the ABIM and the National Board of Medical Examiners, under the direction of Dr. Richard Friedman, of the University of Wisconsin.

6. The Task Force on Evaluation, appointed in 1975, was defining the content of internal medicine and a report would be forthcoming in early 1977.

The FCIM met twice in 1976, on January 23 and on September 28, and there was a high level of unanimity among the organizations represented on a number of issues.

1. The position paper on the training of internists was unanimously endorsed and published in October, 1976.
2. The manpower study sponsored by the FCIM was proceeding in good order.

The Council, in the very short time since its formation, was also tackling a number of other problems:

1. The ASIM proposed that preceptorship assignments in graduate medical education be made part of the medical school curriculum. The Council decided that such assignment should not be made compulsory but did adopt a motion "encouraging local ASIM component societies to provide directors of departments of medicine a list of individuals willing and capable of servicing as preceptors".
2. In matters of recertification and relicensure, ASIM announced its endorsement of the ACP's position that recertification in internal medicine should meet state requirements for relicensure or reregistration as one method of fulfilling state requirements for continuing medical education. The Council did not take an official stand on the matter, since the ABIM could not support linking recertification to relicensure because of possible legal controversies.
3. A conference for program directors in internal medicine was proposed and the FCIM agreed to sponsor and organize the meeting in the Spring of 1977.

4. The Council decided to create a task force under ASIM leadership to study extensively the complex problem of the cost of medical care.
5. The formation of state councils of internal medicine was under consideration. Dr. Alvin Tarlov reported that such a council was already being formed in Illinois. After discussion, FCIM approved in principle the concept of a mode of interface among the Association of Professors of Medicine [APM], the ACP and component societies of ASIM. They requested, however, that the term "federated" not be used in the name of any such state councils, particularly since the ABIM had no regional components.

The AMA House of Delegates, Dr. Julius E. Stolfi reported, was not ready to accept the idea of direct specialty representation. Interestingly, a number of specialty societies represented at the annual meeting also concurred with the AMA in this sentiment. A welter of current political issues in medicine were tackled in the June meeting; at the top of the list was the reorganization of the AMA, with final approval of the Constitution and Bylaws, incorporating eight councils. The House of Delegates then took positions on the following subjects:

1. Five specialty Boards still did not consider osteopaths eligible for certification. The AMA wanted them to reconsider their policies, for they generally favored the admission of qualified osteopathic physicians to specialty board examinations.
2. The AMA Council on Medical Education favored the reinstatement of the postdoctoral year in the training programs for physicians who provide primary care for patients.
3. The CCME presented a report on "The Specialty and Geographic Distribution of Physicians" being developed for the AMA Clinical Convention in 1976.
4. The AMA reaffirmed its position to assist in conflict resolution between hospital administrations and physicians in training on an advisory basis, stressing that this did not constitute endorsement of collective bargaining through trade unions.
5. The AMA strongly objected to violence on television and urged physicians, their families and their patients to refrain from viewing such programs.
6. The House urged the AMA forcefully to oppose inaccurate articles on "unnecessary surgery" currently appearing in the communications media.
7. The House also adopted a resolution that a private patient's care not be delegated to a house officer without permission from the responsible physicians.
8. Several resolutions on medical ethics were passed, and the House asserted that decisions concerning life support treatment, as in the Quinlan case, do not belong in the courts. The matter was referred to the Judicial Council.
9. A "second opinion" resolution was approved, with the qualification defending the right of patient refusal and stressing that the second opinion might not necessarily be the correct one.

10. The Medical Liability Commission was given temporary life by the delegates with the stipulation that it avoid participation in the political arena.

## JCAH "All or None" Accreditation Policy

The JCAH, at its last meeting in 1976, modified the "all or none" accreditation policy to specify that all programs in a given institution surveyed by the Joint Commission or its councils must be included in the survey, but no program that qualified for approval would be disapproved because of the failure of one program, unless that program did not meet the requirements after four years. The Joint Council also accepted the permissive position of local option in the matter of admission of podiatrists to hospital medical staffs.

The Medical Liability Commission, which was given tentative continued support at the AMA annual meeting, had had a rocky beginning, I reported to the Board of Regents. Formed in response to the HEW's Commission on Medical Malpractice, which wanted a large ongoing commission, including all kinds of professionals, the Medical Liability Commission was an attempt to foster self-policing among the providers of care. The AMA initiated the Commission, but one of the pathologists on the Commission appeared before a congressional committee, speaking as if he were representing the opinion of the Medical Liability Commission and its 22 represented societies. His comments, however, were his own opinion about the intrusion of government into the practice of medicine which was very disturbing to the other members of the Commission. The AMA's Board of Trustees gave notice that it would discontinue support of the Commission, an action which would quickly force it out of existence. The AMA and the American Hospital Association [AHA] were its largest financial supporters. The Commission forestalled this action at its September meeting by revising its bylaws to recognize the objections of the AMA regarding political appearances in Washington.

I also updated, for the Board of Regents' information, the activities of the CMSS. In April, the CMSS redefined its purposes as follows:

1. To participate in and provide representation to the liaison committees, CCME, American Board of Medical Specialties [ABMS] and other appropriate medical educational organizations.
2. To provide a forum for the discussion of problems of national and mutual interest in the medical specialties.
3. To initiate studies and discussions of problems of national importance confronting American medicine. To implement these objectives they adopted three goals:
   a. to foster excellence in the education and competence of physicians;
   b. to improve the quality of medical care; and
   c. inform and advise the American public regarding the progress of constructive activities in medicine. Committees were to implement these goals.

## Annual Session 1977

A special historic note of the Annual Session held in Dallas, from April 18-21,

1977, was the formal organization of the Council of Subspecialty Societies in Internal Medicine.

The work of the Ad Hoc Committee to Establish Liaison with Subspecialty Societies in Internal Medicine, and the efforts of Dr. Jeremiah Barondess, its Chairman, came to fruition on this occasion. Dr. Jack Myers' introductory statement emphasized the potential advantages of the construction of the Council of Subspecialty Societies in terms of overarching issues involving all the subspecialties, including responsibilities of all these societies to work together on manpower and increasing governmental attention to manpower and financial issues, challenges to internal medicine in accreditation and certification, and the disadvantageous position held by internal medicine relative to surgical specialties, especially in CMSS and in ABMS.

Dr. James Clifton, President-Elect, emphasized the importance of maintaining the identity of internal medicine and the protection of both general internal medicine and its subspecialties. Illustrating a series of potential inputs and support services which the College was prepared to provide, he suggested ways in which liaison arrangements could be structured to assist ongoing activities of the Council.

1. From the College to the Council: One member of the Board of Regents and one member of the Board of Governors could sit with the Council. These would be individuals knowledgeable about College policy and initiatives and about issues arising for consideration. In addition, College officers could attend at least a portion of each Council meeting to facilitate discussion and planning. Another possible arrangement might be for the Council, together with a College liaison representative, to meet in closed session for a half day and then meet with the College officers.

2. From the Council to the College: Dr. Clifton suggested that two to three Council members be designated to sit with the Board of Regents and the Board of Governors at their regular meetings. These individuals in turn would report to the Council, which could select items for inclusion in its own agenda for discussion. Reactions could be brought from the Council to the College by these representatives or by the Regents and Governors sitting with the Council or by both groups.

The ensuing discussion among the representatives revealed widespread acceptance and even enthusiasm for the concept, but some organizational problems which related to individual subspecialty societies were apparent. The sense of the meeting was that a "Letter of Intent" should be provided by the College, officially inviting the subspecialty societies to form a Council, which would be presented to their respective Boards. The Committee met again the next day and concluded decisions on representation. From those subspecialties already convened at the initial meeting, representation would be as follows:

One representative each: Allergy; Endocrinology and Metabolism; Hematology; Infectious Diseases; Nephrology (probably representing two societies); Oncology; Rheumatology.

Two representatives each: Cardiology; Gastroenterology/ Liver Diseases; Pulmonary Diseases.

When the Board of Regents met on April 20, the Committee presented the following actions for approval, on which the Board agreed:

1. The establishment of the Council of Subspecialty Societies in accordance with the above description;
2. Procedures as above outlined for the formation and structuring of the Council; and
3. That the College take on the secretarial expenses and administrative functions of the Council.

The 1977 Annual Session, featured a special lecture by ACP President, Dr. Jack D. Myers, on "The Computer-Artificial Intelligence and Medical Diagnosis." Dr. Myers' program developed at the University of Pittsburgh, called the INTERNIST/CADUCEUS utilized high level computerized technology as a consultant to the internist in complex and difficult diagnostic problems.

The Dallas Meeting drew 3,360 registrants, a disappointing attendance when compared with 5,640 in San Francisco in 1975, and 5,179 in Philadelphia the 1976, Bicentennial session. However, the State of the Art lectures and the panels were especially successful, and attendance at the scientific sessions had improved. The quality of the papers was good, with the added input from the subspecialty societies attending. Dr. Barondess, Chairman of the Scientific Program Committee, said the Committee members agreed that the College should continue to tap these societies for papers. The societies should, however, not be requested to screen papers. The Committee wished to avoid any imposition on those groups, and any implication that the ACP would be obliged to accept a certain number of abstracts from societies.

The Postgraduate Workshop Mini-courses were extremely successful. There were two courses: 88 subscribed to "Topics in Clinical Hematology", on the subject of hemostasis; 150 subscribed to "Modern Uses of Antimicrobial Agents". Symposium attendance was fairly good. Approximately 85 percent of the Workshop tickets were sold, and 93 percent of Meet the Professor session tickets were sold.

At the Spring meeting of the Board of Regents, the President, Dr. Myers applauded the work of the Steering Committee, saying it had become an effective part of the organization. He was also very pleased that the FCIM was doing a good job. Thanking the Executive Vice President for the work he had done during the year, he commented that his own responsibilities had been easy because of his support and because nothing very radical had been introduced during Dr. Rosenow's last year.

The President-Elect, Dr. James A. Clifton, looked forward to the coming year and recounted events at the annual meeting of the ASIM which he, Dr. Jack Myers and I had attended. There had been approximately 230 attendees. Dr. Clifton spoke on the panel, "The Views of Various Parents of the Federated Council". Not having a proposal that would represent the views of the Board of

Regents, he stressed, he made his remarks as a Fellow of the College. Dr. Clifton also expressed his concern that member organizations were discouraged over the AMA's secretariat functions for the LCGME and that open hostility was developing within the Committee and elsewhere over the problem. He warned the Board that they could expect to hear a great deal more about it in the near future.

The Secretary-General, Dr. Richard W. Vilter, reported the total membership of the College as of that date to be 35,871, of which 137 were Masters; 13,825 Fellows; 10,260 Members; 192 Affiliate Members; 123 Honorary Fellows and 11,334 Associates.

In his report, President Jack Myers, now outgoing Chairman of the Steering Committee, presented a very important document from the ABIM, titled "Attributes of the General Internist and Recommendations for Training", which the Committee had approved for publication. This statement which appeared in the *ACP Bulletin* in February, 1977, and in the *Annals* in April, 1977, was developed by the ABIM's Council on General Internal Medicine and approved by the ABIM Board of Governors on December 8, 1976.

> [It characterized the effective training program as producing] an internist who is proficient in the basic skills of data gathering, clinical reasoning, diagnosis and in planning diagnostic studies and management; [who has] a scholarly understanding of disease, ability in self-education and is able to meet the human needs of the patient.

Describing further attributes in some detail, the statement concluded with some very specific criteria as guidelines in support of residency training programs, covering basic training, teaching and training role models, hospital care, ambulatory and critical care, exposure to subspecialty disciplines, research, and advanced training to produce academic leaders.

Dr. Myers conveyed that the ABIM realized that the LCCME, which accredits training programs in internal medicine, had guidelines (last revised in 1974), for use in conjunction with the accrediting procedure. It was, therefore, not offering this document as a replacement for the guidelines of the RRC-IM. Rather, it had generated these statements to add to its position on the internist and primary care.

Parenthetically, in light of this statement it was interesting to note the findings of the primary care manpower study being conducted at the University of Southern California. It showed that if one looks at the kind of care a patient receives, then five distinct types of care can be identified: first contact, general, specialty, consultative, and episodic. Further, if general care is defined as the care a patient gets 95 percent of the time from one doctor, internists who classified themselves as "general internists" did almost 70 percent general care. Cardiologists did about 60 percent general care, gastroenterologists did abaout 53 percent, and all of the other subspecialists except infectious disease specialists, did 40 percent or more of general care. Infectious disease specialists are predominantly hospital based, and thus would not be likely to provide as much general care as the previously mentioned practitioners. These facts suggested that residency training designed to develop primary care capabilities was paramount in internal medicine and its subspecialty disciplines.

The *Self-Learning Series,* Dr. Neal J. Elgee announced, had been accepted for Category I credit for the AMA Physicians' Recognition Award. Completion of each monthly unit in this series conferred eligibility for three hours of credit. Approximately 1,500 physicians had subscribed to this new audio-visual service.

Dr. Marcus M. Reidenberg, Chairman of the Clinical Pharmacology Committee, presented a letter from Dr. Nottingale of the Food and Drug Administration [FDA] to Dr. Moser concerning drug abuse and amphetamine labeling. The Committee had considered the letter and concluded that additional continuing education activities for physicians in the treatment of obesity was warranted. They had strong doubts that removing the labeled indication of adjunctive treatment of obesity from amphetamines would aid in solving drug abuse problems in the US. They recommended that the American College of Physicians:

1. continue to include therapy of obesity in its continuing education programs;
2. urge the Editor of the *Annals of Internal Medicine* to solicit and publish a critical review paper on the drug therapy of obesity; (The format of this could be similar to the papers currently published in the "Drugs: Five Years Later" series); and
3. not support efforts to prevent physicians from prescribing amphetamines for medically valid indications. The Committee took the position, however, that long-term treatment for obesity with amphetamines was ineffective and, therefore, not a valid indication.

The Committee also anticipated the development of patient package inserts and their use in an increasing number of prescription drug packages. They recommended that the ACP participate in the development of guidelines concerning the nature of information to be included in these documents, especially the specific wording of patient package inserts included in drugs prescribed as a part of the practice of internal medicine and its subspecialties. The Board of Regents approved these measures.

The Credentials Committee of the College announced some new criteria which the Board approved. For a number of years it had been very difficult to evaluate properly the quality of written material submitted by candidates advancing to Fellowship. There had always been a variety of acceptable ways in which a physician could demonstrate scholarly activities; written material was only one of them. In order to make it more understandable to the Governors, the Committee recommended that there be a weighting of the quality of written material based on the following alternative criteria:

1. The written material would provide 100 percent of the evidence of scholarly activity;
2. The written requirement would fulfill 75 percent of the scholarly activity;
3. 50 percent of this activity would be fulfilled by the written material;
4. 25 percent could be fulfilled in this way and,
5. All scholarly activity might be accomplished aside from written material.

The Committee then reported reviewing the credentials of a total of 831 physicians who had been proposed for Membership and election to Fellowship.

The Educational Activities Committee asked the Board for action to initiate preparation of *MKSAP V*. Dr. Ralph R. Tompsett, Chairman, requested and received approval to 1) initiate *MKSAP V*, 2) convene the Ad Hoc Editorial Committee to develop the program, and 3) to constitute subspecialty committees immediately to prepare the syllabus for each subspecialty subject.

The Committee also recommended that the "Library for Internists" be updated on a three-year basis correlated with the timing and publication of the *MKSAP* "Annotated Bibliography". This was approved.

## Library for Internists II

The "Library for Internists II" was distributed gratis, and 789 were distributed. The *Annals* Editorial Office had combined this with the "Annotated Bibliography" for *MKSAP IV* in a special reprint which was sold for three dollars. Approximately 1,600 of these were sold and costs were recovered to about $4,600.

The Committee had recently analyzed the patterns of Regional Meeting attendance and again found that individual state meetings always showed a larger percentage of the regional members in attendance. In combined meetings the majority of registrants were from the state in which the meeting was held, with clearly low attendance from those in other participating regions. Total regional meetings registration for 1976-77 was 5,471.

Postgraduate Courses for the year of 1974-75 had 4,784 registrations in 40 courses, with five of the courses oversubscribed. The year 1975-76 showed a striking increase to 5,385 in 46 courses, with six oversubscribed. The year 1976-77 looked very promising, with 4,259 registrants already, as of April 11, and additional courses still scheduled. Four of these had already been oversubscribed.

Continuing medical education publication sales were impressive. The *MKSAP III* finally ended with 28,949 programs sold. The new *Self-Learning Series* had received 1,875 subscriptions to date. In order to promote the *Medical Skills Library*, a letter was sent to 400 medical directors in the US, offering an "on-approval" opportunity to receive and review any two topics for a two-week period at no charge. Forty-five replies were received, with five direct purchases. A similar letter sent to 575 members of the Association for Hospital Medical Education resulted in receipt of 10 direct orders. Since the College had taken over the distribution, approximately $1,600 worth of medical skills films and books had been sold.

The Fellowships and Scholarships Committee, chaired by Dr. Daniel S. Ellis, recommended that the Board of Regents create a fifth scholarship to be funded in the same amount as the existing scholarships, Dr. Ellis further recommended that the Board give special consideration in selecting candidates for scholarships to those who indicated a definite commitment to the goal of obtaining full faculty positions in teaching general internal medicine and of developing research programs in the management of patients in general internal medicine. The Board concurred with the special consideration and approved the fifth scholarship.

The Medical Practice Committee, as usual, had a wide array of activities to review with the Board. Dr. John R. Gamble, Chairman, reported some special new developments which promised to engage the College's attention closely in the near future.

1. Development of Procedure Evaluation Criteria

   Already involved in medical procedure evaluation, the Medical Practice Committee recommended the appointment of ad hoc committees composed of members of the College representing the subspecialties of internal medicine for the purpose of evaluating medical procedures that have been identified as current problems, i.e., obsolete, or future problems, new procedures that become popular before much experience is documented. Discussions had begun following the California Medical Association's adoption of a description of procedures to evaluate established medical procedures of dubious or experimental nature.

   A second model was developed at the Harvard Medical School, in which intensive one-year studies evaluated the scientific justification for particular aspects of medical practice. This activity was later to become an established grant-supported project under the auspices of the College, the Clinical Efficacy Assessment Program.

2. Anti-Microbial Usage Evaluation

   The ISCAMU was formed in order to evaluate the inappropriate use of drugs in hospitals and to develop corrective PSRO Guidelines. The Department of HEW awarded a contract to the ACP to implement this project. The study analyzed over 5,000 charts in 20 randomly selected Pennsylvania short-term acute care hospitals and identified several areas of inappropriate antimicrobial usage. The Medical Practices Committee agreed that certain subscription practices and behaviors should be changed in order to insure better use of antimicrobials. ISCAMU had provided data by which to test the effectiveness of a program directed toward modifying physician/prescription behavior.

3. ACP's Statement Concerning HEW's Proposal for Accrediting Health Manpower

   The Board of Regents approved the statement of this Committee on the Accreditation of Health Manpower. The College representatives then presented it to the CMSS where it was favorably received and incorporated in its official position. Some revisions were made in the statement on national health insurance.

4. The Medical Necessity Project

   Eight procedures had recently been evaluated.

   a. The project had determined that reimbursement for surgical sympathectomy used for the treatment of hypertension was justifiable in lumbar unilateral indications, but that lumbar bilateral sympathectomy should be reimbursed only upon submission of a satisfactory report.

b. Basal metabolic rate should almost never be reimbursed; there was some discussion that occasionally physicians do use this procedure in what is called an "open method". If this should occur, a satisfactory report might be accepted.

c. Protein-bound iodine, ballistocardiograms, angiocardiography using carbon monoxide methods, and icterus index should never be reimbursed.

d. Phonocardiograms were deemed reimbursable with interpretation in the report, but when performed with indirect carotid artery tracing and similar study, they should never be reimbursed.

e. Angiography A, (coronary unilateral selective injection, single-view, supervision and interpretation only,) might be paid upon submission of a satisfactory report. The Committee remained undecided about reimbursement for Angiography B, (extremity unilateral-view supervision and interpretation only).

This continued as an ongoing program under the auspices of Blue Cross/Blue Shield in conjunction with the College, reviewing myriad procedures which had significant implications in the cost of medical care.

After reviewing the questions regarding Patient Package Inserts, the Board of Regents resolved that, if properly designed, written and effectively distributed, PPI's could assist patients in achieving a safe recovery. A detailed statement was released to the press and subsequently published in the June, 1977 issue of the *ACP Bulletin*.

## H.R.-2222: House Staff as "Employees"

Simultaneously published with this statement was another major statement approved by the Board on a very important developing legislative issue, House Bill 2222, entitled "House Staff as 'Employees'. In part, the statement regarding H.R.-2222 read:

> The American College of Physicians expresses its strong opposition to House Bill 2222 amending the National Labor Relations Act to include interns, residents, and other housestaff physicians as 'professional employees' for the purpose of organizing and collective bargaining. The 37,000-member College, which consists of practitioners of internal medicine, clinical investigators, and medical educators, believes that this proposed legislation would have a deleterious effect upon graduate medical education in the United States. It would have as its ultimate impact the deterioration of patient care.

> Interns and residents are graduate medical students preparing for their professional careers and not employees primarily engaged in medical practice.

The remaining portion of the statement placed the physician in training in the context of undergraduate medical education, residencies and fellowship programs as an integral part of medical education and in continuity with all other aspects of graduate medical education, emphasizing that the student/teacher relationship could not yield to managerial egilaterianism.

An educational model rather than employee/employer relationship is mandatory to preserve this system. The American College of Physicians strongly advises that the proposed amendments be rejected.

Dr. Robert G. Petersdorf, Chairman of the ABIM, announced that the Board was sponsoring and staffing, along with the College, the ASIM and the APM, a conference for program directors who are not members of the APM. The ABIM remained the largest single constituency on the ABMS. It is the ambience of the ABIM to attempt to provide Certificates of Special Competence in Emergency Medicine and Critical Care Medicine if this is acceptable to the ABMS.

The Board had authorized a document which reviewed the history of accreditation of residency programs, which had been approved by the ABIM and endorsed by the APM and ASIM. Inadvertently it had not been presented to the Steering Committee at its last meeting. The Board of Regents approved the document.

In a final warmly bestowed gesture, the Board approved the title of Executive Vice President Emeritus on me at my last meeting with them.

### Executive Vice President's Final Report

My final report as the Executive Vice President could very well be titled "Unfinished Business". I reviewed the legacy of continuing problems and opportunities which the Board and my successor would have to try in every possible way to resolve or develop. My long-time concerns were a predictable list:

The ASIM

A number of recent developments made me more optimistic about a final solution in the reasonably near future.

1. Relations had improved since the failure of the merger attempt five years previously. Increasingly, the Society and the College were taking similar positions on a variety of subjects.
2. The creation of FCIM offered an opportunity for cooperative action in concert with two other organizations.
3. The ASIM leadership had approached ACP leaders with the possibility of interdigitating annual meetings.
4. In general, the formation of chapters had not been threatening to ASIM. In some areas, it had certainly brought the two societies closer together.
5. The ASIM had named me as "Internist of the Year" in 1977. I thought this was indicative of the growing goodwill of the ASIM toward the College and I would leave the Executive Vice Presidency feeling that I had helped to promote new cooperation and mutual support.

As more Chapters were being formed, I believed another opportunity for ACP-ASIM merger might present itself. If it did, I urged the College and the ASIM to do what was suggested five years ago, namely, to seek outside, expert advice in the design of an informative questionnaire which would be sent out jointly to the members of both societies. I believed it to be an essential element in determining the attitudes of each of the constituencies toward the merger. Any kind of survey should consider the constituencies involved:

1. ACP members who are also ASIM members.
2. ACP members who do not belong to ASIM.
3. Academically oriented physicians.
4. ACP members who are not internists.
5. ASIM members who do not belong to ACP.

Coordinating Council on Medical Education

The College was still not officially represented on the Coordinating Council on Medical Education and LCGME. Though many ACP Regents were on the CCME and LCGME, they were appointed by other organizations, such as CMSS, Association of American Medical Colleges [AAMC], AMA, etc., and not by the College. In the LCGME this fact posed a very difficult problem.

I questioned the benefit of having the RRC-IM evaluate a program, recommend accrediting and then submitting it to another body for official approval. This might be all right as a due process procedure, but it could be handled more effectively in some other way. When LCGME was first formed, I understood it would do much more than be an accrediting body. It was intended as a body which would study procedures, policies and regulations of all Residency Review Committees and then recommend more uniform operational procedures for all accrediting bodies.

It was also interesting to note that the CMSS and AHA only had two representatives each on the LCGME and the other groups had four each. I believed that this body could be more effective in an advisory or coordinating capacity if it were made up of representatives from each of the RRC's, instead of being represented by the parent bodies. Then reporting to and working with the CCME would be more appropriate. In this system, accreditation responsibility would revert to the RRC and the CCME could easily serve as a body for appeal to provide due process. Unless some mechanisms like this were adopted, I was convinced that the days of the LCGME would be limited.

In other groups in which the College had direct representation, such as in the JCAH, RRC-IM and now in FCIM, I believed we could be satisfied that our work was very effective.

The Medical Liability Commission

Since the meeting of the Regents in November, the Medical Liability Commission had gone out of business, illustrating how difficult it was for a consortium to do very much about the issue. As an alternative the American Medical Association had pledged a good deal of additional work in liability matters.

Subspecialty Societies

The representatives of the Subspecialty Society were holding a third meeting during the current Annual Session. I suggested that the allied specialty societies might also be included, if the Council of Subspecialty Societies proved to be successful.

The Steering Committee

The combined efforts of the Governors and Regents as an executive body was growing in effectiveness. I hoped that it would become even more active in decision-making and would handle many detailed matters between meetings of the Boards of Governors and Regents. I did not feel, however, that it should replace the policy decision-making which was the prerogative of the Board of Regents. For actions on many already established policies previously needing Board approval, the Steering Committee could certainly expedite without such approval.

Family Practice

A number of years previously, the ACP had supported the formation of the American Board of Family Practice [ABFP]. Three classes of young physicians with three years of training in approved residency programs had taken the ABFP examinations. In 1977, there were just over 300 approved family practice programs and even though some had not yet recruited any residents, there were enough to have certified approximately 1,600 from the residency qualifying route, representing the number who had taken three years of formal training and passed the certifying examination. In July, 1977, there were 2,000 in first year positions. At that time, about 90 medical schools had distinct visible divisions or departments of family practice. Some of these young physicians wanted to become members of the ACP. I again urged the Board to consider them eligible for membership for the following reasons:

1. They were going to be providing primary care along with internists.
2. They had had three years of formal training, a good part of which was in internal medicine.
3. The ABFP was established in the same way as other boards including the ABIM. The College was on record as having given support for the establishment of this board.
4. These physicians would benefit from ACP's excellent educational programs and would be more likely to participate as members of the College.
5. ACP allows all other medical specialties with a board to be members.
6. Currently, according to ACP rules, anyone who takes the ABIM, either passing or failing, is eligible for Membership in the College, and exclusion of this group was tenuously arbitrary.

There are residents from some marginally approved medical residency programs who had never passed the ABIM, yet were eligible for College membership. I agreed they should be; they could continue their education better inside the ACP than outside.

Over the next few years, I asserted, there would be increasing demands for more physicians to provide primary care. Currently, the College was promoting general training in internal medicine as essential to developing good primary care physicians. This would require more training in the ambulatory setting; a point specifically emphasized in family practice programs. The likelihood existed that over time, family practice programs would move toward additional training in the hospital setting. It seemed clearly in the public interest that family physicians and internists should work as closely together as possible.

In parting, I discussed the pleasure of the Rosenow travels and celebrations during the past year. In January, Esther and I went to Maracaibo, Venezuela, where I was made an honorary professor of the Zulia University. Following the current Annual Session, we were invited to Santiago, Chile, where the local Society of Internal Medicine would present to me a medal, the Southern Cross of the Grand Cross of Chile, signifying that I had contributed substantial good to the people of Chile through the education of their physicians.

At the current College meeting, the President of the Royal Australasian College of Physicians made me an Honorary Fellow of that College.

The AMA presented me a special plaque for distinguished service and the CMSS also presented a plaque for my contributions to that organization. Dr. and Mrs. Bryan Williams hosted a farewell dinner at their beautiful home in Dallas. This was a gala event and all present and many past Officers, Regents and Governors and their wives honored Esther and me with their presence. A beautiful silver tray was given with the stipulation that we could exchange it for something Chinese to add to our collection. We did so, and two beautifully carved wooden panels from the Wang Li Period of the Ming Dynasty (1573-1620 A.D.) now hang on our living room wall.

College employees had given us a heart-warming farewell party and we were very pleasantly surprised, particularly, by some of the presentations made. I received a First Edition of Osler's *Textbook of Medicine* and a new miniature camera. The greatest surprise I think I ever experienced was the gift from the Staff of a lovely oil painting of Esther, painted by Diana Dawson, a former student of Nelson Shanks, who had done my portrait which hangs in the Board Room. I announced that we planned to stay in Philadelphia and hoped that many of the Regents would stop by and see us.

### Epilogue

Through almost 18 years I enjoyed serving the College in its many activities. Over this time one of the original objectives has been very much fulfilled. This was to convert the College from an excellent educational organization dominated by academic leaders into a truly national medical organization which will increasingly take an important role in all aspects related to providing the public with high quality care through education.

Under new leadership, the College can be expected to continue its reorganization so that all forces influencing its "Core Mission" can be understood and managed. Social trends, governmental activities, relations to other societies, and economic forces will be better understood so internal medicine will be increasingly effective in providing the people of the country with the highest quality of medical care.

# Bibliography of Published Statements and Resolutions of the Board of Regents*

1. "Report" [in] Important Actions of the Board of Regents and Board of Governors, ACP-ASIM Liaison Committee, *ACP Bulletin* 4(4), 1963, 215-216. [Statement adopted April, 1963, regarding amendments to the ACP position on ASIM functions.]

2. "The Urgent Need for Federal Support of Programs to Provide More Physicians," *ACP Bulletin* 11(6), 1970, 279. [Adopted April, 1970.]

3. "Community Planning for Comprehensive Health Service," *ACP Bulletin* 11(6), 1970, 280. [Adopted April, 1970.]

4. "Organization and Functions of a Department of Internal Medicine in Community Hospitals," *ACP Bulletin* 11(6), 1970, 281-282. [Adopted April, 1970, as suggested by the Committee on Hospitals.]

5. "Physicians' Assistant," *ACP Bulletin* 12(5), 1971, 220-221. [Adopted April, 1971.]

6. "Delivery of Health Services," *ACP Bulletin* 12(5), 1971, 221. [Adopted April, 1971]

7. "Statement on Alcoholism," *ACP Bulletin* 12(5), 1971, 225. [Adopted April, 1971.]

8. "A Resolution Adopted by the Assembly of the AAMC on the Fight Against Cancer," [endorsement in] Important Actions of the Board of Regents and Board of Governors, April, 1971, *ACP Bulletin* 12(7), 1971, 365-366.

9. Residency Review Committee for Internal Medicine, "Special Requirements for Residency Training Programs in Internal Medicine," [in] Important Actions of the Board of Regents and Board of Governors, Executive Committee, April, 1971, *ACP Bulletin* 11(7), 1971, 362-363.

   For text of "Special Requirements . . . ", see:

   Barondess, Jeremiah, "A Summary Statement of the Views of the RRC-IM Concerning the Proposed Revision of 'Essentials of Approved Residency Programs' Pertaining to Residencies in Internal Medicine," *ACP Bulletin* 11(8), 1970, 412-413. ['Essentials' adopted by the AMA, ABIM and ACP also published in *ACP Bulletin* 11(12), 1970, 607-610.

10. Allyn, Richard, "Visiting Professors to Hospitals," *ACP Bulletin* 12(6), 1971, 279-281. [Project of the Committee on Hospitals, approved November, 1970 and April, 1971.]

* Resolutions referenced or quoted in the text, but not listed in the bibliography, are unpublished and taken from the Minutes of the Board of Regents. Unless specified as statements of other organizations endorsed by the Board, listed statements are those of the ACP.

11. "Meeting at HEW with Dr. Roger Egeberg" [in] Important Actions of the Board of Regents and Board of Governors, Committee on Governmental Activities, April, 1971, *ACP Bulletin* 12(7), 1971, 367-368. [Statement on 'Accessibility of Quality Health Care'.]

12. "The Internist's Role in Emergency Medical Care," *ACP Bulletin* 12(12), 1971, 618-619. [Adopted November, 1971.]

13. "Statement Regarding Proposed Amalgamation of ACP and ASIM" [in] Executive Vice President's Rounds, *ACP Bulletin* 13(5), 1972, 219.

14. McGill, Douglas B. "Delineating Hospital Privileges for the Medical Staff," *ACP Bulletin* 13(7), 1972, 348-352. [Prepared for the ACP Hospital Committee].

15. "Cardiopulmonary Resuscitation" [in] Actions of the Board of Regents, Hospitals Committee, April, 1972, *ACP Bulletin* 13(8), 1972, 446.

16. "Statement from the Committee on Venereal Diseases," *ACP Bulletin* 12(11), 1972, 590. [Adopted as recommended by the Committee on Community Services, November, 1972.]

17. "ACP Asks Administration to Restore Medical School Funds," *ACP Bulletin* 14(6), 1973, 350. [Adopted April, 1973.]

18. "Detection of Cancer" [and] "Physical Examination" [in] Actions of the Board of Regents, Cancer Committee, April, 1974, *ACP Bulletin* 14(7), 1973, 410.

19. "San Joaquin Foundation Project"[in] Actions of the Board of Regents, April, 1973, *ACP Bulletin* 14(7), 1973, 415-416. [Resolution to establish PSROs, endorsing statement of the Association of American Medical Colleges on PSROs.]

    For text of AAMC Statement, see:

    Council of Academic Societies, Report of Special Representative, "Policy Statement on PSROs, i.e., Quality Control of Medical Care - A Standard Setting Mechanism" [in] Actions of the Board of Regents, April, 1973, *ACP Bulletin* 14(7), 1973, 419. [Adopted by the AAMC Executive Council, March, 1973.]

20. Frommeyer, Walter B., Jr., "Recertification, A Status Report," *ACP Bulletin* 14(8), 1973, 475-476. [Includes statement adopted April, 1973.]

21. "ACP Speaks Out on PSRO Legislation," *ACP Bulletin* 15(7), 1974, 10-12. [Congressional testimony, Truman G. Schnabel, Jr. Resolution adopted by the Board of Regents, April, 1973.]

22. "AHA Statement Regarding Microbiologic Sampling in Hospitals," [in] Actions of the Board of Regents, Medical Practice Committee, March, 1974, *ACP Bulletin* 15(7), 1974, 29. [Endorsement of American Hospital Association Summary Statement, March, 1973.]

23. "Letter from Dr. Bertram Bell regarding Ambulatory Care Service and the Utilization of Nurses Trained as Surrogate Physicians" [in] Actions of the Board of Regents, Medical Practice Committee, March-April, 1974. *ACP Bulletin* 15(7), 1974, 29-30. [includes approved resolution.]

25. Joint Commission on Accreditation of Hospitals, "Listing Program for Specialized Clinical Service" [endorsement in] Actions of the Board of Regents, Medical Practice Committee, November, 1974, *ACP Bulletin* 16(2), 1975, 17-18.

26. American Board of Internal Medicine, "Training and Certifying the Primary Care Physician," *ACP Bulletin* 16(1), 1975, 53. [ABIM adopted September, 1974; Regents approved, November, 1974.]

27. "Policies of the American College of Physicians," *ACP Bulletin* 16(1), 1975, 10-12, 22-28. [Adopted November, 1974.]

28. "Statement on Primary Care," *ACP Bulletin* 16(6), 1975, 13. [Endorsement in April, 1975, of the Coordinating Council on Medical Education Report: "Physician Manpower and Distribution: The Primary Care Physician," June 3, 1974.]

29. "Delineating Hospital Privileges by the Medical Staff," *ACP Bulletin* 16(6), 1975, 13-15. [Adopted April, 1975.]

30. Residency Review Committee in Internal Medicine, "Primary Care Statement" [in] Actions of the Board of Regents, Steering Committee, *ACP Bulletin* 16(6), 1975, 13-15. [Approved April, 1975.]

31. "Statement on National Health Insurance," *ACP Bulletin* 16(12), 1975, 6-8. [Adopted November, 1975.]

32. "Recertification and Relicensure," *ACP Bulletin* 17(5), 1976. [Adopted April, 1976.]

33. Federated Council for Internal Medicine, "Specialty Distribution of Physicians: Congressional Statement," *ACP Bulletin* 17(1), 1976, 12-13.

34. Federated Council for Internal Medicine, "Position Papers on the Internist and Primary Care," *ACP Bulletin* 17(2), 1976, 10-12. [FCIM endorsements of statements by the American Board of Internal Medicine, American College of Physicians and American Society of Internal Medicine.]

35. Federated Council for Internal Medicine, "Position on an Integrated Health Manpower Policy for Primary Care," *ACP Bulletin* 17(3), 1976, 4-5. [Presented at the Conference on Primary Care, Institute of Medicine, Washington, DC, January 9, 1976.]

36. World Medical Association, "Declaration of Tokyo", October 10, 1975, *ACP Bulletin* 17(6), 1976, 15. [Endorsement by Board of Regents, April, 1976.]

37. "Determining Patterns of Care in Cancer," *ACP Bulletin* 17(7), 1976, 9.

38. "JCAH 'All or None Policy' " [in] Actions of the Board of Regents, Joint Commission on Accreditation of Hospitals, April, 1976, *ACP Bulletin* 17(7), 1976, 18-19.

39. Federated Council for Internal Medicine, "Training More Primary Care Internists," *ACP Bulletin* 17(10), 1976, 4-5.

40. Council on General Internal Medicine, American Board of Internal Medicine, "Attributes of the General Internist and Recommendations for Training," *Annals of Internal Medicine* 86(4), 1977, 472-473. Also in *ACP Bulletin* 18(2), 1977, 14-15. [Board of Regents endorsed November, 1976.]

41. "Patient Package Inserts" [in] Regents Voice Policy on Two Issues, *ACP Bulletin* 18(6), 1977, 9.

42. "House Staff as 'Employees' " [in] Regents Voice Policies on Two Issues, *ACP Bulletin* 18(6), 1977, 8-9.

# APPENDIXES

# A. Officers and Governing Boards

## A.1 *Officers*

### President

(President-Elect in preceding year)
1959-60 Howard P. Lewis
1960-61 Chester S. Keefer
1961-62 Chester M. Jones
1962-63 Franklin M. Hanger
1963-64 Wesley W. Spink
1964-65 Thomas M. Durant
1965-66 A. Carlton Ernstene
1966-67 Irving S. Wright
1967-68 Rudolph H. Kampmeier
1968-69 H. Marvin Pollard
1969-70 Samuel P. Asper
1970-71 James W. Haviland
1971-72 Hugh R. Butt
1972-73 William A. Sodeman
1973-74 Walter B. Frommeyer, Jr.
1974-75 Truman G. Schnabel, Jr.
1975-76 Robert G. Petersdorf
1976-77 Jack D. Myers

### First Vice President

(Vice President 1968- )*
1959-60 Wesley M. Spink
1960-61 J. Murray Kinsman
1961-62 Joseph D. McCarthy
1962-63 Marshall N. Fulton
1963-64 Elsworth L. Amidon
1964-65 William C. Menninger
1965-66 Carl V. Moore
1966-67 Wright Adams
1967-68 Samuel P. Asper
1968-69 Richard P. Stetson
1969-70 Walter B. Frommeyer, Jr.
1970-71 W. Philip Corr
1971-72 Kenneth G. Kohlstaedt
1972-73 Julius E. Stolfi
1973-74 John A. Layne
1974-75 Harrison J. Shull
1975-76 Maxwell G. Berry
1976-77 Lawrence E. Young

### Second Vice President*

1959-60 Walter de M. Scriver
1960-61 Carter Smith
1961-62 John C. Leonard
1962-63 Paul H. Revercomb
1963-64 Fuller B. Bailey
1964-65 Howard Wakefield
1965-66 Thomas Findley
1966-67 Edward C. Klein, Jr.
1967-68 Stacy R. Mettier

### Third Vice President*

1959-60 Garfield G. Duncan
1960-61 Karver L. Puestow
1961-62 Carl V. Moore
1962-63 Willis M. Fowler
1963-64 Frederick W. Madison
1964-65 Theodore J. Abernethy
1965-66 Charles M. Caravati
1966-67 John A. Layne
1967-68 Victor Grover

### Secretary-General

1959-1968 Wallace M. Yater
1968-1974 R. Carmichael Tilghman
1974-1978 Richard W. Vilter

### Treasurer

1958-1963 Thomas M. Durant
1963-1969 William A. Sodeman
1969-1975 William F. Kellow
1975-1981 Edward J. Stemmler

*Offices of Second and Third Vice President discontinued April, 1968.

## Staff Officers

1926-1959 Edward R. Loveland, Executive Secretary
1960-1977 Edward C. Rosenow, Jr., Executive Director (1960-
    1970), Executive Vice President, (1970-1977)
1977-    Robert H. Moser, Executive Vice President
1972-1978 Calvin F. Kay, Deputy Executive Vice President
1960-1980 Fred C. Dauterich, Jr., Director, Finance and
    Administration

### Editors, *Annals of Internal Medicine*

1932-1960 Maurice C. Pincoffs
1960-1970 J. Russell Elkinton
1970-    Edward J. Huth

## Chairmen of the Board of Governors

1959-1962 Marshall N. Fulton, Providence, Rhode Island
1962-1964 George C. Griffith, Los Angeles, California
1964-1966 John A. Layne, Great Falls, Montana
1966-1968 Roberto F. Escamilla, San Francisco, California
1968-1971 Maxwell G. Berry, St. Louis, Missouri
1971-1973 John R. Gamble, San Francisco, California
1973-1975 Jeremiah A. Barondess, New York, New York
1975-1977 Bryan Williams, Dallas, Texas

## A.2 *Regents*

| | |
|---|---|
| Theodore J. Abernethy, Washington, DC | [1964-65†] 1965-1971 |
| Wright Adams,Chicago, IL | 1968-1974 |
| Thomas P. Almy, Hanover, NH | 1968-1973 |
| Ellsworth L. Amidon, Burlington, VT | 1957-1963 [1963-64†] |
| Samuel P. Asper, Baltimore, MD | [1967-1970†] 1970-1972 |
| Fuller B. Bailey, Salt Lake City, UT | 1954-1962 [1963-64†] |
| Jeremiah A. Barondess, New York, NY | [1973-1975*] 1975-1977 [1977-1980†] |
| Maxwell G. Berry, Kansas City, MO | [1969-1971*] 1972-1975 [1975-76†] |
| Stuart O. Bondurant, Jr., Albany, NY | 1973-1978 [1978-1981†] |
| G. Malcolm Brown, Ottawa, ON | 1965-1972 |
| Hugh R. Butt, Rochester, MN | 1965-1970 [1970-1972†] 1972-73 |
| Charles M. Caravati, Richmond, VA | 1959-1965 [1965-66†] |
| Thomas L. Carr, Albuquerque, NM | 1975-1980 |
| James A. Clifton, Iowa City, IA | 1972-1976 [1976-1978†] 1979-80 |
| Robert C. Dickson, Halifax, NS | 1968-1974 |
| Thomas M. Durant, Philadelphia, PA | [1958-1965†] 1965-1968 |

† Officer
* Chairman, Board of Governors
‡ Ex Officio, Staff Officer

| | |
|---|---|
| Neil J. Elgee, Seattle, WA | 1973-1978 |
| J. Russell Elkinton, Philadelphia, PA | [1960-1966‡] |
| Daniel S. Ellis, Boston, MA | 1973-1978 |
| A. Carlton Ernstene, Cleveland, OH | 1963-64 [1964-1966†] 1966-1969 |
| Roberto F. Escamilla, San Francisco, CA | [1966-1968*] 1968-1973 |
| John R. Evans, Toronto, ON | 1974-75 |
| | |
| Ray F. Farquharson, Toronto, ON | 1960-1966 |
| Thomas Findley, Augusta, GA | 1958-1965 [1965-66†] |
| Edmund B. Flink, Morgantown, WV | 1971-1976 |
| Thomas F. Frawley, Clayton, MO | 1976-1980 [1980-1982†] |
| Walter B. Frommeyer, Jr., Birmingham, AL | 1966-1969 [1969-70†] 1970-1972 |
| | [1972-1974†] 1974-75 |
| Marshall N. Fulton, Providence, RI | [1959-1962*] [1962-63†] 1963-1969 |
| | |
| John R. Gamble, St. Helena, CA | [1971-1973*] 1973-1977 |
| John R. Graham, Boston, MA | 1969-1974 |
| George C. Griffith, Los Angeles, CA | [1962-1964*] 1964-1970 |
| Dale Groom, Oklahoma City, OK | 1970-1975 |
| | |
| Franklin M. Hanger, New York, NY | 1957-1961 [1961-1963†] 1963-1966 |
| James W. Haviland, Seattle, WA | 1965-1969 [1969-1971†] 1971-72 |
| W. Lester Henry, Jr., Washington, DC | 1974-1980 |
| | |
| Wallace N. Jensen, Washington, DC | 1975-1980 |
| | |
| R. H. Kampmeier, Nashville, TN | 1961-1966 [1966-1968†] 1968-1971 |
| Robert M. Kark, Chicago, IL | 1976-1981 |
| Chester S. Keefer, Boston, MA | 1953-1959 [1959-1961†] 1961-1964 |
| Richard A. Kern, Philadelphia, PA | [1951-1958†] 1958-1961 |
| J. Murray Kinsman, Louisville, KY | 1954-1960 [1960-61†] |
| Edward C. Klein, Jr., So. Orange, NJ | 1959-1966 [1966-67†] |
| Kenneth G. Kohlstaedt, Indianapolis, IN | 1964-1971 (1971-72†] |
| | |
| John A. Layne, Great Falls, MT | [1964-1966*] [1966-67†] 1967-1973 |
| John C. Leonard, Hartford, CT | [1961-62†] 1962-1966 |
| Howard P. Lewis, Portland, OR | [1951-52†] 1952-1958 [1958-1960†] 1960-1963 |
| Victor W. Logan, Rochester, NY | 1967-1970 |
| E. Hugh Luckey, New York, NY | 1965-1968 |
| | |
| Thomas W. Mattingly, Bethesda, MD | 1970-1973 |
| Joseph D. McCarthy, Omaha, NE | 1955-1961 [1961-62†] |
| Thomas M. McMillan, Philadelphia, PA | [1958-59†] [1960-1964‡] |
| William C. Menninger, Topeka, KS | 1957-1964 [1964-65†] |
| Stacy R. Mettier, San Francisco, CA | 1961-1967 |
| Carl V. Moore, St. Louis, MO | [1961-62†] 1962-1965 [1965-66†] 1966-1969 |
| Jack D. Myers, Pittsburgh, PA | 1971-1975 [1975-1977†] |
| | |
| Walter L. Palmer, Chicago, IL | 1937-1944; 1947-1955; 1957-1960 |
| George W. Pedigo, Jr., Louisville, KY | 1974-1979 |

† Officer
* Chairman, Board of Governors
‡ Ex Officio, Staff Officer

Robert G. Petersdorf, Seattle, WA · 1968-1974 [1974-1976†] 1976-77
Maurice C. Pincoffs, Baltimore, MD · [1959-60‡]
Herbert W. Pohle, Milwaukee, WI · 1974-1977
H. Marvin Pollard, Ann Arbor, MI · 1959-1966 [1967-1969†] 1970-1972
Karver L. Puestow, Madison, WI · 1954-1960 [1960-61†]

Charles H. Rammelkamp, Jr., Cleveland, OH · 1972-1977

Truman G. Schnabel, Jr., Philadelphia, PA · 1968-1973 [1973-1975†] 1975-76
Harrison J. Shull, Nashville, TN · 1969-1974
Carter Smith, Atlanta, GA · 1954-1957 [1960-61†] 1966-1972
William A. Sodeman, Philadelphia, PA · [1963-1969†] 1969-1971 [1971-1973†] 1973-74
William B. Spaulding, Dundas, ON · 1975-1981
Wesley W. Spink, Minneapolis, MN · [1959-60†] 1960-1962 [1962-1964†] 1964-1967
Richard P. Stetson, Chestnut Hill, MA · [1958-59*] 1964-1967 [1968-69†] 1969-70
Julius E. Stolfi, Brooklyn, NY · [1972-73†] 1973-1978

R. Carmichael Tilghman, Baltimore, MD · 1960-1968 [1968-1974†]
Ralph R. Tompsett, Dallas, TX · 1974-1979

Richard W. Vilter, Cincinnati, OH · 1971-1974 [1974-1980†]

Howard Wakefield, Chicago, IL · 1957-1964 [1964-65†]
Dwight L. Wilbur, San Francisco, CA · 1951-1957 [1957-1959†] 1959-1962
Bryan Williams, Dallas, TX · [1975-1977*] 1979-
Robert Wilson, Charleston, SC · 1956-1963
Theodore E. Woodward, Baltimore, MD · 1974-1979
Irving S. Wright, New York, NY · 1959-1965 [1965-1967†] 1967-1970

Lawrence E. Young, Rochester, NY · 1972-1976 [1976-77†]

## A.3 *Governors*

### ALABAMA

D. O. Wright, Birmingham . . . . . . . . . . . . . . . 1954-60
Walter B. Frommeyer, Birmingham . . . . . . . . 1960-66
Howard L. Holley, Birmingham . . . . . . . . . . . 1966-72
Alwyn A. Shugerman, Birmingham . . . . . . . . 1972-75
Thomas N. James, Birmingham . . . . . . . . . . . 1975-79

**ALASKA To 1977, SEE Washington/Alaska**

### ARIZONA

William R. Hewitt, Tucson . . . . . . . . . . . . . . . 1957-63
Hayes W. Caldwell, Phoenix . . . . . . . . . . . . . . 1963-69
Arie C. van Ravenswaay, Tucson . . . . . . . . . . 1969-72
Ashton B. Taylor, Phoenix . . . . . . . . . . . . . . . 1972-76
Charles A. L. Stephens, Jr., Tucson . . . . . . . . 1976-80

### ARKANSAS

John N. Compton, Little Rock . . . . . . . . . . . . . 1956-62
Jerome S. Levy, Little Rock . . . . . . . . . . . . . . 1962-71
Robert S. Abernathy, Little Rock . . . . . . . . . . 1971-75
Joseph H. Bates, Little Rock . . . . . . . . . . . . . . 1975-79

### CALIFORNIA (Northern) and NEVADA

Stacy R. Mettier, San Francisco . . . . . . . . . . . 1951-62
Roberto F. Escamilla, San Francisco . . . . . . . 1962-68
John R. Gamble, San Francisco, St. Helena . . . 1968-72
Maurice Fox, Palo Alto . . . . . . . . . . . . . . . . . . 1972-77

† Officer
* Chairman, Board of Governors
‡ Ex Officio, Staff Officer

## CALIFORNIA (Southern)

George C. Griffith, Los Angeles............1955-64
W. Philip Corr, Sr., Riverside..............1964-70
Edward W. Boland, Los Angeles...........1970-72

### Region I

Edward W. Boland, Los Angeles...........1972-73
Walter P. Martin, Long Beach; Carson......1973-76
Phil R. Manning, Los Angeles.............1977-81

### Region II

Varner J. Johns, Jr., Loma Linda..........1972-76
J. Edward Berk, Laguna Hills.............1976-80

### Region III

David B. Carmichael, Jr., La Jolla.........1972-76
John C. McCall, Jr., La Jolla.............1976-80

## COLORADO

Constantine F. Kemper, Denver...........1952-61
Charley J. Smyth, Denver.................1961-67
William A. H. Rettberg, Denver...........1967-73
Robert V. Elliott, Denver................1973-77

## CONNECTICUT

John C. Leonard, Hartford...............1952-61
Wilson Fitch Smith, Hartford.............1961-67
Benjamin V. White, West Hartford.........1967-73
Howard M. Spiro, New Haven............1973-77

## DELAWARE

Ward W. Briggs, Wilmington.............1957-66
A. Henry Clagett, Jr., Wilmington..........1966-72
Herbert M. Baganz, Jr., Wilmington.......1972-75
Robert W. Frelick, Wilmington............1975-80

## DISTRICT OF COLUMBIA

Theodore J. Abernethy, Washington........1958-64
Thomas W. Mattingly, Washington........1964-70
Henry D. Ecker, Washington.............1970-76
Frank G. MacMurray, Washington.........1976-80

## FLORIDA

Karl B. Hanson, Sr., Jacksonville..........1957-66
Donald F. Marion, Miami................1966-72
Chester Cassel, Miami..................1972-75
Charles K. Donegan, St. Petersburg........1975-80

## GEORGIA

T. Sterling Claiborne, Atlanta.............1957-66
Tully T. Blalock, Atlanta.................1966-72
Edwin C. Evans, Atlanta.................1972-76
Nicholas E. Davies, Atlanta..............1976-80

## HAWAII

Hastings H. Walker, Honolulu............1958-64
Morton E. Berk, Honolulu................1964-70
John L. Bell, Honolulu..................1970-73
Bernard W.D. Fong, Honolulu............1973-77

## IDAHO

Richard P. Howard, Pocatello.............1951-60
Paul F. Miner, Boise....................1960-66
Charles C. Johnson, Boise................1966-72
Maurice M. Burkholder, Boise............1972-76
Bernard L. Kreilkamp, Ketchum...........1976-80

## ILLINOIS (Northern)

Wright Adams, Chicago.................1957-66
Eliot E. Foltz, Winnetka.................1966-72
Robert M. Kark, Chicago................1972-76
Armand Littman, Hines..................1976-80

## ILLINOIS (Downstate)

Thomas D. Masters, Springfield...........1958-64
Edward W. Cannady, East St. Louis.........1964-70
Richard Allyn, Springfield................1970-76
Earl R. Ensrud, Urbana..................1976-80

## INDIANA

Kenneth G. Kohlstaedt, Indianapolis.........1958-64
Glenn W. Irwin, Jr., Indianapolis..........1964-70
Donald E. Wood, Indianapolis............1970-76
George T. Lukemeyer, Indianapolis.........1976-80

## IOWA

Willis M. Fowler, Iowa City..............1953-62
William B. Bean, Iowa City..............1962-64
Elmer L. DeGowin, Iowa City............1964-71
Atlee B. Hendricks, Davenport...........1971-75
Leslie W. Swanson, Mason City..........1975-79

## KANSAS

Fred J. McEwen, Wichita................1958-64
Sloan J. Wilson, Mission; Kansas City......1964-70
John L. Morgan, Emporia................1970-76
Ernest W. Crow, Wichita................1976-80

## KENTUCKY

Sam A. Overstreet, Louisville.............1954-63
Carl H. Fortune, Lexington...............1963-69
George W. Pedigo, Jr., Louisville..........1969-74
Franklin B. Moosnick, Lexington..........1974-78

## LOUISIANA

Marion D. Hargrove, Shreveport..........1954-61
G. Gordon McHardy, New Orleans........1961-68
A. Seldon Mann, New Orleans...........1968-74
Marion D. Hargrove, Jr., Shreveport.......1974-78

## MAINE

Elton R. Blaisdell, Portland . . . . . . . . . . . . . . . 1957-66
William C. Burrage, Portland . . . . . . . . . . . . . 1966-67
Albert Aranson, Portland . . . . . . . . . . . . . . . . 1967-74
Philip P. Thompson, Jr., So. Portland . . . . . . 1974-78

## MARYLAND

R. Carmichael Tilghman, Baltimore . . . . . . . . 1951-60
Samuel P. Asper, Baltimore . . . . . . . . . . . . . . 1960-66
Martin L. Singewald, Baltimore . . . . . . . . . . . 1966-72
Theodore E. Woodward, Baltimore . . . . . . . . 1972-74
Richard B. Hornick, Baltimore . . . . . . . . . . . . 1974-78

## MASSACHUSETTS

John R. Graham, Boston . . . . . . . . . . . . . . . . . 1959-67
Daniel S. Ellis, Boston . . . . . . . . . . . . . . . . . . 1967-73
Roger B. Hickler, Worcester . . . . . . . . . . . . . . 1973-77

## MICHIGAN

Noyes L. Avery, Jr., Grand Rapids . . . . . . . . . 1959-68
Muir Clapper, Detroit . . . . . . . . . . . . . . . . . . . 1968-74
Beverly C. Payne, Ann Arbor . . . . . . . . . . . . . 1974-78

## MINNESOTA

Hugh R. Butt, Rochester . . . . . . . . . . . . . . . . . 1959-65
James C. Cain, Rochester . . . . . . . . . . . . . . . . 1965-71
Howard L. Horns, Minneapolis . . . . . . . . . . . . 1971-75
Richard J. Reitemeier, Rochester . . . . . . . . . . 1975-79

## MISSISSIPPI

Laurance J. Clark, Sr., Vicksburg . . . . . . . . . . 1951-60
William K. Purks, Vicksburg . . . . . . . . . . . . . . 1960-66
Wesley W. Lake, Sr., Pass Christian . . . . . . . . 1966-72
Guy D. Campbell, Jackson . . . . . . . . . . . . . . . 1972-76
Thomas M. Blake, Jackson . . . . . . . . . . . . . . . 1976-80

## MISSOURI

Paul O. Hagemann, St. Louis . . . . . . . . . . . . . 1959-65
Maxwell G. Berry, Kansas City . . . . . . . . . . . . 1965-71
Thomas F. Frawley, St. Louis . . . . . . . . . . . . . 1971-75
Thomas W. Burns, Columbia . . . . . . . . . . . . . 1975-79

## MONTANA/WYOMING

John A. Layne, Great Falls . . . . . . . . . . . . . . . 1959-66
Alfred M. Fulton, Jr., Billings . . . . . . . . . . . . . 1966-72
Allan L. Goulding, Billings . . . . . . . . . . . . . . . 1972-76
Francis J. Allaire, Great Falls . . . . . . . . . . . . . 1976-79

## NEBRASKA

Edmond M. Walsh, Omaha . . . . . . . . . . . . . . . 1955-64
Henry J. Lehnhoff, Jr., Omaha . . . . . . . . . . . . 1964-70
John D. Hartigan, Omaha . . . . . . . . . . . . . . . . 1970-76
Robert L. Grissom, Omaha . . . . . . . . . . . . . . . 1976-80

## NEVADA 1951-1980 SEE CALIFORNIA (Northern)

## NEW HAMPSHIRE

Sven M. Gundersen, Hanover . . . . . . . . . . . . . 1953-62
Jarrett H. Folley, Hanover . . . . . . . . . . . . . . . . 1962-68
J. Dunbar Shields, Jr., Concord . . . . . . . . . . . 1968-74
Maurice L. Kelley, Jr., Hanover . . . . . . . . . . . 1974-78

## NEW JERSEY

LeRoy W. Black, Rutherford . . . . . . . . . . . . . . 1959-65
James F. Gleason, Atlantic City . . . . . . . . . . . 1965-71
Harvey E. Nussbaum, Millburn . . . . . . . . . . . 1971-75
Norval F. Kemp, Perth Amboy . . . . . . . . . . . . 1975-79

## NEW MEXICO

Robert Friedenberg, Albuquerque . . . . . . . . . . 1954-63
Reginald H. Fitz, Albuquerque . . . . . . . . . . . . 1963-69
Thomas L. Carr, Albuquerque . . . . . . . . . . . . 1969-75
Fred H. Hanold, Albuquerque . . . . . . . . . . . . . 1975-79

## NEW YORK

### Eastern

E. Hugh Luckey, New York . . . . . . . . . . . . . . 1959-63

### Downstate I

William J. Grace, New York . . . . . . . . . . . . . . 1963-69
Jeremiah A. Barondess, New York . . . . . . . . . 1969-75
Felix E. DeMartini, New York . . . . . . . . . . . . 1975-78

### Downstate II

Victor Grover, Brooklyn . . . . . . . . . . . . . . . . . 1963-66
Julius E. Stolfi, Brooklyn . . . . . . . . . . . . . . . . 1966-72
Leon M. Levitt, Brooklyn . . . . . . . . . . . . . . . . 1972-76
Lawrence Scherr, Manhasset . . . . . . . . . . . . . . 1976-80

### Upstate (Western)

Lawrence E. Young, Rochester . . . . . . . . . . . . 1959-61
Victor W. Logan, Rochester . . . . . . . . . . . . . . 1961-67
Paul A. Bunn, Syracuse . . . . . . . . . . . . . . . . . 1967-70
Stuart O. Bondurant, Jr., Albany . . . . . . . . . . 1970-73
Marshall Clinton, Buffalo . . . . . . . . . . . . . . . . 1973-77

## NORTH CAROLINA

Robert L. McMillan, Winston-Salem . . . . . . . . 1959-65
Monroe T. Gilmour, Charlotte . . . . . . . . . . . . 1965-68
Joseph B. Stevens, Greensboro . . . . . . . . . . . . 1968-74
John T. Sessions, Jr., Chapel Hill . . . . . . . . . . 1974-78

## NORTH DAKOTA

Lester E. Wold, Fargo . . . . . . . . . . . . . . . . . . . 1959-65
Robert M. Fawcett, Devils Lake . . . . . . . . . . . 1965-71
P. Roy Gregware, Bismarck . . . . . . . . . . . . . . 1971-75
Robert J. Ulmer, Fargo . . . . . . . . . . . . . . . . . . 1975-79

## OHIO

A. Carlton Ernstene, Cleveland . . . . . . . . . . . . 1957-63
Richard W. Vilter, Cincinnati . . . . . . . . . . . . . 1963-69
Charles Rammelkamp, Jr., Cleveland . . . . . . . 1969-72
William H. Bunn, Jr., Youngstown . . . . . . . . . 1972-76
Richard P. Lewis, Columbus . . . . . . . . . . . . . . 1976-80

## OKLAHOMA

Bert F. Keltz, Oklahoma City . . . . . . . . . . . . . 1955-64
William W. Rucks, Oklahoma City . . . . . . . . . 1964-70
Robert M. Bird, Oklahoma City . . . . . . . . . . . 1970-74
Ceylon S. Lewis, Jr., Tulsa . . . . . . . . . . . . . . . 1974-79

## OREGON

Merl L. Margason, Portland . . . . . . . . . . . . . . 1951-60
Daniel H. Labby, Portland . . . . . . . . . . . . . . . 1960-66
Franklin J. Underwood, Portland . . . . . . . . . . 1966-72
Wayne R. Rogers, Portland . . . . . . . . . . . . . . . 1972-76
J. David Bristow, Portland . . . . . . . . . . . . . . . 1976-77

## PENNSYLVANIA (Eastern)

William A. Jeffers, Philadelphia . . . . . . . . . . . 1958-61
Truman G. Schnabel, Jr., Philadelphia . . . . . . 1961-67
George D. Ludwig, Philadelphia . . . . . . . . . . . 1967-69
Francis J. Sweeney, Jr., Philadelphia . . . . . . . 1969-76
George L. Jackson, Harrisburg . . . . . . . . . . . . 1976-80

## PENNSYLVANIA (Western)

Frank J. Gregg, Pittsburgh . . . . . . . . . . . . . . . 1955-64
William M. Cooper, Pittsburgh . . . . . . . . . . . . 1964-70
Donald W. Bortz, Greensburg . . . . . . . . . . . . . 1970-76
John B. Hill, Pittsburgh . . . . . . . . . . . . . . . . . . 1976-80

## RHODE ISLAND

Marshall N. Fulton, Providence . . . . . . . . . . . 1953-62
Irving A. Beck, Providence . . . . . . . . . . . . . . . 1962-68
William J.H. Fischer Jr., Providence . . . . . . . 1968-74
Milton W. Hamolsky, Providence . . . . . . . . . . 1974-78

## SOUTH CAROLINA

Orlando B. Mayer, Columbia . . . . . . . . . . . . . 1956-65
Dale Groom, Charleston . . . . . . . . . . . . . . . . . 1965-68
Vince Moseley, Charleston . . . . . . . . . . . . . . . 1968-74
Roy A. Howell, Jr., Bennettsville . . . . . . . . . . 1974-78

## SOUTH DAKOTA

Donald L. Kegaries, Rapid City . . . . . . . . . . . 1958-64
Theodore H. Sattler, Yankton . . . . . . . . . . . . . 1964-67
Gordon S. Paulson, Rapid City . . . . . . . . . . . . 1968-73
Robert F. Thompson, Yankton . . . . . . . . . . . . 1973-77
Everett W. Sanderson, Sioux Falls . . . . . . . . . 1977-

## TENNESSEE

Rudolph H. Kampmeier, Nashville . . . . . . . . . 1954-61
Harrison J. Shull, Nashville . . . . . . . . . . . . . . 1961-67
Hall S. Tacket, Memphis . . . . . . . . . . . . . . . . . 1968-73
Gerald I. Plitman, Memphis . . . . . . . . . . . . . . 1973-77

## TEXAS ( Northern)

Alfred W. Harris, Dallas . . . . . . . . . . . . . . . . . 1964-66
Ralph R. Tompsett, Dallas . . . . . . . . . . . . . . . 1966-73
Bryan Williams, Dallas . . . . . . . . . . . . . . . . . . 1973-77

## TEXAS (Southern)

Victor E. Schulze, San Angelo* . . . . . . . . . . . 1957-63
Hatch W. Cummings, Jr., Houston* . . . . . . . . 1963-69
Robert A. Hettig, Houston . . . . . . . . . . . . . . . 1969-75
Don W. Chapman, Houston . . . . . . . . . . . . . . 1975-79
(*Statewide Governor to 1964)

## UTAH

Theodore C. Bauerlein, Salt Lake City . . . . . . 1954-60
Drew M. Petersen, Ogden . . . . . . . . . . . . . . . . 1960-67
James R. Miller, Salt Lake City . . . . . . . . . . . 1967-73
Donald E. Smith, Salt Lake City . . . . . . . . . . . 1973-77

## VERMONT

Elbridge E. Johnston, St. Johnsbury . . . . . . . . 1956-65
Sinclair T. Allen, Jr., Burlington . . . . . . . . . . . 1965-71
Robert E. O'Brien, Winooski . . . . . . . . . . . . . 1971-75
Porter H. Dale, Montpelier . . . . . . . . . . . . . . . 1975-78

## VIRGINIA

Kinloch Nelson, Richmond . . . . . . . . . . . . . . . 1959-65
William Parson, Charlottesville . . . . . . . . . . . . 1965-66
Julian R. Beckwith, Sr., Charlottesville . . . . . 1966-71
W. Taliaferro Thompson, Richmond . . . . . . . . 1971-75
Edward W. Hook, Charlottesville . . . . . . . . . . 1975-79

## WASHINGTON & ALASKA

James W. Haviland, Seattle . . . . . . . . . . . . . . . 1956-65
Neil J. Elgee, Seattle . . . . . . . . . . . . . . . . . . . . 1965-71
William E. Watts, Seattle . . . . . . . . . . . . . . . . 1971-74
Alvin J. Thompson*, Seattle . . . . . . . . . . . . . . 1974-78
(*1977-78 Washington, only)

## WEST VIRGINIA

Robert U. Drinkard, Jr., Wheeling . . . . . . . . . 1959-65
Edmund B. Flink, Morgantown . . . . . . . . . . . . 1965-71
Jack H. Baur, Huntington . . . . . . . . . . . . . . . . 1971-75
John E. Jones, Morgantown . . . . . . . . . . . . . . 1975-79

## WISCONSIN

Frederick W. Madison, Milwaukee . . . . . . . . . 1954-63
J. Le Roy Sims, Madison . . . . . . . . . . . . . . . . . 1963-69
Herbert W. Pohle, Milwaukee . . . . . . . . . . . . . 1969-74
George E. Magnin, Marshfield . . . . . . . . . . . . 1974-78

## PUERTO RICO

Federico Hernandez-Morales, San Juan . . . . . . 1957-66
Jose A. De Jesus, Caparra Heights . . . . . . . . . 1966-72
Eli A. Ramirez-Rodriguez, Bayamon . . . . . . . 1972-76
Jose M. Torres-Gomez, San Juan . . . . . . . . . . 1976-80

## CANADA

### ALBERTA

Percy H. Sprague, Edmonton............1954-63
Stephen B. Thorson, Calgary.............1963-69
Allan M. Edwards, Edmonton............1969-75
G. Sigurd Balfour, Lethbridge............1975-79

### ATLANTIC PROVINCES

Clyde W. Holland, Halifax, N.S...........1953-62
Robert C. Dickson, Halifax, N.S...........1962-68
Lea C. Steeves, Halifax, N.S............1968-74
G. Ross Langley, Halifax, N.S............1974-78

### BRITISH COLUMBIA

H. Archibald Des Brisay, Vancouver.......1953-63
Russell A. Palmer, Vancouver............1963-70
Donald S. Munroe, Vancouver............1970-74
F. W. B. Hurlburt, Vancouver............1974-79

### MANITOBA/SASKATCHEWAN

Francis A. L. Mathewson, Winnipeg.......1957-66
John M. Kilgour, Winnipeg...............1966-72
Robert E. Beamish, Winnipeg.............1972-76
John P. Gemmell, Winnipeg..............1976-80

### ONTARIO

W. Ford Connell, Kingston...............1958-64
O. Harold Warwick, London.............1964-70
William B. Spaulding, Hamilton...........1970-75
Ramsay W. Gunton, London..............1975-79

### QUEBEC

W. H. Philip Hill, Jr., Montreal...........1959-65
Douglas G. Cameron, Montreal...........1965-71
Stuart R. Townsend, Montreal............1971-75
deGuise Vaillancourt, Montreal............1975-79

## LATIN AMERICA

### REPUBLICS OF CENTRAL
### AMERICA/CANAL ZONE

Rolando A. Chanis, Panama..............1957-63
Mario Rognoni, Panama.................1963-70
Eduardo de Alba, Balboa Heights..........1970-76
Rudolfo V. Young, Balboa Heights.........1976-80

### CUBA

Carlos F. Cardenas, Havana..............1956-65
(Region discontinued 1965)

## MEXICO

Ignacio Chavez, Mexico City.............1951-61
Salvador Zubiran, Mexico City............1961-67
Jose Baez-Villasenor, Mexico City.........1967-70
Eduardo Barroso, Mexico City............1970-76
Luis R. Velasco-Candano, Mexico City......1976-80

## US GOVERNMENT SERVICES

### US AIR FORCE

Oliver K. Niess........................1958-63
Richard L. Bohannon....................1963-67
Kenneth E. Pletcher.....................1967-68
Robert B.W. Smith......................1968-71
Ernest J. Clark.........................1971-73
Dana G. King, Jr.......................1973-76
Ernest J. Clark.........................1976-78

### US ARMY

Leonard D. Heaton.....................1959-68
William G. Dunnington..................1968-70
Joseph A. Hawkins.....................1970-72
Nicholas F. Conte......................1972-75
Edward J. Huycke......................1975-78

### US NAVY

Bartholomew W. Hogan..................1955-61
Edward C. Kenney......................1961-65
Robert B. Brown.......................1965-68
Robert O. Canada......................1968-69
George M. Davis, Jr.....................1969-73
William J. Jacoby, Jr....................1973-78

### VETERANS ADMINISTRATION

William S. Middleton....................1955-63
Joseph H. McNinch.....................1963-66
H. Martin Engle........................1966-69
Charles A. Rosenberg...................1969-75
Herbert M. Baganz, Jr...................1975-81

### US PUBLIC HEALTH SERVICE

Leroy E. Burney.......................1956-61
Luther L. Terry........................1961-65
William H. Stewart.....................1965-69
Jesse L. Steinfeld......................1970-73

### US DEPARTMENT OF HEALTH,
### EDUCATION & WELFARE

(continued USPHS Governorship)
Henry E. Simmons......................1973-75
Robert Van Hoek.......................1975-76
Donald S. Fredrickson...................1976-80

# B. Awards, Fellowships and Scholarships

## B.1 *Awards of the American College of Physicians*

**The John Phillips Memorial Award.**

Established on October 27, 1929, for distinguished contributions in internal medicine.

1932 Oswald T. Avery, New York, NY
1933 William B. Castle, Brookline, MA
1935 Leo Loeb, St. Louis, MO
1936 Eugene Markley Landis, Boston, MA
1937 Richard E. Shope, Princeton, NJ
1938 Harry Goldblatt, Cleveland, OH
1939 Tom Douglas Spies, Birmingham, AL
1940 Rene J. Dubos, New York, NY
1941 William Christopher Stadie, Philadelphia, PA
1942 John R. Paul, New Haven, CT
1942 James D. Trask, New Haven, CT
1946 Edwin Joseph Cohn, Boston, MA
1947 Fuller Albright, Boston, MA
1948 Ernest W. Goodpasture, Nashville, TN
1949 Edwin B. Astwood, Hamilton, Bermuda
1950 Edward C. Kendall, Rochester, MN
1952 Andre F. Cournand, New York, NY
1953 Charles H. Best, Toronto, Ontario, Canada
1954 Donald Dexter Van Slyke, Upton, NY
1956 Linus Pauling, Pasadena, CA
1957 Cecil James Watson, Minneapolis, MN
1958 Amos Christie, Nashville, TN
1959 C. Sidney Burwell, Boston, MA
1960 Dickinson W. Richards, New York, NY
1961 Armand J. Quick, Milwaukee, WI
1962 Irvine H. Page, Cleveland, OH
1963 John A. Luetscher, Jr., Palo Alto, CA
1964 Jesse L. Bollman, Rochester, MN
1965 Jerome W. Conn, Ann Arbor, MI
1966 Helen B. Taussig, Baltimore, MI
1967 Maxwell M. Wintrobe, Salt Lake City, UT
1968 Sol Sherry, Philadelphia, PA
1969 James A. Shannon, Washington, DC
1970 Carl V. Moore, St. Louis, MO
1971 Maxwell Finland, Boston, MA
1972 Victor A. McKusick, Baltimore, MD
1973 Willem J. Kolff, Salt Lake City, UT
1973 Belding H. Scribner, Seattle, WA
1974 Oscar D. Ratnoff, Cleveland, OH
1975 Leon O. Jacobson, Chicago, IL
1976 Paul B. Beeson, Seattle, WA
1977 Grant W. Liddle, Nashville, TN

## The James D. Bruce Memorial Award

Established October 20, 1946 for distinguished contributions in preventive medicine.

1948 James Stevens Simmons, Boston, MA
1949 Stanhope Bayne-Jones, New York, NY
1950 Karl F. Meyer, San Francisco, CA
1951 Rolla E. Dyer, Atlanta, GA
1952 James H. S. Gear, Johannesburg, South Africa
1953 Thomas Francis, Jr., Ann Arbor, MI
1954 David Marine, Rehoboth, DE
1955 Sir Howard Walter Florey, Oxford, England
1956 John F. Enders, Boston, MA
1957 Alvin F. Coburn, Chappaqua, NY
1957 Caroline Bedell Thomas, Baltimore, MD
1958 Jonas E. Salk, Pittsburgh, PA
1959 Joseph E. Smadel, Bethesda, MD
1960 John H. Dingle, Cleveland, OH
1961 Albert B. Sabin, Cincinnati, OH
1962 Joseph Stokes, Jr., Philadelphia, PA
1963 Charles H. Rammelkamp, Jr., Cleveland, OH
1964 Robert J. Huebner, Bethesda, MD
1965 Luther L. Terry, Philadelphia, PA
1966 Robert A. Phillips, Dacca, East Pakistan
1967 David T. Smith, Durham, NC
1968 Walsh McDermott, New York, NY
1969 Colin M. MacLeod, New York, NY
1970 Theodore E. Woodward, Baltimore, MD
1971 Lowell T. Coggeshall, Foley, AL
1972 Saul Krugman, New York, NY
1973 Alexander D. Langmuir, Boston, MA
1974 Vincent P. Dole, New York, NY
1975 Dorothy M. Horstmann, New Haven, CT
1976 Gordon Meiklejohn, Denver, CO
1977 Edward D. Freis, Washington, DC

## The Alfred Stengel Memorial Award

Established April 17, 1947 for outstanding service to the
the American College of Physicans.

1948 Charles F. Martin, Montreal, Quebec, Canada
1950 James E. Paullin, Atlanta, GA
1951 George Morris Piersol, Philadelphia, PA
1952 George H. Lathrope, Morristown, NY
1953 A. Blaine Brower, Dayton, OH
1954 Thomas M. McMillan, Philadelphia, PA

1955 Maurice C. Pincoffs, Philadelphia, PA
1956 Cyrus C. Sturgis, Ann Arbor, MI
1957 William D. Stroud, Philadelphia, PA
1958 Alex M. Burgess, Sr., Providence, RI
1959 Hugh J. Morgan, Nashville, TN
1960 Edward R. Loveland, Philadelphia, PA
1961 T. Grier Miller, Philadelphia, PA
1962 William S. Middleton, Madison, WI
1963 Walter L. Palmer, Chicago, IL
1964 Richard A. Kern, Philadelphia, PA
1965 Robert W. Williams, Seattle, WA
1966 Howard P. Lewis, Portland, OR
1967 Chester M. Jones, Boston, MA
1968 Thomas Findley, Augusta, GA
1969 Wallace M. Yater, Washington, DC
1970 Dwight S. Wilbur, San Francisco, CA
1971 Marshall N. Fulton, Providence, RI
1972 Irving S. Wright, New York, NY
1973 Rudolf H. Kampmeier, Nashville, TN
1974 R. Carmichael Tilghman, Baltimore, MD
1975 Hugh R. Butt, Rochester, MN
1976 Edward C. Rosenow, Jr., Philadelphia, PA
1977 Walter B. Frommeyer, Jr., Birmingham, AL

## The American College of Physicians Award

Established in 1958 for distinguished contributions in science as related to medicine

1960 Philip S. Hench, Rochester, MN
1961 Arthur Kornberg, Palo Alto, CA
1962 Murray L. Barr, London, Ontario, Canada
1963 Arnold R. Rich, Baltimore, MD
1964 A. Baird Hastins, La Jolla, CA
1965 Vincent DuVigneaud, New York, NY
1966 Charles P. Leblond, Montreal, Quebec, Canada
1967 Marshall A. Nirenberg, Bethesda, MD
1968 Philip Bard, Baltimore, MD
1969 William B. Kouwenhoven, Baltimore, MD
1970 Robert F. Pitts, New York, NY
1971 Solomon A. Berson, Bronx, NY
1971 Rosalyn S. Yalow, Bronx, NY
1972 Robert A. Good, Minneapolis, MN
1973 H. Sherwood Lawrence, New York, NY
1974 George C. Cotzias, Upton, NY
1975 Henry G. Kunkel, New York, NY
1976 Donald S. Frederickson, Bethesda, MD
1977 Julius H. Comroe, Jr., San Francisco, CA

## The Edward R. Loveland Memorial Award

Established in 1961 for outstanding contributions by a layman or lay organization to community service in the field of health improvement.

1962 E. A. VanSteenwyk, Philadelphia, PA
1963 Robert L. Stearns, L.L.D., Denver, CO
1965 University of Pennsylvania, Philadelphia, PA
1966 Mrs. Albert D. Lasker, New York, NY
1967 John M. Russell, New York, NY
1968 Senator Lister Hill, Washington, DC
1969 John W. Gardner, Washington, DC
1970 W. K. Kellogg Foundation, Battle Creek, MI
1971 Western Interstate Commission for Higher Education, Boulder, CO
1972 The National Institutes of Health, Bethesda, MD
1973 The Commonwealth Fund, New York, NY
1974 American Cancer Society, New York, NY
1975 American National Red Cross, Washington, DC
1976 Robert Wood Johnson Foundation, Princeton, NY
1977 Henry J. Kaiser Family Foundation, Palo Alto, CA

## The William C. Menninger Memorial Award

Established on April 9, 1967 for distinguished contributions to the science of mental health.

1968 George L. Engel, Rochester, NY
1969 Howard P. Rome, Rochester, MN
1970 Dana L. Farnsworth, Cambridge, MA
1971 Ewald W. Busse, Durham, NC
1972 Theodore Lidz, New Haven, CT
1973 John Romano, Rochester, NY
1974 Ephraim T. Lisansky, Baltimore, MD
1975 Daniel X. Freedman, Chicago, IL
1976 Seymour S. Kety, Boston, MA
1977 David A. Hamburg, Washington, DC

## The Distinguished Teacher Award

Established on April 5, 1968, for physicians demonstrating "enobling qualities of a great teacher as judged by the acclaim and accomplishments of his former students who have been inspired and have achieved positions of leadership in the field of medical education primarily as teachers of succeeding generations of students".

1969 Eugene A. Stead, Jr., Durham, NC
1970 Duncan Graham, Toronto, Ontario, Canada
1970 Tinsley R. Harrison, Birmingham, AL
1971 George C. Griffith, LaCanada, CA
1972 Thomas M. Durant, Philadelphia, PA

1973 Thomas Hale Ham, Cleveland, OH
1973 Robert F. Loeb, New York, NY
1974 William S. Middleton, Madison, WI
1975 Franz J. Ingelfinger, Boston, MA
1976 Francis C. Wood, Philadelphia, PA
1977 A. McGehee Harvey, Baltimore, MD

### Richard and Hinda Rosenthal Foundation Award

Established in 1976 to be awarded to a scientist or scientific group for notable contributions to improve clinical care in the field of internal medicine and to an individual or organization whose recent approach in the delivery of health care will increase its clinical and economic effectiveness.

1977 Area Health Education Centers, Chapel Hill, NC
1977 Baruch S. Blumberg, Philadelphia, PA
1977 WAMI Program (Washington, Alaska, Montana, Idaho), Seattle, WA

## B.2 *Fellowships & Scholarships*

To promote and advance clinical research, the Regents of the College first established Research Fellowships on April 15, 1934, which were "designed to benefit young physicians in the early stages of preparation for teaching and investigative careers in medicine." In 1961, these one year awards were changed to three year Fellowships. In 1965, the Research Fellowships, which had supported to that date 91 scholars, were discontinued and, in their place, Teaching and Research Scholars were appointed for a term of three years and stipends were gradually increased. In 1967, in memorial honor to the 11th President of the ACP, the leading candidate was designated the George Morris Piersol Scholar.

Additional Teaching and Research Scholarships in Medical Nutrition were established in 1974 by the Nutrition Foundation, Inc., with two scholarships awarded each year for three year terms. These scholarships were continued until 1981.

The College also supports numerous other physicians in training through its Traveling Scholarships and Latin American Scholarships programs, and for limited periods, special programs supported by foundations.

The A. Blaine Brower Traveling Scholarships
Willard O. Thompson Memorial Traveling Scholarships
Alfred Stengel Traveling Scholarships
Dr. James H. and Dorothy S. Hutton Traveling Scholarships
George C. Griffith Traveling Scholarships
Latin American Scholarships

In 1948, the W. K. Kellogg Foundation and the College established a program to prepare academicians for teaching medicine in Latin American countries. From 1948 to 1969, 167 physicians from 16 Central and South American countries, designated "Kellogg Fellows", received graduate medical training in the United States and Canada. In 1964, these physicians, many of whom later assumed major professional leadership roles in their own countries, were received as "Affiliate" members of the College. In 1981, these scholars became eligible for full Membership in the College and by proposal, for direct election to Fellowship.

### Teaching and Research Scholars

#### 1965-1968

Robert Dean Conn (FACP), University of Washington, Seattle, WA
Ann Miller Lawrence (FACP), University of Chicago, Chicago, IL

#### 1966-1969

Lawrence M. Lichtenstein (FACP), Johns Hopkins University, Baltimore, MD
Philip W. Majerus (FACP), Washington University, St. Louis, MO

#### 1967-1970

Robert Lee Barenberg (Member), University of New Mexico, Albuquerque, NM and
  University of Miami, Miami, FL
* John Smith Barrett (Member), University of Pennsylvania, Philadelphia, PA
  Victor Samuel Behar (FACP), Duke University, Durham, NC

#### 1968-1971

John D. Hines (FACP), Case Western Reserve University Cleveland, OH. First George
  Morris Piersol Scholar.
* Herbert Savel, University of Vermont, Burlington, VT
  Stuart James Updike (FACP), University of Wisconsin, Madison, WI

#### 1969-1972

Oliver Elon Owen (FACP), Temple University Health Sciences Center, Philadelphia,
  PA. George Morris Piersol Scholar.
Alan Lester Bisno (FACP), University of Tennessee, Memphis, TN
Philip Felig (FACP), Yale University School of Medicine, New Haven, CT

#### 1970-1973

Timm A. Zimmermann (Member), University of Washington, Seattle, WA. George
  Morris Piersol Scholar.
W. Dallas Hall, Jr. (FACP), Emory University, Atlanta, GA
Alan S. Keitt (FACP), University of Florida College of Medicine, Gainesville, FL

#### 1971-1974

* George Reliford Spooner, III, Medical College of Georgia, Augusta, GA. George Morris
  Piersol Scholar.
  Philip Eugene Cryer (FACP), Washington University, St. Louis, MO
  Robert Charles Griggs (FACP), University of Rochester, Rochester, NY

* Term not completed.

## 1972-1975

Gino V. Segre (FACP), Massachusetts General Hospital, Boston, MA. George Morris
   Piersol Scholar.
Michael G. Rosenfeld (Member), University of California, San Diego, CA
* Stephen Waasa Spaulding (FACP), Yale University School of Medicine, New Haven, CT

## 1973-1976

Jerry Thomas Guy (FACP), Ohio State University, Columbus, OH. George Morris
   Piersol Scholar.
Robert S. Wigton (FACP), University of Nebraska Medical School, Omaha, NE
Frederick R. DeRubertis, Jr. (FACP), University of Pittsburgh, Pittsburgh, PA

## 1974-1975

Elizabeth Jansson Ziegler, University of California, San Diego, CA. (One year special
   Teaching and Research Scholar).

## 1974-1977

Richard Littleton Guerrant (FACP), University of Virginia Medical Center, Charlottes-
   ville, VA. George Morris Piersol Scholar.
Robert James Anderson (FACP), University of Colorado, Denver, CO
Jan Henrick Tillisch (Member), University of California, Los Angeles, CA

## 1975-1978

Eli Chester Ridgeway, III (FACP), Harvard University, Boston, MA. George Morris
   Piersol Scholar.
Charles Henry Scoggin (FACP), Duke University, Durham, NC
Caroline Armistead Riely (FACP), Yale University, New Haven, CT

## 1976-1979

Nicholas Francis LaRusso (Member), Rockefeller Institute, New York, NY. George
   Morris Piersol Scholar.
Mitchell DeWayne Andrews (Member), University of Oklahoma, Oklahoma City, OK
Beverly J. Williams (FACP), University of Tennessee, Memphis, TN

## 1977-1980

Alexandra Mary Levine (Member), University of Southern California, La Canada, CA.
   George Morris Piersol Scholar.
* Jeffrey Allen Sandler (FACP), University of California Medical Center, San Diego, CA
Jane Elizabeth Mahaffey (Member), Massachusetts General Hospital, Boston, MA

* Term not completed.

**Nutrition Teaching and Research Scholars (Nutrition Foundation)**

**1974-1975**

Lawrence Jay Brandt (FACP), Montefiore Hospital, Bronx, NY
James Victor Miller, Albuquerque, NM

**1975-1976**

Gary Melvin Brittenham (Member), Cleveland Metropolitan General Hospital, Cleveland, OH
Valerie Charleton Char (Member), University of California, San Francisco, CA

**1976-1977**

\* Robert Ethan Burr (Member), Rockefeller University, New York, NY
Jesus H. Dominquez (Member), University of Connecticut Health Center, Farmington, CT

\* Term not completed.

## C. Membership

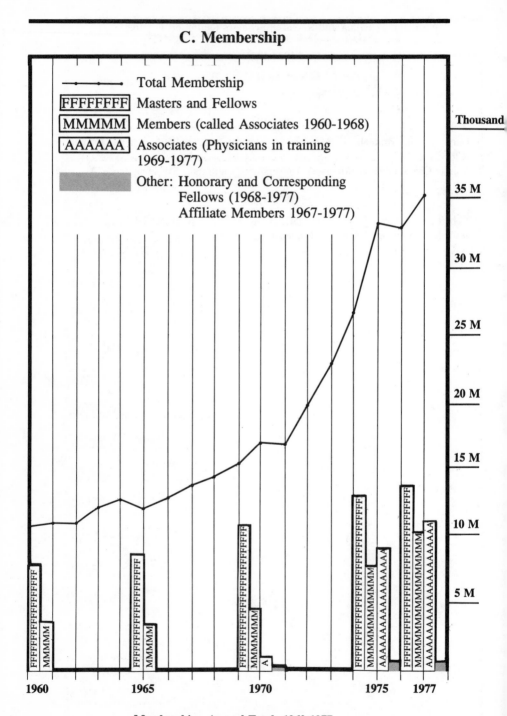

Membership—Annual Totals 1960-1977
Annual Membership by Classes at 5-Year Intervals
1960-1975 and 1977

## D. Publications and Financial Growth

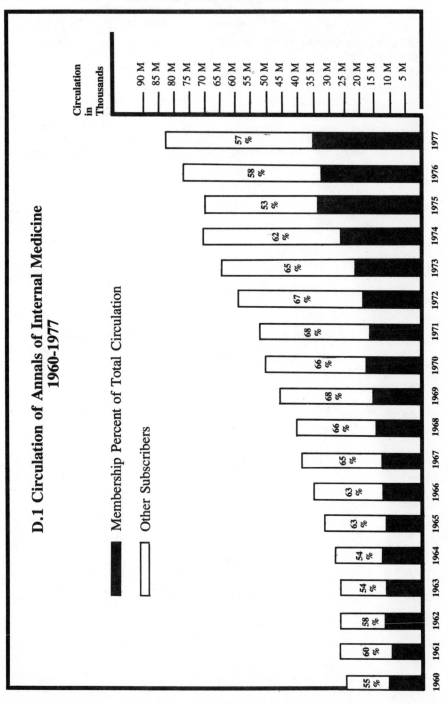

### D.1 Circulation of Annals of Internal Medicine 1960-1977

■ Membership Percent of Total Circulation

□ Other Subscribers

Circulation in Thousands: 90 M, 85 M, 80 M, 75 M, 70 M, 65 M, 60 M, 55 M, 50 M, 45 M, 40 M, 35 M, 30 M, 25 M, 20 M, 15 M, 10 M, 5 M

1977: 57 %
1976: 58 %
1975: 53 %
1974: 62 %
1973: 65 %
1972: 67 %
1971: 68 %
1970: 66 %
1969: 68 %
1968: 66 %
1967: 65 %
1966: 63 %
1965: 63 %
1964: 54 %
1963: 54 %
1962: 58 %
1961: 60 %
1960: 55 %

**D.2** *Medical Knowledge Self Assessment Program (MKSAP) Participation*

|  | ACP Physicians | Other Physicians | Total Participants |
|---|---|---|---|
| MKSAP I    (1968-1970) | 4,936 | 7,194 | 12,130 |
| MKSAP II   (1971-1973) | 13,839 | 5,253 | 19,092 |
| MKSAP III  (1974-1976) | 20,586 | 8,437 | 29,023 |
| MKSAP IV  (1976-1978) | 28,966 | 9,634 | 38,600 |

**D.3** *Financial Growth*

| Year | Operating Costs | Endowment | Property |
|---|---|---|---|
| 1960 | $  720,000 | 1,243,000 | 172,000 |
| 1970 | $2,510,000 | 3,892,000 | 1,973,000 |
| 1977 | $7,523,000 | 5,750,000 | 2,633,000 |

# E. Continuing Medical Education Participation

## E.1 *Regional Meetings Attendance*

| 1961-62 | 27 meetings | 3,276 |
|---|---|---|
| 1970-71 | 36 meetings | 4,991 |
| 1976-77 | 44 meetings | 6,773 |

## E.2 *Postgraduate Courses Participation*

| 1959-60 | 12 courses | 1,237 |
|---|---|---|
| 1969-70 | 24 courses | 2,726 |
| 1976-77 | 47 courses | 5,066 |

## MKSAP Courses first offered

| 1976-77 | 23 courses | 6,118 |
|---|---|---|

### E.3 *Annual Session Attendance*

| | Total | ACP Members | | | Total | ACP Members |
|---|---|---|---|---|---|---|
| **Philadelphia** | | | | **San Francisco** | | |
| 1962 | 7,217 | (3,176) | | 1960 | 5,243 | (2,039) |
| 1970 | 7,719 | (2,991) | | 1967 | 7,230 | (2,991) |
| 1976 | 8,360 | (5,179) | | 1975 | 8,724 | (4,226) |

| | Total | ACP Members | | | Total | ACP Members |
|---|---|---|---|---|---|---|
| **Chicago** | | | | **Denver** | | |
| 1965 | 6,026 | (2,441) | | 1963 | 4,609 | (1,918) |
| 1969 | 6,704 | (2,614) | | 1971 | 5,624 | (2,413) |
| 1973 | 5,765 | (2,712) | | | | |

| | Total | ACP Members | | | Total | ACP Members |
|---|---|---|---|---|---|---|
| **Atlantic City** | | | | **New York** | | |
| 1964 | 5,347 | (2,483) | | 1966 | 2,580 | (3,373) |
| 1972 | 5,759 | (2,681) | | 1974 | 7,077 | (3,895) |

| | Total | ACP Members | | | Total | ACP Members |
|---|---|---|---|---|---|---|
| **Miami Beach** | | | | **Dallas** | | |
| 1961 | 4,922 | (1,974) | | 1977 | 5,401 | (2,303) |

**Boston**
| | | |
|---|---|---|
| 1968 | 8,184 | (3,159) |

# F. Group Insurance Administrators, Inc.

## A History of the ACP Group Insurance Plans for Members

The American College of Physicians initiated an insurance program in 1953 as a membership service. The Board of Regents first discussed the question of providing such a service in 1937. Piersol *(Gateway of Honor)* relates that the "Board . . . directed the Executive Secretary to investigate . . . liability insurance for members of the College . . . " He reported in 1938 that "lack of enthusiasm on the part of liability companies and marked differentiation of liability insurance rates [made it] impractical to make any arrangements . . . at that time. The matter was raised again in 1952, and after a year and a half study, the plan was initiated.

The Board of Regents desired to have the management of the program in the hands of administrators who were experienced in insurance, rather than administrating the program as a staff function. The original administrator was the Association Service Office of Philadelphia, under the direction of Ralph O. Claypoole, Sr. and F. Wells McCormack. The administration was reassigned on April 15, 1955, to Group Insurance Administrators [GIA], under the management of Ralph O. Claypoole, Sr. and Ralph O. Claypoole, Jr. GIA located their offices, as tenants of the College, at 404 S. 42nd Street, Philadelphia, next door to the Headquarters in a building which had been a farmhouse predating the Civil War.

From the appointment of GIA until the present time, the insurance programs sponsored by the College have been their sole business. Therefore, they are responsible to the College for the efficient administration of the insurance plans purchased by the members.

Their work includes soliciting participation of members and answering their inquiries; processing applications and issuing certificates of insurance; billing and collecting premiums; and receiving and processing claims and paying benefits. In addition to these member related services, the GIA creates descriptive literature pertaining to the plans; deals with insurance companies selected as underwriters; and reports to the College officers on their stewardship responsibilities. Throughout the years of the program, the Claypooles, as administrators, have also faithfully maintained an interested membership relations program, attending College Regional Meetings to display materials, and staffing a booth in the exhibit area at every College Annual Session.

In 1971, GIA located their offices in the expanded College Headquarters building, and in 1978 they relocated to Havertown, in the suburbs of Philadelphia, because of College staff space requirements. Their staff consists of nineteen persons who work under the direction of Ralph O. Claypoole, Jr.

### Professional Liability Insurance

The first insurance plan sponsored by the College, Professional Liability (Malpractice) Insurance, was offered to members on January 1, 1953. The initial plan was underwritten by Lloyds and/or British Insurance Companies. After six years, 3,500 members were participating. In 1958, the underwriters requested rate increases which were higher than the premiums charged by local insurance companies which covered county and state medical association plans. The College did not believe the loss experience warranted the rate increases.

The Liberty Mutual Insurance Company [LMIC], Boston, Massachusetts, became the underwriter in 1959. The new plan offered limits from $25,000/$75,000 up to $1 million/$3 million. In addition to members of the College, physicians associated with members were eligible to be insured under the plan. In 1967, the LMIC was authorized to offer a Personal

Catastrophe protection or "umbrella" liability policy with a $1 million limit to College members who held the Professional Liability Insurance.

In 1974, LMIC asked the College to approve their plan to request a 200 percent increase in the premium rates; the alternative was cancellation of the policies to be issued to members. Because 3,003 policies were involved, College approved the request. However, the rates had to be approved by the insurance regulatory officials of each of the 50 states, and when the new rates were not approved in whole or in part by several key states LMIC requested the College to increase the rates in the states which were approved and to terminate the policies of members residing in states where the rate increase was not approved. The College refused to permit this selective procedure, insisting that the insurance offered to members of the College should be available to all members, and not only some members.

In addition, the College Insurance Committee noted several trends in the liability insurance business which were affecting the College Plan. The premium schedules were being raised rapidly by many insurance companies underwriting state and county society plans. The Committee was aware that LMIC would find it more and more difficult to reserve adequately for future losses. The possibility of increasing the participation in the plan was unlikely, because so many members were insured by state and county medical societies, through medical schools and hospitals.

In view of the decision by the College to deny LMIC the right to select states where the company could provide the plan, the insurance company gave notice that each policy with a renewal date of March 1, 1975 and thereafter would not be renewed on the policy annual renewal date. The last policy was not renewed on February 23, 1976. The College was unable to secure a replacement insurance carrier, so the College discontinued sponsoring a Professional Liability Plan. The LMIC continues to honor claims made against insured members, when the alleged incident occurred while the member was insured.

## Disability Insurance

The second plan of insurance for College members, which became effective April 15, 1953, was a Disability Income Protection Plan. The underwriters, Educational Mutual Life Insurance Company [EMLIC], Lancaster, Pennsylvania, initially enrolled 3,000 members. This enabled the company to guarantee insurance to each applicant regardless of his personal health history. The initial coverage was Lifetime Accident and Five Year Sickness protection.

A second disability plan was introduced in 1955, with a Sickness Benefit term of 10 years. In 1962, the 10-year benefit was extended to age 65, if a disability began prior to the 55th birthday, with a 10-year benefit payable for sickness disabilities beginning after age 55, and with any benefit ending on the 75th birthday. The Accident Benefit remained a lifetime coverage.

The Disability Insurance Protection Plan required the termination of individual certificates of insurance following a member's 70th birthday. Since there was a need for continuing protection against loss of income after age 70, as many members continued to work and did not retire, a separate Disability Plan for Senior Age Members was devised, and after August 1, 1956 the individuals who attained age 70 were invited to transfer their disability coverage to the Senior Age Plan. Although limited in amount and in the term of benefits, this Senior Age plan was unique for many years as a part of a professional organization's group disability insurance program, since other group insurance plans of this nature terminated the insurance of individuals automatically at age 70.

In 1963 the College approved extension of the Disability Income Protection Plan to the members of the American Society of Internal Medicine who were not already members of the College. Thereafter, each plan adopted was made available to that group.

In 1969 a major revision instituted premium rates based on the age of the member in place of the previous standard rate for all members. A special rate was included for members age 70 and over.

A major change in the insurance contract was the elimination of the termination requirement after attaining age 70, and the revised policy provided for the continuation of insurance regardless of age as long as the member worked a minimum of 20 hours a week. By 1969 the number of members participating in the Disability Insurance Plan had reached 5,700. The benefits paid to members in the first year of the plan had been in excess of $8 million.

In 1976, as more females entered College membership and became active in the insurance program, the Pregnancy Exclusion in the Disability Plan was amended to provide for the payment of benefits when the pregnancy was complicated by a concurrent disease or abnormal conditions affecting the usual medical management of the pregnancy.

College members on active duty status in the Armed Forces had been ineligible to be insured under the Disability plan, but, after discussions with several members in the Armed Forces and determining the extent of civilian incomes being earned outside of their regular work, the insurance company agreed to insure the civilian income of such members.

At the end of 1981 this Plan insured 6,000 members and more than 12,000 members had participated in the plan since 1953. With each revision of the plan, weekly benefit rates were adjusted and maximum benefits increased from $100 in 1953 to $600 in 1981. The benefits paid to members or in their behalf during the 28 years the plan had been in force were in excess of $23 million.

### Dread Disease Insurance

A third plan of insurance became effective June 15, 1954, which is known today as the Cancer-Specified Disease Plan. The insurance was originally designed to reimburse the medical expenses which a member might incur when he or a family member suffered one of the listed dreaded diseases. This plan was modeled after the "polio" policies being sold to the public at the time, and included not only polio but other dreaded diseases. Other than leukemia, cancer was not included on the original list of diseases. The maximum benefit for any one disease was $10,000. In 1957 cancer in all forms was added to the Plan, with a $5,000 limit for cancer losses.

The American Casualty Company decided to non-renew the more than 2,500 uninsured members in 1964, as losses mounted, with the bulk of the claims stemming from cancer cases. The EMLIC, underwriter of the College Disability Income Protection Plan took over the Plan and continues to insure the Plan to date.

In 1967, the Plan was amended to include a Coordination of Benefits provision, making the insurance supplemental to other group and government medical reimbursement insurance. It was further revised in 1969 to permit widows and dependent children of deceased members to remain insured under the Plan.

From 1954 through 1981, the insured members received more than $900,000 in reimbursement of the medical expenses incurred by the dreaded disease, with cancer representing the bulk of claims. Participation gradually dropped to less than 1,500 members as broader forms of Major Medical and Major Hospital Insurance became available.

### Life Insurance

After a survey of the College members indicated sufficient interest, the College Insurance Committee selected John Hancock Mutual Life Insurance Company [JHMLIC] to underwrite a Group Life Insurance Plan. The Plan, made effective March 1, 1960, had an initial enrollment of over 1,800 members. It offered one amount of life insurance of $20,000 for members up to age 41, under a Reducing Term Insurance, reducing after age

41 to $1,000 in force at age 71 and thereafter. Protection was also included for death by accident or loss of limb through dismemberment, acting as a double indemnity feature.

In 1960 the insurance laws of New Jersey, Wisconsin and Texas did not permit sale of Group Life Insurance to members of a professional association. However, New Jersey and Wisconsin permitted the Group Life Plan to be sold to the members resident in those states in 1976. Originally the members in these states could only purchase on an individual term life insurance policy, including the accidental death and dismemberment feature. Texas still prohibits the sale of the Group Plan to the residents of that state. In 1963 a Supplemental Plan of Life and Accidental Death-Dismemberment Insurance was added for insured members between age 41 and 65. The Plan earned a dividend after all losses had been paid for nine out of the first thirteen policy years. The financial success of the Plan permitted further expansion in 1969 and maximum coverage was increased to $25,000, without any change in the premiums. By this time, the participation by College members had reached 2,700.

In 1972 the Plan was revised to offer three additional coverage plans. Plans II and III offered $50,000 of insurance, on a reducing term basis; Plan II beginning at age 40 and reducing at five year intervals to age 70, with $2,500 remaining in force; Plan III to remain in force to age 65, when the amount reduced to $25,000 until age 70, and to $12,500 thereafter. An optional Survivor Income Benefit was offered which could be endorsed upon any of the Life Insurance Plans.

The amounts of all plans of coverage were increased by 20 percent in 1975 without any change in premiums. Plan IV was added to offer a $120,000 amount of insurance. The value of each plan was increased again in 1978, 1979 and in 1981, when two additional plans, Plan V at $200,000 and Plan VI at $250,000, were offered. By the end of 1981, the total life and accidental death and dismemberment benefits paid on behalf of insured members had reached $9,000,000. Enrollment was 3,837 at the end of the twenty-second policy year.

## Major Hospital Expense Insurance

A Major Hospital Expense Insurance Policy was introduced in 1963, underwritten by EMLIC. In 1966, however, EMLIC requested a $1,000 deductible amendment to the plan and a 100 percent premium rate increase because of loss payments of more than $500,000. A Coordination of Benefits provision was also requested. Though adjustments were obviously necessary, the College believed these provisions were unreasonable and GIA sought the advice of other health insurance companies. The JHMLIC offered a Major Hospital Expense Plan with a $500 deductible, a Coordination of Benefits provision and 50 percent premium rate increase. The plan was adopted on January 1, 1966, and pre-insured members were issued replacement policies without regard to their past medical history. Other members under age 60 were also accepted by open enrollment.

Continued adjustments to the plan were necessary in the succeeding years. The rapid increase in hospital expenses nationwide was reflected in benefits payments. In 1969, rates were age adjusted and graded daily hospital room allowances introduced. The advent of Medicare changed the need for the plan by members age 65 and over and the loss experience had proven that the age span from 45 to 59 was too long to maintain one rate. The allowances were revised in 1971 and 1973. Also in 1973, the plan was expanded to make the maximum benefit for each cause of injury or disease $50,000, instead of the original $15,000. For the first time, outpatient expenses were added and up to $150 was allowed for emergency room use.

The plan was improved in 1974 to include 1) increase in maximum benefits for hospitalization to $100,000; 2) a co-insurance ratio requirement under which the plan would cover 80 percent of the first $5,000 and then 100 percent of the balance of covered expenses; and

3) the Hospital Emergency Care Benefit was expanded to include ambulance service. Reimbursement for professional services performed in a hospital was also added.

Maximum benefits for both organic and non-organic diseases were again raised in 1975. Both the co-insurance requirement and the pregnancy exclusion were eliminated. Newborn children were automatically insured at birth. Pre-admission testing expenses in a hospital were to be paid and an outpatient Hospital Expense Benefit of $150 was added in 1976. Adjustments and increases were required again in 1979 and in 1981.

Participation in the plan peaked in 1978 and then declined to 2,605 members by 1981. Hospitals, medical schools, clinics and medical groups were increasingly purchasing hospitalization insurance for their employees, including physicians, and the need for the College Plan diminished.

### High Limit Accidental Death and Dismemberment Plan

The Insurance Committee adopted a High Limit Accidental Death and Dismemberment Plan in 1967, with the Bankers Life and Casualty Company, of Chicago, as underwriters. Over 1,500 members enrolled, and chose from six plan options ranging from $25,000 to $200,000, and including personal life or family coverage options. Insurance for members attaining age 70 was reduced to $10,000 with the same provisions for family coverage.

The Plan provides 24-hour protection worldwide under all circumstances, including travel, for those covered. By 1981, benefits amounting to $1,104,900 had been paid on 30 presented claims. The loss record since 1970 has not required any increases or adjustments in premium rates.

### Insurance for Employees of Members

Employees of members of the insurance program were first included in 1971. The ACP Insurance Trust amended the definition of "members" to include employees of College members. The policies of EMLIC were amended to provide Disability Insurance and Cancer-Specified Disease Insurance. The Major Hospital Expense Plan under the JHMLIC and the Bankers Life and Casualty Company's High Limit Accidental Death and Dismemberment Plan were also amended to be extended to employees.

In order to fulfill the requirements of the Federal Employee Retirement Income Security Act of 1974 [ERISA], a new insurance trust was established in 1976, known as the American College of Physicians Members' Employees Group Insurance Trust. All contracts were then issued to all employees of members under this trust. Because legal requirements vary in many states, applying differently to employees and to professional associations, life insurance is not offered to employees of members.

By 1981, the number of members who have used this plan to provide for their employees was 248, with the Major Hospital Expense Plan being the primary coverage purchased. There has been $83,000 paid in benefits under the Disability Plan and $205,000 in hospital expense reimbursements.

The Claypooles have operated a very successful insurance program for the College members. The fact that they work only for College members has meant that insured members have always had them "in their corner" to straighten out problems which arise from misunderstandings between insurance carriers and the members. They have always been an actively participating part of the College, attending Regional Meetings and Annual Sessions where they are personally available to members. The Claypooles have always been cooperative and helpful far beyond merely handling the insurance needs of members.

In 1979, following the death of Ralph O. Claypoole, Sr., his son offered to establish and finance an annual award in his name. The Board of Regents accepted and the established Ralph O. Claypoole, Sr., Award is given "in recognition of distinguished achievements in the clinical practice of internal medicine".

# G. Memorandum of Intent

## Background

The AMERICAN COLLEGE OF PHYSICIANS is a nonprofit membership Delaware Corporation, consisting of physicians who specialize in the practice of internal medicine or other related fields of medicine. The principal purposes of ACP are:

a. Maintaining and advancing the highest possible standards in medical education, medical practice and medical research.
b. Preserving the history and perpetuating the best tradition of medicine and medical ethics.
c. Maintaining both the dignity of internal medicine and the efficiency of its function in relation to public welfare.

The AMERICAN SOCIETY OF INTERNAL MEDICINE is a nonprofit membership California corporation, consisting of physicians who specialize in the practice of internal medicine. The principal purposes of ASIM are:

a. To study the scientific, economic, social and public aspects of the practice of medicine at a national level in order to secure and maintain the best patient care and the highest standard of practice in the medical specialty known as Internal Medicine.
b. To maintain a federation of state, District of Columbia, United States Territorial and United States Commonwealth Societies of qualified doctors of medicine specializing in the practice of internal medicine, and for the coordination of their efforts in furthering the practice of internal medicine.
c. To complement and supplement the aims and activities of ACP.
d. To encourage the development of strong State, District of Columbia, United States Territorial and United States Commonwealth Societies of Internal Medicine.

It is deemed by the governing boards of ACP and ASIM to be in the best interest of both organizations and their respective memberships to create a new, separate and distinct national organization whose goals and purposes shall be in accord with the goals and purposes of ACP and ASIM, and whose membership shall initially consist of the membership of ACP and ASIM.

## Agreement:

IT IS HEREBY AGREED by and between THE AMERICAN COLLEGE OF PHYSICIANS and the AMERICAN SOCIETY OF INTERNAL MEDICINE as follows:

1. ACP and ASIM shall create under the laws of the State of Delaware a new national nonprofit membership corporation to be known as AMERICAN COLLEGE OF PHYSICIANS-AMERICAN SOCIETY OF INTERNAL MEDICINE, which name will not be altered without a two-thirds (2/3) vote of the Council provided for hereinafter. Its principal place of business shall be in the City of Philadelphia, State of Pennsylvania.
2. The principal purposes, goals and aims of ACP-ASIM shall be:
   a. To maintain both the dignity of internal medicine and efficiency of its function in relation to public welfare.
   b. To maintain and advance the highest possible standards of medical education, medical practice and medical research.
   c. To study the scientific, economic, social and legislative aspects of medicine at a

national level in order to secure and maintain the best patient care, and highest standard of practice in internal medicine.

d. To maintain a federation of state, territorial, and Canadian provincial societies composed of qualified doctors of medicine specializing in the practice of internal medicine or other related fields of medicine for the coordination of their efforts in furthering the practice in internal medicine.

e. To preserve the history and perpetuate the best tradition of medicine and medical ethics.

f. To preserve the history and perpetuate the traditions and practices of the AMERICAN COLLEGE OF PHYSICIANS and the AMERICAN SOCIETY OF INTERNAL MEDICINE.

3. The organizational structure of ACP-ASIM shall be in conformance with the following requirements:

a. ACP-ASIM shall be composed of component societies and their individual members.

b. The component societies of ACP-ASIM shall be chartered by ACP-ASIM and shall:

i. Subject to membership criteria set by ACP-ASIM, elect and admit their own individual members.

ii. Elect their own officers and representatives to the national organization, who, however, must be members of respective component societies by which they are elected as officers or representatives.

iii. Set their own policies within the goals and purposes set by ACP-ASIM, including the determination of local dues and local assessments.

c. Membership in ACP-ASIM shall consist of the individual members of the component societies, which have been chartered by ACP-ASIM.

d. The respective classes, rights, and privileges of individual members shall be set and determined by ACP-ASIM.

e. The membership criteria for each class of individual membership shall be determined by ACP-ASIM.

f. All of the members of ACP and ASIM on the effective date of the reorganization shall automatically be admitted to membership in ACP-ASIM and to membership in the component society representing the area in which they practice, provided such individuals have not resigned from membership from ACP or ASIM subsequent to March 1, 1972. For the purpose of reorganization, all of the component societies of ASIM on the effective date of reorganization shall automatically be chartered by ACP-ASIM.

g. Subsequent to the effective date of reorganization, new Members in ACP-ASIM shall be elected to the membership of the component society of ACP-ASIM representing the area in which the applicant carries on his professional activities.

h. All active members shall have equal rights, including the right to hold office locally and nationally.

i. ACP-ASIM shall have a Council which shall:

i. Be composed of councillors from each of the component societies, with each component society having at least one councillor and some proportionate numerical representation.

ii. Councillors shall be elected by the component society of which they are member.

iii. The Council shall elect the officers and the Board of Directors of ACP-ASIM.

    iv. Nominations for the Board of Directors and officers shall be by a nomination committee appointed by the president; however, nominations may be made from the floor of the Council.

    v. The Council may initiate, recommend and review policies set by the Board of Directors.

    vi. Each Councillor shall be elected for a term of three years, but shall in no instance serve more than a total of six years.

    vii. The Council shall approve or disapprove dues, and assessments recommended by the Board of Directors.

    viii. The Council shall meet at least annually.

  j. ACP-ASIM shall be governed by a Board of Directors which shall consist of the officers of ACP-ASIM and the Directors of ACP-ASIM elected by the Council.

  k. Each member of the Board of Directors shall be elected for a term of three years, but in no instance shall serve for more than a total of six years.

  l. The Board of Directors shall adopt the policies to carry out the purposes of ACP-ASIM, which policies shall be subject to review by the Council.

  m. The Board of Directors shall appoint the chief administrative officer of ACP-ASIM.

  n. The Board of Directors shall adopt and recommend to the Council the dues, assessments for ACP-ASIM, for final approval by the Council.

  o. Any action by the Board of Directors may be rescinded by a two-thirds (2/3) vote of the Council.

  p. The nomination committee shall consist of six individual members, two each from the Council, the Board of Directors, and the membership at large.

4. ACP and ASIM hereby agree that upon the effective date of reorganization, all of the assets and rights of both organizations shall be transferred to or consolidated into ACP-ASIM, and ACP-ASIM shall thereupon assume all of the liabilities and responsibilities of both organizations.

5. ACP and ASIM hereby agree to create a joint committee to meet as often as necessary to implement the terms and conditions of this agreement. As of April 20, 1972, the joint committee shall consist of the President, President-Elect, and the Immediate Past President of each organization.

6. ACP and ASIM hereby further agree and covenant to execute all documents and to enter into all other necessary negotiations, contracts or agreements to effect the purposes and intent of this agreement.

7. ACP and ASIM further agree not to change substantially their respective present methods of operation, conduct of business, or criteria or procedures for election to membership prior to the effective date of the reorganization.

8. ACP and ASIM hereby further agree and covenant that this agreement shall be placed on the agenda of the next scheduled meeting of the Board of Regents of ACP, which is to be held on April 15, 1972, and the House of Delegates of ASIM, which is to be held on April 14-16, 1972, for approval and ratification thereof. This agreement shall not become binding until such approval has been secured.

9. ACP and ASIM further agree that the reorganization contemplated by this agreement shall be placed on the agenda of the annual meeting of the members of ACP and the House of Delegates of ASIM scheduled for April, 1973. After such approvals are secured, the reorganization shall become effective as soon thereafter as practical.

DATED: March 9, 1972

# INDEX

# NAME INDEX

# SUBJECT INDEX

A key to acronyms used in the text is found at the end of the Index.

Numerals in bold face type are (1) dates; (2) publication editions in Roman; and (3) tables, graphs and lists in the appendix.

## A

Academic regalia, 21

Academic physicians, in ACP, 2-3, 12, 90-92

Accreditation of, animal facilities, 97, 117-118, 145, 184; extended care facilities, 77, 135; health manpower, 297, 390; hospitals, 76-77, 266-267; 340-341, 384; physicians' assistants, 260-261, 335, 344; psychiatric facilities, 226; rehabilitation facilities, 144, 335; See Also Joint Commission on Accreditation of Hospitals; Residency Review Committee in Internal Medicine

Accreditation Council for Psychiatric Facilities, 226

ACP/ABIM Joint Committee on Osteopathy (ad hoc), 204

ACP/APA Task Force, 142, 173, 184, 200, 214, 262, 274-275, 360

ACP/ASIM amalgamation, failure of, 278; plan for, 267-268, 427-429; proposed, 172-173, 213

ACP/ASIM Liaison Committee, 33-34, 60-61, 81-82, 93, 94, 153, 172-173, 189, 194, 200, 214, 238, 267-268, 316

*ACP Bulletin, See Bulletin of the American College of Physicians*

Administrative affairs, 6, 10-11

Administrative committees, 14; on executive search, 24-25, 35; on personnel, 14; on structure, 10, 14, 23, 294

Administrative officer, chief, 3, 10-11; qualifications of, 13

Advertising, Committee on Journal (*Annals*), 71

Advisory Board of Medical Specialties (ABMS), 5

Affiliate Members, 96, 142-143

Aged, homes for, accrediting of, 77, 135

Alcoholism, statement on, 245-246

Alfred Stengel Memorial Award, establishment of, 8; to Edward Loveland, 23, 29

Alfred Stengel Research Fellowship, 31

Allied health professionals, 10, 151, 234, 315; See Also Physicians' Assistants

Ambulatory care, physician education in, 345

American Academy of Family Physicians, relationship of College with, 330

American Academy of General Practice, 154, 234

American Academy of Pediatrics, 65, 167, 133, 234

American Association for the Accreditation of Laboratory Animal Care, 118, 145, 184

American Association of Medical Legal Consultants, and malpractice cases, 280

American Board of Family Practice, 193, 260, 394; examinations of, 280

American Board of Internal Medicine, 5-6, 8, 52, 57, 73-74, 89, 99, 112, 129, 141, 145-146, 150, 158-160; 185-186, 204-205, 246-247, 298-299, 338-339, 363-364, 381-382;
certifying boards of, 99, 115, 145-146, 157, 159, 160, 185-186, 204-205, 246-247, 298-299, 327, 338, 381; ACP membership requirements and, 8, 57, 115, 204-205, 238, 338; analysis of, 73-74, 185-186, 381; family practice certification compared with, 112; foreign medical graduates and, 160, 185-186; oral examination for, 52, 99, 145-146, 157, 160, 185-186, 246-247; residency training and eligibility for, 129, 157, 158-159
clinical competence assessment program of, 299, 319, 382
functions and procedures of, revised, 319, 381
General Internal Medicine, Council of, 338-339
headquarters of, 89, 146-147
in-training examinations of, 267, 299, 318-319
National Board of Medical Examiners, collaboration with, 185-186; and computer evaluation of examinations, 319, 382
policy positions of, on graduate medical education, 112, 185-186; on manpower and health care delivery, 381; on osteopathy, 185, 204-205; on primary care, 129, 338-339
recertification, plan for, 289-290, 318-319, 363-364;
reorganization of, 359-360
subspecialty boards of, 150, 204-205, 213, 246-247, 298-299, admission of Canadian physicians to, 185-186
Subspecialty Medicine, Council on, 338-339

American Board of Pediatrics, 159

American College of Obstetricians and Gynecologists, 125

American College of Physicians, anniversary of (25th), 7, (50th) 111, 113-

## ACRONYMS USED IN THE INDEX

| | |
|---|---|
| AAMC | Association of American Medical Colleges |
| ABIM | American Board of Internal Medicine |
| ACP | American College of Physicians |
| AHA | American Hospital Association |
| AMA | American Medical Association |
| APA | American Psychiatric Association |
| ASIM | American Society of Internal Medicine |
| CPHA | Commission on Professional and Hospital Activities |
| FCIM | Federated Council for Internal Medicine |
| HEW | Health, Education and Welfare, US Department of |
| JCAH | Joint Commission on Accreditation of Hospitals |
| MKSAP | Medical Knowledge Self-Assessment Program |
| PSRO | Professional Standards Review Organizations |
| WMA | World Medical Association |

# LIST OF ACRONYMS

## MEDICAL SOCIETIES AND OTHER ORGANIZATIONS

Other organizations not listed below are referenced in the text by full name only.

| | |
|---|---|
| AAALAC | American Association for the Accreditation of Laboratory Animal Care |
| AAFP | American Academy of Family Physicians |
| AAGP | American Academy of General Practice |
| AAMC | Association of American Medical Colleges |
| AAMI | Association for the Advancement of Medical Instrumentation |
| AAP | American Academy of Pediatrics |
| AAPA | American Academy of Physicians' Assistants |
| ABFP | American Board of Family Practice |
| ABIM | American Board of Internal Medicine |
| ABMS | Advisory Board of Medical Specialties |
| ABP | American Board of Pediatrics |
| ACEP | American College of Emergency Physicians |
| ACOG | American College of Obstetrics and Gynecology |
| ACP | American College of Physicians |
| ACS | American College of Surgeons |
| AEMB | Alliance for Engineering in Medicine and Biology |
| AFAB | Animal Facilities Accreditation Board |
| AHA | American Hospital Association |
| AJCC-SERR | American Joint Committee on Cancer Staging and End Results Reporting |
| AMA | American Medical Association |
| ANHA | American Nursing Home Association |
| APA | American Psychiatric Association |
| APDIM | Association of Program Directors in Internal Medicine |
| APM | Association of Professors of Medicine |
| APTA | American Physical Therapy Association |
| ARPT | American Registry of Physical Therapists |
| ASIM | American Society of Internal Medicine |
| | |
| CARF | Commission on Accreditation of Rehabilitation Facilities |
| CAS | Council of Academic Societies (of AAMC) |
| CCME | Coordinating Council on Medical Education |
| CMSS | Council of Medical Specialty Societies |
| CSS | Council of Subspecialty Societies (of ACP) |
| CPHA | Commission on Professional and Hospital Activities |
| | |
| DRB | Drug Research Board (of NRC) |
| | |
| ECFMG | Educational Commission for Foreign Medical Graduates |

| | |
|---|---|
| SMA | Southern Medical Association |
| TCC | Tri-College Council |
| UNESCO | United Nations Educational, Social and Cultural Organization |
| VA | Veterans' Administration |
| WMA | World Medical Association |